ADOLESCENT PSYCHIATRY

DEVELOPMENTAL AND CLINICAL STUDIES

VOLUME 17

Annals of the American Society for Adolescent Psychiatry

ADOLESCENT PSYCHIATRY

DEVELOPMENTAL AND CLINICAL STUDIES

VOLUME 17

Edited by
SHERMAN C. FEINSTEIN
Editor in Chief

Senior Editors
AARON H. ESMAN
JOHN G. LOONEY
GEORGE H. ORVIN
JOHN L. SCHIMEL
ALLAN Z. SCHWARTZBERG
ARTHUR D. SOROSKY
MAX SUGAR

The University of Chicago Press
Chicago and London

The University of Chicago Press, Chicago 60637
The University of Chicago Press, Ltd., London

© 1990 by The University of Chicago
All rights reserved. Published 1990
Printed in the United States of America

International Standard Book Number: 0-226-24063-0
Library of Congress Catalog Card Number: 70-147017

The paper used in this publication meets the minimum requirements of American National Standard for Information Sciences—Permanence of Paper for Printed Library Materials, ANSI Z39.48-1984. ∞ ™

CONTENTS

THE RESEARCH EXPERIENCE

EPILOGUE

PART III. DEVELOPMENTAL ISSUES IN ADOLESCENT PSYCHIATRY

PART IV. PSYCHOPATHOLOGY AND PSYCHOTHERAPY OF ADOLESCENT EMOTIONAL DISORDERS

PRESIDENT'S PREFACE

Adolescent Psychiatry, the Annals of the American Society for Adolescent Psychiatry, has been a source of great pride to the Society. It has become one of the preeminent forums for clinical adolescent psychiatry, providing information for and enhancing the skills of the thousands of psychiatrists who work with adolescents. The Annals has been particularly rich in articles about psychotherapy, the main therapeutic vehicle for the adolescent psychiatrist.

Adolescents, striving for their freedom, for their individuality, for their own identity, do not take kindly to establishment-chosen mind-controlling drugs. Psychotherapy offers an enhancement of one's own powers, implicit in greater self-control and in better understanding of others. To adolescents, this is an appealing choice of treatment for their difficulties.

Psychotherapy, today, is an endangered form of treatment—"endangered" because, wherever one turns, one hears of insurance programs that are either cutting the funding for psychotherapy or not paying for it at all. In addition, many government-funded health schemes do not pay for psychiatrists to do psychotherapy. In the current high tide of biological psychiatry, there are many who believe that the future of psychiatry lies in the biological field and that psychotherapy will disappear. It is worthwhile to listen to the wisdom of some prominent members of our profession.

Keith Brodie, past president, American Psychiatric Association, and chair, Department of Psychiatry, Duke University, recommends (1983) that "psychiatry must emphasize that its union of medical knowledge with psychotherapeutic skill provides the patient with optimal expertise in the treatment of mental illness." Herbert Pardes, president,

American Psychiatric Association, and chair, Department of Psychiatry, Columbia University, predicts (1986), "The mental health field will increasingly require professional medical expertise that combines psychological and biological knowledge, in order to deal simultaneously with psychological and biological issues, to understand the use of psychopharmacological agents, and, simultaneously, to treat patients psychologically." Toksos Karasu, chair of the American Psychiatric Association Commission on Psychotherapeutic Research, concludes (1982), "Ideally, then, psychotherapy and pharmacotherapy would work both separately and sequentially in a total therapeutic regimen." Mark Aveline, Nottingham, England, states (1984), "Psychotherapists treat the walking wounded, many of whom have long histories of psychiatric treatment, with repeated admissions, diagnoses of psychiatric illness, and expensive and palliative medication. . . . Psychotherapy provides an effective, appropriate, and inexpensive treatment for major problems of relationships, which otherwise might be inappropriately and expensively treated with medication and/or admission." The Canadian Psychiatric Association believes that the psychiatrist of today must be competent in both psychotherapy and psychopharmacology.

Psychotherapy is an essential tool, necessary for the treatment of trait disorders, necessary in the combined therapy of many trait and state disorders, necessary as the treatment of choice for a number of specific psychiatric disorders, and necessary as an essential component of the treatment of the chronic psychosis (Katz 1986). Fred Grunberg (1986), in his Canadian Psychiatric Association presidential address, reviewed many of the biological discoveries of the last few decades. He pointed out that they have had very little effect on the treatment of psychiatric disorders and that most of the advances have come from the serendipitous discoveries of clinical practitioners. Finally, Leon Eisenberg (1986), Harvard University, pointed out that, just at the time that the rest of medicine is becoming much more aware of the psychosocial determinants of illness, psychiatry is being swept into a biological current that carries the danger of the reification of disease that has characterized the other medical specialities.

As one can see in these brief examples of current comments on the role of psychotherapy, psychiatry has progressed past the split between biological and psychological psychiatry, between what has been described as mindless and brainless psychiatry. The split originated in the ignorance of the functioning of the mind and the brain and led to an either/or approach, which in the light of current knowledge is outdated. One need only look at the developments in the field of psychoneuroimmunology to see how outdated that split is.

The practice of psychiatry without psychotherapy is bad practice, and we should not let insurance companies, politicians, or civil servants push us into practicing bad psychiatry. ASAP is committed to the study, development, and enhancement of psychotherapy while staying abreast of new developments in the biological aspects of psychiatry. The Annals of the American Society for Adolescent Psychiatry are the proof of this commitment.

PHILIP KATZ
President

REFERENCES

Aveline, M. 1984. What price psychiatry without psychotherapy? *Lancet* 13(October): 856–858.

Brodie, H. K. 1983. Presidential address: psychiatry—its focus and its future. *American Journal of Psychiatry* 140:965–968.

Eisenberg, L. 1986. Mindlessness and brainlessness in psychiatry. *British Journal of Psychiatry* 148:497–508.

Grunberg, F. 1986. Presidential address: reflections on the specificity of psychiatry. *Canadian Journal of Psychiatry* 31:799–805.

Karasu, T. B. 1982. Psychotherapy and pharmacotherapy: toward an integrative model. *American Journal of Psychiatry* 139:1102–1113.

Katz, P. 1986. The role of the psychotherapies in the practice of psychiatry: the position paper of the Canadian Psychiatric Association. *Canadian Journal of Psychiatry* 31:458–465.

Pardes, H. 1986. Neuroscience and psychiatry: marriage or coexistence? *American Journal of Psychiatry* 143(10): 1205–1212.

PART I

ADOLESCENCE: GENERAL CONSIDERATIONS

EDITORS' INTRODUCTION

Psychiatry, which has ties to the biological and social, has been deeply affected by economic, societal, and political forces that are changing the face of medical practice. As a recent Group for the Advancement of Psychiatry report points out, the practice of psychotherapy is most vulnerable to these pressures, and the future of the physician psychotherapist is endangered. The chapters in this part reflect the wide range of psychiatric involvement in all areas from unfamiliar business aspects to sensitive efforts to put difficult adolescents in touch with themselves.

Frank T. Rafferty reflects on the history of recent programs for the prevention of mental disorders in children and adolescents. It became clear that the state governments could not finance, operate, and sustain comprehensive systems of mental health services and, finally, reduced their efforts to being the provider of last resort for the poor and chronically ill. While physicians prefer the free market system to state controlled medicine, they have been uncomfortable with the notion of medical services distributed as commodities. Examination of the developing delivery systems reveals an increasing delineation of those groups emphasizing the least expensive and most efficient services and those groups presenting the highest quality, the highest value, the most recent technology, the most convenience, and the freedom of choice. Rafferty documents that relentless market forces of supply and demand will move health care ever closer to the concerns that the nation will develop a two-tiered health care based on the ability to pay.

Richard A. Gardner discusses the existence of extremes in the American educational system and, especially, the lack of appreciation that differences exist at the various levels. He focuses on the erosion of our educational systems and its relevance to the therapist of adolescent psychiatric patients. He criticizes the elementary schools where egalitarianism, report cards, and deterioration of quality in the schools are indications of educational chaos. At the high school level, the author describes informational deficits, impaired motivation, and regression as consequences of parental and educational overprotection. In college, Gardner sees a bastardization of the system that contributes to psychopathologic trends toward superficial learning and identity confusion. Gardner concludes that many young people are being shortchanged in their educational experiences.

Lillian H. Robinson believes that parental failings are not always the cause of troubled children—many started with good intentions. Parents learn to parent through early experiences with their own parents. Not feeling accepted, tolerating poor care, being denied privacy by intrusive parents, are areas in which children need to assume responsibility—parents may vie with them for controls. Robinson reviews research literature to conclude that parents change significantly after participating in parent discussion groups or individual therapy. She emphasizes that some of the disturbance is the effect rather than the cause of the child's illness—parents need understanding and support.

Nicholas Putnam identifies a mild, nonautistic form of pervasive developmental disorder, better known as the "nerd" syndrome. This disorder is characterized by impairment in the development of reciprocal social interaction, verbal and nonverbal communication skills, and imaginative activity. Putnam describes the mild pervasive developmental disorder's (MPDD) adolescence as a period of great risk because of the deficits in socialization skills, language skills, and identity formation. The author further illustrates facets of developmental difficulties such as holistic versus sequential thinking, MPDD and computers, the appearance of MPDDs, and speech and language of MPDDs. Putnam suggests that the diagnosis of mild pervasive developmental disorder should allow for a number of interventions.

Philip Katz presents a sensitive view of the first few minutes in the engagement of difficult adolescents in psychotherapy. The engagement, right from the opening moment, tests the psychiatrist's skill, creativity, empathy, and tenacity. Professor Katz recommends planning an approach: clarify your role as a stranger; analyze the situation to the patient; seek opportunities to empathize with the patient; offer immediate help to the patient. Katz notes that the work should begin prior to the arrival of the patient. The psychiatrist should be prepared to deal with the fear and anger that the patient brings to the interview. The psychiatrist should have a strategic plan for the opening moments: understanding, knowledge, empathy, and a warm and positive prognosis. The author believes that proper preparation will enable the psychiatrist to engage the adolescent in distress.

Derek Miller conceptualizes the termination of treatment as a phase in the psychotherapeutic process. An initial goal of treatment is the creation of a therapeutic alliance that leads to the abandonment of primitive defenses. The end of treatment implies the dissolution of this alliance without the destruction of the internalized attitudes and feelings that it has helped create. When an adolescent behaves in a symptomatic way that is developmentally destructive, dangerous to self and others, and reflective of a psychonoxious environment, psychotherapeutic intervention may be indicated. The indications for treatment determine both the goals of therapy and its likely termination. Miller discusses the timing of termination; psychological growth of the patient and family; the availability of a cascade of treatment programs from inpatient to partial hospital to outpatient; and psychopharmacological approaches. The author concludes that successful termination depends on the acceptance by the adolescent and the family of a mutually satisfactory balance of mastery over problems, during which secondary individuation continues.

1 THE EVOLUTION OF TWO-TIERED HEALTH CARE

FRANK T. RAFFERTY

The title of this symposium, "Adolescent Psychiatric Needs: Criteria for a Healthy Society," is one that appeals to the humanitarian instincts of all practicing psychiatrists. When caring for mentally disordered adolescents, there is the perception that the world must be totally populated with these unfortunate creatures. It is impossible not to be aware of the missed opportunities to have addressed the needs of these youngsters; our entire society would certainly be healthier if we had. Unfortunately, the historical landscape is littered with the wreckage of plans for the prevention of mental disorders in children and adolescents, including those that were planned, seemingly adequately funded, and well executed.

The 1988 national election calls to mind one of the best of these—the Joint Commission on the Mental Health of Children. This 1968 study was well funded by Congress and had been in progress for three years. It had been extended a fourth in order to report to the new president, Richard Nixon. However, Nixon refused to receive the report, and thus one of the best comprehensive plans to meet the needs of children and adolescents was consigned to the graveyard of unread, unremembered reports and unimplemented plans.

The Johnson administration is now perceived as a sharp marker for the end of large-scale federal social planning, but it was not so clear then. Prevention and early childhood education and intervention were at a peak of popularity. Earl Schaefer of the National Institute of Mental Health (NIMH) had reported on research establishing that the enrichment of infants' lives by play could raise their IQ by eleven points (Schaefer and Aaronson 1972). Although a few major cities were aware of the problems of the War on Poverty and of community mental health center programs, much of the country was still in the process of planning or starting their community action or community mental health programs.

Task Force V of the joint commission had consisted of working papers planning a system for the future. One paper written for the task force proposed that, since the school system served children from age four through adolescence, there should be a computerized system of longitudinal monitoring and evaluating of selected indicators of the biological, emotional, social, intellectual, and communication systems of each child from age four through high school. Medical, educational, psychiatric, and social interventions would be made when appropriate. Many services were to have been provided by referral, but most services, including those involving families, would have been organized around the school as the primary community institution (Rafferty 1968).

More than half that task force paper was devoted to reviewing and analyzing the problems of planning in a democratic society. The emphasis on the rights of the individual, with severe limitations on governmental power and authority to intrude on the privacy of family life and the many competing, powerful, and articulate interest groups, seems to have ensured the failure of the plan. The differences between a planned, controlled economy and the relatively free market economy of the United States were reviewed in detail:

> Contrasting the problems of the private therapist who must be selective to be effective with the problems of the social engineer who cannot implement his insights, highlights the difficulties of the planning task. The private therapist selects children to treat who have their major dependency needs at least potentially satisfied, whose families have the minimum requirements of energy, money, and information, and whose biological, intellectual, and communicative skills can support the treatment process. On the other hand the social engineer finds himself confronted with sets of variables that will not stand still for corrections. . . . if he focuses on health services, ill advised or defective education defeats the effort. If he tries for a measure of control over education, then

inadequate family income sabotages the effort. If he supports the family income and establishes jobs for parents, deficiencies in health and education turn temporary support into the permanent dole. [Rafferty 1968, pp. 18–19]

The problem of meeting the needs of all children and adolescents was described thus: "No previous goal of the society has ever approached this degree of complexity—will have ever sought to control as many variables—and in particular have ever tried to deal with values, causes, rights, etc., so intimately associated with each citizen" (Rafferty 1968, pp. 19–20).

Over the next ten years, a few of the better state governments, while trying to implement ambitious plans, demonstrated that even excellent, well-financed state departments of mental health could not finance, operate, and sustain comprehensive systems of mental health services. Today, only a few states still try to provide comprehensive services. Most states have reduced their efforts to being the provider of last resort for the poor and the chronically ill.

Meanwhile, the unplanned and uncontrolled forces of the relatively free market have continued to function in their own mysterious way. A free market consists of individuals free to make their own decision to buy and sell their goods to anyone in fair exchange for a price determined by the ongoing auction that balances the supply of a particular good against the demand for that good. Although physicians have clearly preferred the free market system to state-controlled medicine, they have been resistant to thinking of their services as commodities distributed on the basis of price. Since the health-care industry was a growth industry and presented a seller's market, price did not seem to be a major factor in regulating health services until this last decade.

In 1983, the federal government introduced diagnostic related groups (DRGs) as a price-setting and volume-regulating mechanism. One common justification for this action to control the cost of health care was that Medicare is the largest single customer of the health-care industry and has a right to use its market clout in determining hospital prices. That, of course, does not explain the use of federal legislation, regulations, cancellation of licensure, and criminal penalties for violations or refusal to participate. Neither the medical nor the hospital organizations effectively opposed government regulation of hospitals through the DRG system.

9

The advocates of government-regulated medicine also justify the intrusion into the market by noting that the very essence of diagnosis and treatment of those in pain, in sickness, and with various handicaps violates the principles of the free market and warrants the intrusion of government into the transaction in order to protect the weak patients from their stronger opponents and sometime oppressors, the physicians and other providers of health-care services.

In a recent article about the resource-based relative-value scale, William Hsiao, director of the Harvard study, wrote,

> The market for physician services does not satisfy the conditions that define a reasonably competitive market. First, widespread health insurance coverage reduces patients' sensitivity to fees. Patients generally choose physicians and services with little concern for price. Second, patients often lack adequate knowledge on which to base their choice of medical services and judgements about technical quality; they typically rely on their physicians for advice in making medical decisions. Physicians are often not subject to the checks and balances generated by traditional competitive forces. Finally, legal restrictions specify who can provide medical services, admit patients to hospitals, and prescribe drugs. Although such restrictions protect patients from unqualified providers, they also tend to grant monopoly power to the medical profession. [Hsiao, Braun, Ynteman, and Becker 1988]

Physicians and health-care providers are likely to believe that government and corporate sponsors are working both sides of the street. On the one hand, they treat health-care services as if they were the same as any other commodity and the physicians were like any other sellers of service in the competitive marketplace. But, on the other hand, they assume the mantle of protector of the weak, sick, and handicapped and impose centrally determined regulations, controls, and prices.

Advocates for a more free health-care market would suggest that a completely free market does not exist in any industry, that most consumers are far from fully informed about any product, that buyers are particularly vulnerable when in a crisis of any kind, and that most sellers have a short-term advantage over most initial or one-time buyers, especially as the technological content of the product rises.

Obviously, there are powerful economic forces, such as supply and demand, that govern the exchange of goods between individuals in any large population. These forces influence the market regardless of the extent of government control and frequently defeat government efforts to regulate prices and total cost.

In any event, the most powerful influence on the shape of the industry over the past ten years has been the single-minded determination of government and corporate sponsors to control the growth of the total cost of health-care services. The unplanned, dynamic, and continuously reorganizing health-care industry has responded with two major formats: the true managed-care, capitated institution as reflected in the closed-staff health maintenance organizations (HMOs) and in the preferred provider organizations (PPOs) and the multihospital system funded primarily by tightly managed, indemnification insurance with unavoidable transfers from the PPOs. The multihospital systems incorporate not only inpatient beds but many components of ambulatory medicine. There are other systems such as nursing homes, medical groups, and the long-term care providers. Health care for the poor, the uninsured, and the underinsured remains an unaddressed but worrisome and tragic problem.

Examination of the array of facilities and payment mechanisms reveals an increasing delineation of those groups emphasizing the least expensive and most efficient services and those groups emphasizing the highest quality, the highest value, the most recent technology, the most convenience, and freedom of choice. Relentless market forces of supply and demand will undoubtedly continue to sort these groups out and move health care ever closer to the realization of the frequently verbalized fears that the nation will develop multiple layers of health care based on the ability to pay.

In fact, there never has been single-class, egalitarian medical care in the United States. Those without money and those with money have always received different care. The majority of the poor did not receive any medical care. In the big cities, medical care for the poor was provided at the large municipal hospitals and clinics, where doctors in training had primary responsibility for the care of patients. Much of that care was excellent, but some of it was not, and it was spottily delivered.

The 1960s were exciting years for the egalitarians in this society. Social movements to reduce discrimination against individuals on the basis of race, sex, and age achieved much success. Campaigns to decrease stigma attached to the handicapped, to cancer, to homosexuality, and to the mentally ill gained ground. The medical aspects of the War on Poverty were among the most successful programs. Medicare and Medicaid addressed two major segments of those disadvantaged for health care. Programs such as the Community Health and Mental Health grants targeted other segments of the needy population. Individual rights were expanded from the traditional inalienable rights of the constitution to include access to certain positive services that were supportive of the traditional rights. These included the right to education, to special education, to legal services, to housing, to treatment, and of course to medical care. Physicians were proud and elated that they could provide the same services to everyone who needed them without regard to cost or ability to pay.

For example, as late as 1979, over half the 550 patients in the Brown Schools of Austin, Texas, were poor. Their treatment was paid for by over 120 public agencies across the country. The poor youngsters received the same definitive, tertiary, inpatient care as the children of movie stars and professional athletes. Line staff were formally unaware of the economic status of anyone.

Yet in the 1960s and 1970s, there were still thousands of people who were not receiving adequate treatment. During those decades, for every well-funded and -staffed child and adolescent program in the inner-city catchment area, there would be five other catchment areas that had only nominal services. Physicians suffered from the clinician's illusion and knew only about the patients they saw. They had no way of knowing how many patients they did not see or how many were not seen by anyone. Long before DRGs or managed care, public psychiatric inpatient programs of necessity limited the length of stay. For example, in 1972, the Illinois Department of Mental Health operated a twenty-one-day program for Medicaid-eligible youngsters. That was rationing of mental health services. Although many of those programs provided superb care for the twenty-one days, no one could begin to compare the value of those services with that provided in the private sector.

The thrust of this chapter is to suggest that, as economic forces continue to affect the health-care market, including the governmental components, there will inevitably be a slow delineation and structuring of at least a two-tier health-care system. The care of the mentally disordered adolescent will be a central component of that system. The industrialization of health care inevitably results in different levels of service similar to the different levels of service in the food, housing, clothing, and transportation industries. The public is accustomed to different price levels when buying food, housing, and transportation.

There are four major trends to watch as this layering of health care develops. These are HMOs and PPOs, multihospital systems, the Champus reform initiatives, and, finally, physician's fees and patterns of practice. The effective moving force of these trends is the government using its market clout as the largest single customer of the health-care industry.

Health maintenance organizations, PPOs, and independent professional associations (IPAs) are prepaid, capitated systems that provide comprehensive health care to a population of subscribers in the most efficient, least expensive manner. An HMO is a closed-staff model in which the physicians and staff are on salary and work in physical locations that belong to the HMO. Preferred provider organizations are contracted networks of physicians and hospitals without extensive physical plants belonging to the PPO. These are favored by physicians since they can participate without changing their practice substantially and they can be organized with a minimum of capital outlay. In principle, a PPO provides incentives for a more efficient, economical form of health care. A typical study of Group Health of Puget Sound in Washington State by the Rand Corporation revealed up to 28 percent savings with a 40 percent reduction in hospital admissions. Despite the recognized ability of managed care to contain hospital costs, there is no reason to believe that the totality of health-care costs will be restrained. In 1987, an extraordinary surge in health-care costs sent many HMOs deeply in debt. Overall, the HMO industry lost $692 million. Three-fourths, or 179 out of 243, of the plans surveyed by National Underwriters lost money. It is generally recognized that a PPO probably will not make money until the third or fourth year. Overall, the Blues plans across the country lost $1.9 billion, with prepaid plans posting some of the major losses (Robinson 1988).

Insolvency of HMOs or PPOs is becoming a multimillion-dollar problem for hospitals and physicians who have been part of their preferred networks. As yet no solution is visible. Approximately 26 percent of the population in the United States is involved with these organizations, and the number is expected to reach 40 percent in another decade. While watching this number grow, pay attention to the HMO membership of Medicare and Medicaid clients. At the moment, HMOs are being very cautious about Medicare. But the marriage of HMOs and Medicare is one made in heaven since it contains the two major ingredients sought by the Health Care Financing Agency (HCFA), namely, capitation and change in physician behavior. Each of these represents a problem to be solved: the HMO and the HCFA must come to an agreement on price-setting and price-changing mechanisms, and the PPOs must be able to manage their physician networks to achieve the same level of control as the closed-staff model.

Multihospital systems are now major players in the health-care industry. There were widespread fears and predictions that all health care would be dominated by a few giant health-care corporations. This is obviously not going to happen. But it is equally obvious that multihospital systems will not disappear, although they are in the midst of major restructuring and downscaling. The following statistics (from Holthaus 1988) are illustrative. Hospitals have closed; since 1981, 320 hospitals have closed—246 between 1984 and 1987. Hospital occupancy rates dropped steadily from 75 percent in 1975 to 63.4 percent in 1986. Out of nearly 1 million staffed hospital beds, 350,000 are empty every day. Hospital operating margins have declined sharply; in 1987, net patient margins were near zero, at .2 percent. Growth in Medicare spending dropped to 4.15 percent in 1986 after ranging from 10.2 to 28.6 percent in the 1970s.

Although inner-city and rural hospitals are closing, new hospitals are opening in other markets. Seventy-nine community hospitals closed in 1987. But forty-five new community hospitals opened. There was a net gain of 125 hospitals in 1987. Hospitals in overbedded, inner-city areas close because of the shift in the insured population to the suburbs and because of insufficient payments by Medicare and Medicaid. In rural areas, where the population is aging and where low Medicare rates do not carry the expense, hospitals are closing (Henderson 1988).

The effort to reduce costs has had a major effect on the organization of health care. Capitation offers the greatest potential opportunity for cost containment leading to the growth of HMOs. But there remains a significant body of American citizens who prefer to choose when, where, and from whom they will receive health care. These people understand that they are not receiving and they are not interested in buying the least expensive medical care any more than they are interested in buying the least expensive housing, food, or transportation. These people choose the high-option health insurance when given a chance and are not deterred by copayments or deductibles. They expect to pay out of pocket for certain technologies such as cosmetic surgery. They will use mechanisms that offer them increased consumer protection. They are high technology and value oriented. They want to be treated by the specialist of their choice and to have immediate access to the best technology, newest drugs, and most convenient facilities.

This higher tier of health care is organized around the multihospital system with little differentiation between profit and nonprofit since both operate with essentially the same economic forces. The medical specialist will be attracted to the hospital system. The generous number of physicians in the educational pipeline will probably assure an adequate supply for all tiers for several decades.

Psychiatry has been on the periphery of these changes because its investment in Medicare, and vice versa, has been weak from the beginning. The exemption of psychiatric units and psychiatric hospitals from DRGs has, in fact, been an incentive for the development of psychiatric units in general hospitals.

Despite all efforts to contain costs, the percentage of the health-care dollar going to mental health care continues to rise, causing problems for both HMOs and the indemnification insurance carriers. Most payors do not appreciate the vast reservoir of unmet needs for psychiatric care. Studies suggest that the prevalence of psychiatric disease is increasing and that, when the public is offered affordable, competent, and effective psychiatric services, the prejudice against psychiatry melts away.

Hospitals adjust to the reduction of length of stay by increasing volume, intensity, and rates. The economic pressure on psychiatric hospitals has indirectly stimulated demand. Hospital management responds to a low census with increased marketing, recruitment of more prestigious psychiatrists, and improvements in services. These reduce the stigma of mental illness and provide consumers with information about treatment for mental illness. The private sector has been sensitive to the principle of treating people close to home and has established hospitals in communities that never would have seen a public facility.

Psychiatrists have survived the recent cost reductions. The major sources of anxiety have been the sense of lack of control and the

15

pervasive competition. The dynamically oriented psychiatrist has been particularly upset with the aggressive competition since he or she would prefer to be independent of both hospital and managed-care systems. But the HMOs and PPOs will offer low-cost systems of mental health services through the use of the primary-care physicians, the nonmedical disciplines, and crisis-oriented interventions. This forces the majority of psychiatric specialists to affiliate with the multihospital systems and forces the dynamically oriented psychiatrist to expand his or her armamentarium of psychiatric procedures.

The Champus reform initiatives will play a major experimental role in the changes taking place in the delivery of health care. There are at least eight of these special programs with differing thrusts and experimental elements that push to the limit the concept of privatization by a public agency. Responsibility for implementation and management is shifted to a private prime contractor, with the public agency retaining the financial responsibility through a contracted total fee. The prime contractor takes on the responsibility of setting up the provider networks from the resources already in place to meet the conditions of the contract.

The message from the first pilot project in the Tidewater area of Virginia is that the Department of Defense is well satisfied with the money saved and can live with the high level of provider dissatisfaction as long as there remains a relatively low level of subscriber complaints. The prime contractor was not renewed after two years, and the contract was put out for bid again. Maybe the major lesson learned is that a community of subscribers and providers can survive with an acceptable level of casualties while a new type of organization tests large-scale mechanisms for managed health care.

The fourth major trend to watch is directly related to the individual practitioner. At the beginning of this decade, the money-saving strategists had two options. They considered the doctor to be the key to controlling expenditures in health care, but they did not have confidence in their ability to control 400,000 individual physicians. The strategic decision was made to control hospital costs. Out of this came the DRGs, the emphasis on reduction of length of stay, the support of ambulatory medicine and surgery, and the restrictive-utilization review practices.

Although DRGs have been successful and have changed hospitals, medical education, and clinical research, the growth in cost of health care is still a problem for government and other financial sponsors. The HCFA and the U.S. Congress have decided that there must be control over physicians' fees. The goal is a national fee scale by fiscal year 1991. The first step is the Harvard study of resource-based relative value scales. The report on the first group of specialties has been submitted. All the medical and specialty societies are trying to evaluate who will win and who will lose. But it is clear that the regulatory bodies, both public and private, are taking direct aim at physicians and do intend to control physician practice patterns. Control of financial incentives for physicians may not control the costs of medical care, which are probably driven by technological development. It is neither possible nor desirable to turn off the development of technology in one segment of society. Nor is it possible to control people's desire for health and longevity once they learn that effective health care is available.

In the near future, psychiatrists will face a concerted attack on the appropriateness of psychiatric treatment for adolescents, with special reference to hospitalization. The utilization review organizations have targeted adolescent hospitalization as a major cause of the increase in costs of psychiatric care. They will attempt to reinvigorate the legal controversy put to rest by the Parham decision and try to mobilize those who would prefer to reinterpret conduct disorders and the personality disorders as social maladjustments that should be managed by the correctional agencies.

The hospitalization of adolescents is a long-term example of the multiple tiers of care determined by economics. Throughout the 1970s, research at the Institute of Juvenile Research revealed an established practice by police when apprehending adolescents. The first question was always, "Where do you live?" When the youngster lived in the affluent suburbs, he or she was taken home, released to custody of parents, and frequently received psychiatric evaluation and care if appropriate. If the youngster lived in the inner city, he or she received up to seven precinct station adjustments and releases before referral to juvenile court, where at best he or she received probation and, if lucky, placement in nonprofessional counseling services. Again psychiatrists saw only the adolescents brought to their offices and were unaware of the thousands managed by the police. Likewise, other social and educational agencies do not identify adolescent pathology and do not provide specific services. These nonmedical agencies justify their failure to use psychiatric technologies on economic grounds.

17

Conclusions

In summary, this chapter has presented the thesis that medical and psychiatric care regulated in a relatively free market is more consistent with the American culture than is the planned, controlled social engineering that would be required to truly meet all the needs of children and adolescents and that the economic forces of supply and demand operating in a relatively free market will naturally force the health-care industry to operate on at least two tiers on the basis of cost.

REFERENCES

Henderson, J. A. 1988. Wave of hospital closings is only one side of healthier story about market adjustment. *Modern Healthcare* (September 9), p. 81.

Holthaus, D. 1988. Election '88: the future of health care. *Hospitals* (October 5), pp. 47–48.

Hsiao, W.; Braun, P.; Ynteman, D.; and Becker, E. R. 1988. Estimating physicians' work for a resource-based relative-value scale. *New England Journal of Medicine* 319:835–841.

Rafferty, F. T. 1968. Task Force V Working Paper: Joint Commission on Mental Health of Children. Typescript.

Robinson, M. L. 1988. Insurers, HMOs hit big recession in '87. *Hospitals* (September 5), pp. 27–28.

Schaefer, E., and Aaronson, M. 1972. Infant education research project: implementation and implication of a home tutoring program. In R. K. Parker, ed. *The Preschool in Action: Exploring Early Childhood Programs*. Boston: Allyn & Bacon.

2 THE AMERICAN EDUCATIONAL SYSTEM AND THE PSYCHOLOGICAL DEVELOPMENT OF THE ADOLESCENT

RICHARD A. GARDNER

In education, as in many other societal functions in this country, there is a coexistence of extremes. On the one hand, we have certain educational institutions that are among the best worldwide. Students from every country come here because of their appreciation that we can provide a superior educational experience. Although many factors have operated in bringing about this situation, one of the most important, I believe, is the freedom of inquiry that we have enjoyed since the days of the founding fathers. In a reasonably classless structure, education has potentially been available to everyone— although there have been times and places where this ideal has been far from realized. Furthermore, areas of poverty notwithstanding, we are basically an affluent country and have had the wherewithal to provide Americans with a high level of education.

But this is only one side of the picture. Coexisting with these superb institutions (sometimes in the same neighborhoods) are schools that hardly justify being referred to as educational institutions. I am referring primarily to school systems in inner-city ghettos where the combination of poverty-stricken children, uncommitted and poorly trained teachers, drugs, and the general atmosphere of violence makes meaningful education almost impossible. And then there is the vast in between. It is this segment that I will focus on in this chapter, with particular emphasis on the erosion of our educational systems in general and the particular relevance of such erosion to the therapist who treats adolescents. I will begin at the elementary school level because it is there that influences begin that affect our adolescent patients at the junior high school, senior high school, and college levels.

Elementary Schools

"ALL MEN ARE CREATED EQUAL"

Ours is seemingly an egalitarian educational system that assumes that all children are created equal and that all children should receive the same educational exposure. This is misguided egalitarianism. The principle blinds itself to the obvious intellectual differences that children exhibit from the time of birth. On the one hand, educators appreciate that every intelligence test has its distribution curve, from the intellectually impaired to the superior. On the other hand, our educational system in the United States does not properly accommodate these differences. I do not claim that there is no appreciation at all of these differences; I claim only that educators do not exhibit enough appreciation of these differences. Although there are special classes for learning-disabled children and technical high schools for those who are not academically inclined, the main thrust and orientation of our educational system is toward preparing youngsters to enter colleges and universities.

Most countries have no problem accepting the fact that not all children should be on a strong academic track. Accordingly, in many countries, somewhere between the ages of nine and eleven children are divided into three tracks. The highest track ultimately leads to the university. The lowest track ends formal, intense academic training at about age eleven or twelve and then emphasizes various trades and skills. The middle track is somewhere between the two. Of course, if the child has been placed in the wrong track, there is still a possibility of switching. We would do well in the United States to institute such a system. It would protect many children from significant grief. To say that all people should be treated equally before the law is certainly reasonable. But to say that all are created equal is absurd. What is more reasonable to say, as Orwell did in *Animal Farm*, is that "some are more equal than others." Because public statements of such inegalitarianism are considered undemocratic in our society at this time, it is extremely unlikely that such changes will be introduced into our system in the foreseeable future—certainly not before the end of this century.

Many of our children who are presently referred to as "learning disabled" are considered to have some kind of a disease, often neurological in etiology. However, when one investigates the specific etiological factors responsible for their disorder, none is found in the vast majority of cases. The assumption is that there is some derangement in cerebral functioning that we have not yet been able to identify by known biological methods but that future research will reveal. As I have described in detail elsewhere (Gardner 1987), I believe that the vast majority of the children so labeled have no particular structural defect in their brains. Rather, they have been unfortunate enough to have been born into a society that places a strong emphasis on certain cognitive skills with which they are not well endowed. Most of these children have WISC-R (Wechsler Intelligence Scale for Children—Revised) IQs in the 80–90 range. Those who consider such children to be suffering with some kind of a neurological disorder are not showing proper respect for the very same distribution curve on which their IQs are recorded. For every child with a 90 IQ, there must be one with a 110 IQ. For every one with an 85, there must be one with a 115. To consider 80–90 IQ children to have a disease is a terrible disservice to them. Significant psychopathology is caused by such labeling, and enormous attempts at educating them to higher levels often proves futile. One of the reasons why such disorders are infrequently diagnosed in other countries is that these children are placed in a lower track, where they do far better. The demands made on them are lesser, their social acceptance is greater, and they do not develop the assortment of secondary psychogenic disorders (including low self-worth, antisocial acting out, and dependency problems) that are seen among such children in this country. Elsewhere (Gardner 1968, 1974a, 1974b, 1975a, 1975b, 1977, 1986, in press), I discuss in detail some of the more common of these problems and approaches to their treatment. The treatment, however, would not be necessary in many other societies, and therapists treating such youngsters should help their patients develop an appreciation of this fact.

REPORT CARDS

In recent years, educators have operated on the assumption that communicating to children anything about deficiencies is going to be devastating to their self-worth. In order to subscribe to this goal, an elaborate system of subterfuge has grown up, the purpose of which is to hide from children information that might prove "upsetting." Report cards demonstrate well this phenomenon, and the therapist does well to familiarize himself or herself with these principles in order better to understand what is going on with patients. The first rule is that words with a pejorative connotation—no matter how slight—are strictly verboten. Checks are given, but not crosses. A child may be "good," but no one is "bad." Students may be "right," but not "wrong." "Tests" are no longer given, only "exercises." In many school systems, the lowest grade the child can get is NI (needs improvement); there is no such thing as a U (unsatisfactory) or an F (perish the thought and bite your tongue!).

Another rule that is rigidly adhered to in such reports is one that I call the rule of the uncompared comparison. Stated briefly the rule is this: in describing a child's performance, never make any references— no matter how subtle—to the baseline or standards by which the student's performance is being judged. In this way, no accurate information about poor performance will be communicated (since the term "poor" has meaning only in relation to its antithesis, "good"), and the child will be spared the painful confrontation with his or her inadequacies. The examples of this are legion: "Jane is doing much better in math." That is the whole sentence. The parent can only wonder, "I guess she must have been doing poorly at first and now she's doing better. Well, that's good to know. But how poorly was she doing at first? And how much better is she doing now? Was she failing then and is she passing now? Or was she failing then and is she still failing now? Did she go from a 10 percent to a 20 percent average [using the now discredited system], from a 30 percent to a 90 percent, or from a 1 percent to a 2 percent?"

Or we are told, "Billy is trying much harder in social studies." Again, the same confusion and frustration is produced. We are glad to learn that, but how far have his efforts got him? No information at all in that department. The real questions that most parents want answered are, Is he passing and failing in comparison to the other kids in the class? Where does he stand? Does he need help? How is he really doing? To spare anyone any hard feelings, no one is told how he is doing. No one's feelings are going to be hurt. All those who do poorly are helped to deny their difficulties. This is supposed to enhance self-esteem. What is enhanced is delusion, procrastination, and the avoidance of painful reality—qualities that have never proved themselves to be particularly effective ways ultimately to enhance anyone's feelings of self-worth or enhance his or her adaptive capacity.

Other devices are commonly used to protect the child from confrontation with inadequacies. Using vague terminology can accomplish this. Words like "slight" and "somewhat" serve this purpose quite well: "Mary is doing somewhat better in spelling," or "Ronald is showing slight improvement in math." Usually, improvement is nonexistent or miniscule, and the teacher believes that it would be devastating to the child's "ego" were he or she told that there was no progress. Another way of accomplishing this is to use a verb form ending in "-ing," in such a way that vague passage of time is implied: "Bobby is doing fractions," "Gail is still learning the three-times table," or "Malcolm is beginning to learn how to organize his time." No one knows exactly how far these children have got in their various pursuits—in fact, one strongly suspects that they have made no progress at all. Another ploy is to avoid focusing at all on academic performance and state, "Virginia is trying very hard," or "Thomas is doing his best." These maneuvers do actually teach children something. They teach them ways to blind themselves to their deficits. In addition, they cannot but lessen their respect for the teacher if they sense his or her duplicity—and they often do.

We need some degree of comparison to ascertain the value of our accomplishments; we cannot judge them in a vacuum. We also need some degree of competition to provide us with the esteem enhancement that comes from excelling others. It is when exceeding others becomes our primary, if not exclusive, source of ego enhancement that we get into difficulty. It is then that we are likely to lose the intrinsic satisfactions of the attainment and become so engrossed in competition that we may deprive ourselves of opportunities for other sources of esteem building. A reasonable degree of excelling others to enhance one's self-worth can be healthy. Used to an excessive degree, it becomes dehumanizing, as one's main purpose in life then becomes beating others down. Competition, used in moderation, can spur us on to work more efficiently toward our goals. Used in excess, however, it may become an end in itself and may then lessen the likelihood that we will reach our goals. We may then become more interested in the winning than in the process and the goal, and this lessens our effectiveness in achieving our aim.

The school can and should be a place that teaches healthy competition, in preparation for the competitiveness of adult life. Because our society is fiercely competitive is no reason to do away with competition completely, as some would attempt to do. Rather, we should tone it down and use it as constructively as possible. Awareness of this progress—as compared to others—can be a useful tool in providing students with healthy competitive impetus. Holmes (1964) provides some excellent examples of this phenomenon in his description of the role of competitive sports in the treatment of his adolescent inpatients.

The main purpose of a teacher's rating or feedback system should be to provide students with information about their level of accomplishment as compared to peers and to pinpoint the steps necessary to correct deficiencies. To say, "Jimmy has how mastered multiplication up to the six-times table, whereas the average student in his grade has, by now, mastered the eight-times table," not only enables everyone to appreciate better the level of accomplishment, but may also serve to encourage Jimmy to work harder to bring up his level. The teacher might add, "Jimmy needs special practice in the seven- and eight-times tables as well as in the addition of three-digit numbers." In addition, no harm is done, and much is to be gained, by utilizing a grading system (A, B, C, D, and F). High grades provide positive reinforcement and enhance motivation. Because children with low grades may feel disappointed should not be a reason for depriving those with the capacity to get higher grades (either via genetic endowment and/or personal and family influences) from enjoying the enhanced self-worth that comes with such accomplishment.

SOME CAUSES OF SCHOOL DETERIORATION

Whereas the home plays the most important role in the child's psychological development during the first three or four years, the schools play an increasingly important if subsidiary role during the next decade or so (at least for most children). Those who are unfortunate enough to be provided with inadequate educational programs are likely to develop psychopathology, both in childhood and in adolescence. There has been a progressive deterioration of our educational systems (both public and private) in the last fifteen to twenty years. A number of factors have contributed to this deterioration. One relates to teachers' salaries. It is unreasonable to expect that schools can attract high-quality, well-educated individuals when other careers provide much greater pay. In most municipalities, garbage men make as much as, if not more than, elementary school teachers. The public sector can generally afford to provide higher salaries than private and parochial schools, yet the public schools seem to be getting the poorest-quality teachers. The more dedicated ones are willing to take positions for lower salaries in order to work in the more academically stimulating atmosphere of the private and parochial schools.

I believe that there has been a general diminution in the commitment of teachers to the educational process. I am not claiming that this is true of all teachers, only that the percentage of teachers who are deeply committed to their profession has been sharply reduced. One manifestation of this trend is the decreased frequency with which children are required to do homework. Giving children homework most often involves homework for the teacher, and less dedicated teachers are not willing to take on this extra responsibility. In previous years, there were many more teachers who were viewed to be somewhat hard nosed and dictatorial, yet their despotism was benevolent, and years later their students have looked back with gratitude on what they were "forced" to do. These days "respect" for the child often involves a degree of permissiveness and indulgence that serves children ill in the course of their education. A good educational experience helps the child learn that there are times when one has to do things that may be unpleasant in order to derive future benefits. "Respecting" the child's wish not to endure such discomforts is basically not in the child's best interests. True respect for children involves the requirement that they do what is best for them, not the indulgence of their avoidance of reasonable responsibilities. The net result of these unfortunate trends is that children learn less during their primary and secondary school years—with the subsequent result that SAT scores have dropped significantly and that, as many studies have demonstrated, the majority of children are abysmally ignorant of basic facts about history, geography, literature, English, and mathematics.

Another factor operative in the deterioration of the educational system has been the growth of a generation of teachers who themselves have not learned very much during their own educational processes. Often, these are teachers who went to college during the 1960s, when students' self-indulgence may have reached an all-time high. Grammar, punctuation, spelling, and foreign languages were dismissed as "irrelevant." Many other subjects that required self-discipline and hard work were also often viewed as irrelevant. Graduates of this era are now teaching our youngsters. Not only do many of these teachers serve as poor models for their students, owing to their impaired commitment to the educational process, but they are compromised as well in what they can teach. I routinely ask parents to bring in my child patients' report cards. Often I see egregious errors in grammar, punctuation, and spelling. I have had secretaries whom I have had to let go after a week or two because of their ignorance of basic English. They were not people who I felt needed time to adjust to a new job; rather, it might have taken years to get them to reach the point at which they could function adequately in a standard secretarial position. They often did not even appreciate how ignorant they were. They did not even recognize that a misspelled word looked misspelled and so had no motivation to consult a dictionary for the correct spelling.

High School

In their book *What Do Our 17-Year Olds Know?* Ravitch and Finn (1987) report a study conducted with approximately 18,000 seventeen-year-olds who were selected to reflect the makeup of the population as a whole regarding region, sex, race, type of school, and type of community. Among their findings are the following. Thirty percent of the students did not know that Christopher Columbus reached the New World before 1750. More than 35 percent were not aware that the Watergate scandal took place after 1950. More than 30 percent believed that one consequence of the Spanish-American War was the defeat of the Spanish Armada. Approximately half the students believed that *Nineteen Eighty-Four* dealt with the destruction of the human race in a nuclear war. Over one-third did not know that Aesop wrote fables. Over 42 percent did not know who Senator Joseph McCarthy was or for what he became infamous. Seventy percent were unable to identify the Magna Carta. The book goes on and on with many more examples of the abysmal ignorance of the average American teenager. These findings should not be surprising, considering the kinds of educational programs these youngsters are being provided.

Some parents bring their adolescents for treatment because of poor academic motivation. Many of these youngsters attend schools where the educational standards are low and where they are automatically moved ahead every year and then dropped off the edge of the system when they complete the twelfth grade. Some, however, are in more demanding high schools, but they still have little commitment to the educational process. Sometimes the youngster's lack of motivation is indeed related to intrafamilial and intrapsychic problems. At other times, the youngster is merely one of a stream of hundreds of thousands who are moving along an educational track that demands little and provides even less. Their teachers are uncommitted and unmotivated, watch the clock, do not give homework, and so do not provide models for their students—models of people who are "turned on" by learning.

Whatever the cause of the youngster's impaired academic motivation, I often tell such parents that my treatment is not likely to be successful as long as the youngster knows that, whatever happens, he or she will still go on to college. I ask them if they have the guts to make a bona fide threat, a threat that will under no circumstances be withdrawn, namely, that if the patient does not show significant improvement in academic motivation, under no circumstances will he or she go to college for four years of nonlearning and self-indulgence. I advise them to warn the youngster that grades themselves will not be the only criterion to ascertain whether the youngster is deserving of college. This is important because of the grade inflation that exists in our school systems as well as the capacity of youngsters to manipulate their teachers into giving them higher grades. Rather, the criteria that will be used will be both SAT scores and the parents' own observations of the youngster's commitment to learning and the educational process. It is best to leave this vague. To use as a criterion a certain number of hours of homework per night is not useful because the youngster may easily satisfy this requirement with feigned commitment to homework. I warn the parents that they should not make this threat unless they intend to follow it through. I generally advise them to think about it for a week or two and discuss it in detail before making it. I tell them also that they do well to have a plan of operation if the youngster does not indeed go to college.

My experience has been that most parents do not make this threat. They just do not have the courage to do it. The notion that their youngster should not go to college is painful, if not impossible, for them to entertain. They would consider it humiliating if their child did not have a "higher education." They do not know how they could face their friends. They point out other youngsters who entered college with the same lack of motivation and then turned around at some point along the program. I agree that such youngsters exist, but my experience has been that they are a minority.

Some parents of unmotivated adolescents believe that the problem lies in the school and that the solution is to transfer to another one. This rarely works. I try to emphasize to such parents that the problem lies in the youngster's head, not in the building in which the nonlearning is taking place. Although stories about people such as Abraham Lincoln and others who learned significantly under conditions of privation may seem trite, they should still be told. Again, many parents do not follow my advice, spend their money in a special private school, and still find that the youngster is not particularly motivated. When I see adolescents who are already in the first year of one of these "colleges" and are getting low marks (even with grade inflation and limited standards), I generally advise the parents to tell their youngsters that they are no longer going to squander their money on them. I advise them to remove their youngsters from school and have them go out into the workplace for six months or a year and then rethink the whole college decision. After having experiences in the "real world," the youngsters are in a better position to make decisions regarding education versus other options. In addition, if they are really motivated to go to school, then they should be willing to work to contribute toward tuition. Regardless of the affluence of the parents, such youngsters do well to contribute a reasonable fraction of their educational expenses. Such a requirement helps separate the truly motivated from the jokers. Unfortunately, most parents with the college disease do not accept this advice.

On occasion, I will see a patient who is a high school or even a college dropout who stays at home and does nothing. The parents are not complaining so much about the fact that the youngster is not getting an education (they are long past that point); they are now complaining about the fact that they have a "parasite" on their hands. Indeed they do. The youngster sits around the house all day, watches television, listens to rock music, and gabs with friends. Although in the late teens, the youngster is functioning at the three-year-old level. Most often (but not always) there has been a long-standing past history of significant indulgence. This indulgence must be dealt with at the present time. The parents have to be advised to make life tough for such youngsters. No services should be provided. Such youngsters should be required to cook their own meals, purchase their own food, do their own laundry, and be made uncomfortable in many other ways. If possible, television sets should be removed and certainly stereo players. As much as possible, the youngster should be provided with an atmosphere of sensory deprivation. Even telephone services should be restricted and cut off when possible. Otherwise, the youngster is going to sink into a chronic state of morbid dependency on the parents. Again, many of these parents are not capable of following through with these recommendations, so deeply entrenched is their overprotectiveness.

College

I believe that many (but certainly not all) colleges in the United States are not serving primarily as educational institutions; rather, they are serving as what I call "winter camps" that alternate with their students' summer recreational (and sometimes work) programs. Most youngsters attending colleges are looking not for an education but for another four years of self-indulgence and prolongation of their dependent state. We have a unique disease in the United States, which I call the college disease. Millions of parents believe that it is crucial that their children attend college and believe that the schools to which they are sending their children are serving educational purposes. When there is a demand for something, there will always be individuals who will be pleased to provide a supply of the item, especially when there is good money to be made in the business. Most college institutions in the United States are basically businesses that cater to a gullible population of parents who believe that it is crucial that their children (no matter how simple or academically unmotivated) have a college education (no matter how specious and inferior).

These institutions have their academic hierarchy, their assistant professors, associate professors, and full professors. They have their college-style buildings (especially red brick and ivy), their alumni associations, their football teams, and their fund-raising campaigns. They even offer formal courses; the "students" take examinations;

and grades are given. Yet the whole thing does not add up to what can justifiably be referred to as an education. The majority of students are not there to learn; rather, they are there primarily to have a "good time"—which often includes significant indulgence in sex, alcohol, and drugs. What they most often learn are some new sexual techniques, what their tolerance for alcohol is, and perhaps the use of some new drugs that they have not tried before. They also learn how easy it is to get a college diploma. When the "students" are not engaged in these activities, they go though the motions of attending classes, but little is learned. Grade inflation fosters the delusion that they are learning something and ensures that even those with borderline intelligence will get high grades. It is rare for someone to fail. And why should they fail? Does one kick a good customer out of the store? If a customer's parents are willing to continue to pay for the services provided, it would be self-destructive of the college in this highly competitive market to cut off a predictable supply of money because of the student's failure to consume the product being offered.

These colleges provide many of their students with gratification of pathological dependency needs. Such colleges also serve as a mechanism for transferring dependency from parents to those who administer these institutions. Thwarting college authorities (especially by antisocial behavior and refusal to study) is often a transfer of rebellion from parents to school authorities—a rebellion in which the dependency-denial element is often operative.

When I attended college, we generally went from 9:00 A.M. to 5:00 P.M. Monday through Friday and a half day on Saturday. Most courses met four or five times a week and laboratory courses two to three afternoons a week. It was expected that one would do four or five hours of homework a night. School began the day following Labor Day and continued right through early June. There was a one-week Christmas vacation, possibly a one-week Easter vacation, and of course national holidays. Otherwise, we went to school. This is no longer the case. Even in the so-called best colleges and universities, the formal academic program is far less rigorous. Most students average two or three hours a day of classes, while professors may only have to come in five to ten hours a week and are otherwise unseen. These days, the academic year, although it may start around Labor Day, generally ends in early May. Some institutions use the Christmas and/or Easter season as an excuse for an extended holiday (two to four weeks).

Others have long vacations (lasting two to four weeks) between semesters. Many need no other excuse for a long break than the season (spring or winter vacation). These students are being shortchanged. "Educations" of this kind may cost $15,000 a year or more.

Recently, a mother of a patient, who teaches at one of the public universities in New York City, related to me an incident that demonstrates well the deterioration of our educational systems, even at the highest level. The woman is a highly intelligent, well-trained, scholarly individual with a Ph.D. in a very demanding field. One day, her chairman called her into his office and told her that he was having a problem with her, namely, that too many of her students were failing. He informed her that a 40 percent failure rate was unacceptable. She informed him that she was actually being quite generous and that, if she had graded in a more honest way, about 60 percent of her students would fail. He told her that he had sat in on a couple of her classes, knew exactly what the problem was, and considered it easily rectifiable. He then went on to explain to her that she was not giving tests in the "correct" manner. What she was doing was to tell students on Friday, for example, that there would be a test on Monday covering the material in certain chapters of the textbook. This he considered "unfair" to the students. Rather, the "correct" way to give a test was to tell the students on Friday exactly what questions would be asked on Monday. Under the new system, the failure rate dropped from 40 to 20 percent, but even then she found herself being quite generous. Such procedures are a manifestation of the bastardization of the educational system. They make a farce of education and, worse, are a terrible disservice to students. The next step, of course, is merely to tell what questions will be asked and give the answers that will be expected. If one extends this further, one might as well give out (or sell) the diplomas in advance and save everybody a lot of trouble.

Things are even worse at some of the two-year colleges. Many of these institutions merely go through the motions of providing an education and are basically a sham. Students are given textbooks that are seemingly rigorous and demanding, yet in actuality the students are required to learn only a small fraction of what is presented therein. Those in charge recognize the travesty but are party to it, even at the highest levels. The net result of all this is that students are not getting a bona fide education and are thereby entering into the workplace ill equipped to handle jobs for which they are ostensibly being trained.

Also, they are being deprived of the feelings of accomplishment and high self-worth enjoyed by those who have acquired skills and talents through years of hard labor and dedication. The situation thereby contributes to psychopathology because feelings of low self-worth are an important contributing factor in the development of psychogenic symptoms. In addition, it contributes to psychopathic trends (I am not saying gross psychopathy) because of the sanctions that the youngsters are given for "cutting corners," taking shortcuts, and otherwise doing shabby work.

Therapists treating adolescents for ego-dystonic homosexuality may find that their patients enter a high-risk situation when they go off to college. Although I believe that homosexuality may very well have congenital and even genetic contributing factors (varying in intensity from patient to patient), I also believe that environmental factors also operate (again varying from patient to patient). Whatever the combination of heredity and environment, I consider obligatory homosexuality to be a psychiatric disorder and try to help patients who come to treatment for this disturbance. DSM-III referred to such individuals as "ego-dystonic homosexuals." DSM-III-R has no diagnostic category that specifically mentions the word "homosexual" and allows the diagnosis of such individuals under "sexual disorder not otherwise specified" (302.90). If such a youngster's treatment extends to the time of college entrance, then a new problem may arise in the therapy. Most colleges today have active gay communities that are not only quite overt about their homosexuality but also involve themselves actively in various campus activities. Although the ostensible function of such groups is political and educational, they proselytize, seduce, and make every attempt to add to their numbers. This is a dangerous situation for the youngster who is ambivalent about homosexuality and trying to "go straight." Because I consider obligatory homosexuality to be a psychiatric disturbance, I view these groups to be examples of misguided liberalism on campus. To me, it is as appropriate to have a homosexual club on a college campus as it is to have a club of drug addicts, people with character disorders, anorexia-bulimics, and so on. If the latter clubs were formed with the recognition that we are dealing with a form of psychopathology and the group's goal is to help one another with their problems ("self-help" groups), then I would have no difficulty supporting these organizations. However, the homosexual groups have no such philosophy.

32

Although I have no objection to homosexuals' getting their civil rights, and although I also believe that a certain amount of education about homosexuality is useful, I believe that the kind of education that these groups provide is erroneous and misguided—especially because it tries to educate others into believing that homosexuality is a normal, healthy human variation. A common maneuver for these proselytizers is to attempt to make straight youngsters feel embarrassed about their heterosexuality. They may try to get them to feel that they are not showing reasonable flexibility in their sexual options and that they are narrow minded. I believe that such need to convert others stems from an underlying insecurity about the alleged normality of their homosexuality and follows the principle that misery loves company. The more straight youngsters homosexuals can convert, the more secure they believe they will be in their rationalization that their homosexuality is a normal human variant and not a form of psychopathology.

In recent years, many unisex colleges have gone coed. There are, however, certain girls' colleges that have remained all female. Not surprisingly, some of these have become attractive to homosexual girls. Heterosexual girls who attend such colleges, often because they are quite prestigious, may then find themselves lured into a lesbian life-style. Some of these heterosexual girls have never entertained notions of lesbianism and, had they not been proselytized, would have proceeded along the heterosexual track. Many of these girls were not particularly successful in their relationships with boys and so became prime targets for conversion. Accordingly, I consider these girls to have been corrupted.

I recognize that the things that I have just said about homosexuality on college campuses put me in a particularly unpopular position in the mid- to late 1980s. I suspect that there are many others on these campuses who share my views but who fear expressing them openly lest they subject themselves to public condemnation, picketing, and even job loss. Although most universities pride themselves on being institutions where there is freedom of expression of ideas, there are still certain ideas not freely expressed—even in the most liberal and open universities. Criticism of homosexuality is one such example. Therapists treating college-bound homosexual youngsters do well to encourage them to avoid attending universities where militant homosexual groups are likely to have influence over their patients. Rather, they do well to encourage their applying only to schools where the gay community is either nonexistent or plays a limited role in college life. Admittedly, such places may be difficult to find, but they do exist.

Conclusions

The primary implications of my comments are that, with the exception of a small fraction of very gifted students who attend excellent colleges and universities, most young people are being shortchanged when it comes to the education that they are receiving. Therapists do well to make every attempt to apprise their patients of the deficiencies in their educational systems because often they are not aware of these defects. Whatever other benefits a patient may receive from treatment, attendance at a specious educational institution ultimately contributes to dissatisfaction in life, feelings of low self-worth, and frustration. Such feelings are at the bedrock of psychogenic psychopathology. No matter how skilled we are as therapists, if our patients are not being adequately prepared to function in the real world, our efforts may prove futile. Furthermore, there are many who pass through these deficient educational systems and somehow appear to be successful in life. By "success" here I refer to the capacity to earn money. But what they have never been exposed to—and may never appreciate having missed—is the richer kind of educational experience that most of these schools are not providing. When the school is not providing teachers who are committed to the educational process, perhaps therapists can (admittedly to a limited degree) serve as models by communicating to their patients their own commitment to the academic process. This touches on the modeling element, so important in treatment. When the school does not promulgate the notion of learning for its own sake, the therapist does well to introduce this notion to the patient—sometimes for the first time. Discussion of intellectual subjects with adolescents (of course, as a reasonably small fraction of the therapeutic program) can be therapeutic and serve to provide the youngster with this experience.

REFERENCES

Gardner, R. A. 1968. Psychogenic problems of brain-injured children and their parents. *Journal of the American Academy of Child Psychiatry* 4:161–177.

Gardner, R. A. 1974a. The mutual storytelling technique in the treatment of psychogenic problems secondary to minimal brain dysfunction. *Journal of Learning Disabilities* 7:135–43.

Gardner, R. A. 1974b. Psychotherapy of minimal brain dysfunction. In J. Masserman, ed. *Current Psychiatric Therapies*. New York: Grune & Stratton.

Gardner, R. A. 1975a. Psychotherapy in minimal brain dysfunction. In J. Massermann, ed. *Current Psychiatric Therapies*. New York: Grune & Stratton.

Gardner, R. A. 1975b. Techniques for involving the child with MBD in meaningful psychotherapy. *Journal of Learning Disabilities* 8(5): 16–26.

Gardner, R. A. 1977. Psychogenic learning disabilities. *Acta Paedopsychiatrica* 42:188–209.

Gardner, R. A. 1986. *The Psychotherapeutic Techniques of Richard A. Gardner*. Cresskill, N.J.: Creative Therapeutics.

Gardner, R. A. 1987. *Hyperactivity, the So-Called Attention-Deficit Disorder, and the Group of MBD Syndromes*. Cresskill, N.J.: Creative Therapeutics.

Gardner, R. A. 1988. *Psychotherapy with Adolescents*. Cresskill, N.J.: Creative Therapeutics.

Holmes, D. M. 1964. *The Adolescent in Psychotherapy*. Boston: Little, Brown.

Ravitch, D., and Finn, C. E. 1987. *What Do Our 17-Year-Olds Know?* New York: Harper & Row.

LILLIAN H. ROBINSON

Scott Peck (1983) made a provocative statement in *People of the Lie*: "If one wants to seek out evil people, the simplest way to do so is to trace them from their victims. The best place to look, then, is among the parents of emotionally disturbed children or adolescents" (p. 107). Unfortunately, many professionals who work with adolescents have this perception of their patients' parents and are pessimistic about the likelihood of helping them improve their parenting. Because the parental role is so important, there is a tendency to assume that, when things go wrong, the parents are responsible. Our social institutions, including schools, courts, and some social agencies, spend much time and energy blaming parents. All this seems unfair because, in my experience, parental failings are not always the cause of troubled youngsters' difficulties and those parents who have behaved destructively and contributed to their children's disturbance have usually had good intentions. Therapists who choose to work with children have an understandable bias in their favor, which can make it difficult to establish rapport with the parents. Some who are empathic and skillful with their young patients are impatient and judgmental with parents. They regard working with them as a necessary evil and are unclear as to how parents can help in the treatment process. Kessler (1966) stated that, "of all the causative factors, the parental influences seem the most susceptible to change." She added that, "in their zeal to cure, professional workers may . . . foster the impression that if parents will only do the right thing, in the right spirit, the children will have no problems" (p. 410). Of course it is not this simple. Environment is important, but organic factors, constitutional sensitivities, chance happenings (such as illness or surgery), fantasies, and genetic factors all contribute both to personality development and to psychopathology.

Our ability to help troubled adolescents depends in part on our ability to make an alliance with their parents. It is usually the parents who recognize that their youngster is having difficulties. Sometimes they come to this realization after a discussion with teachers or others who are involved with their child, but, unless they realize that their child needs help, they are not likely to seek it. Parents who are able to recognize their child's emotional problems generally feel that they have caused them. Accordingly, it is vitally important to help them deal with their guilt.

Parents learn to be parents through their early experiences with their own parents. If they did not feel accepted by their parents, they find it difficult to accept themselves or their children. Parents who did not have good care may find it very difficult to be nurturing. Parents who felt neglected as children may develop compensating patterns of smothering care, doing more for their children than they want to do and feeling resentful. Often these parents are quite instrusive and cannot bear to allow their children any privacy. When they intrude into areas in which children need to assume responsibility, the children become angry and rebellious, and the parents reciprocate in kind, feeling that their devotion and help are unappreciated. They sense that they are contributing to the difficulties and are often eager to understand the part that they are playing.

Parent counseling and education can be an effective method for helping parents who are motivated. By sharing experiences in discussion groups, they feel less alone with their problems. Attending a class and becoming familiar with literature about child development and child rearing affirms for them the importance of the parental role. Information about children's behavior that is usual at different ages makes it possible for them to have more appropriate expectations for their children. Gilberg (1975) suggested that many parents' unrealistic expectations stem from society's fantasy that parenthood is a supremely happy state. When faced with the realities of child rearing, they often feel inadequate because their family life is different from the idealistic models in television dramas. The Group for the Advancement of Psychiatry (GAP) report, *The Joys and Sorrows of Parenthood*

(1973) points out that peace and quiet are often disrupted in normal homes and that parents' disappointment about unrealized expectations tends to be greatest during their children's adolescence. Parents of adolescents often have conflicting expectations as, for example, when they expect their adolescent's independence in some matters but continuing dependence in others.

American parents tend to push their children to achieve in academics, sports or the arts. Some expect their children to make up for their own disappointments and failures. Parent education can help them understand how children look at the world, how they feel about stressful events, and how they think and reason. This awareness often facilitates communication, helps promote a more positive parent-child relationship, and provides the basis for more effective action on the parents' part.

Recommendations of ways of handling children can be made in parenting classes or in individual counseling sessions. This is usually what parents think they want, but there is no foolproof recipe for rearing children, and it can be dangerous to give too much advice. There are only a few things about which there has been general agreement. For the most part, there are a number of options, each of which has advantages and disadvantages. Parents with authority conflicts may feel compelled to defy the therapist. They need to be helped to devise their own child-rearing methods on the basis of increased understanding of their children's needs.

Markowitz (1975) disagrees with the notion that direct statements of the therapist's views will hinder parents' ability to develop their own resources. He feels that, in order for the parents to feel free to take advice or reject it, advice must be clearly labeled as such and therapists should be straightforward about how confident they are of its validity. He recommends dealing gently with parents since those who are treated harshly will be likely to react punitively with their children. He stresses the importance of full discussion and debate about the advice, which should be given only after a careful history is taken and rapport established. The parents' strengths need to be acknowledged, and an important goal is to help guilty, insecure parents feel more confident. Therapists should express interest both in the child and in the family and its concerns, including the stresses created by the child. Without a relationship, the therapist's help, advice, and recommendations count for very little. If one is too quick to make recommendations, parents may become angry and defensive.

Kessler (1966) quotes Slavson, who stated that "the chief function of the therapist is to demonstrate to the parent what a good parent really is by acting it out toward the father and mother of the young patient. . . . Frequently it is the parents' first experience with a person in a parental role who is calm, understanding, sympathetic, and kindly, though firm. The pattern thus set and the example supplied are of immense value in changing (habitual) behavior of parents" (p. 444). Therapists should not exploit parent's feelings of dependency. Kessler states, "One tries to help them feel like effective parents, not like dependent children" (p. 444). It is also important not to compete with parents or criticize them in their children's presence. Markowitz (1975) warns against using guidance groups as a forum for the leader to ventilate accumulated wisdom and states that "it must to some extent be a process group in which the way individuals act toward their fellow group members can be compared with how they say they behave toward their children" (p. 325).

Through interaction and discussion, parents become better able to judge when their child-rearing practices are meeting their children's needs and when they are serving the parents' interests. For example, parents are often greatly relieved if they can be convinced that they do not need to monitor their child's schoolwork and that to do so is often destructive to the parent-child relationship and can lead to a sense of incapability and low self-confidence on the child's part (Robinson and Phillips 1968). The parents may also feel relieved of some stress if they can decide not to intrude too much into the child's peer relationships. Many parents feel that it is up to them to be sure that their child has "nice" friends. It is important to help intrusive parents understand that no one can choose someone else's friends and that having a friend who steals, lies, or uses bad language is better than being friendless. Many parents can be helped to allow their children more autonomy, thus making it possible for them to learn from experience which friends are enjoyable to be with and which friends will get them in trouble. Enabling parents to gain these insights in the context of a trusting relationship can often relieve some of the anxiety that is associated with parenting.

Working with parents of emotionally disturbed youngsters is often a combination of both informing and advising the parents and dealing with their own feelings and conflicts. Although some older adolescents can be treated alone, parental involvement is essential to effective work with a child or a young adolescent. Treatment should always be planned with the parents, not dictated to them. They are entitled to know why certain recommendations are made.

Parents are extremely important members of the team in dealing with hospitalized youngsters. The decision to hospitalize an adolescent is influenced by the psychopathology of the adolescent patient, the family situation, and the availability of resources. Adolescents may require hospitalization because of the severity of their own emotional disturbance or because the parents' psychopathology makes it impossible for them to safeguard the adolescent at home and support outpatient treatment. Ideally, as partners in the therapeutic process, parents can stimulate and help sustain their child's interest in treatment and encourage growth and behavior change. These tasks demand more insight and patience than some parents possess. Children who are self-destructive or unable to relate to others are often poorly tolerated by parents. Most parents react with mixed feelings to the recommendation that their child be removed from their home and hospitalized. Even though they may feel relieved, it increases their feelings of inadequacy. It is extremely important to support the parents and help them regain their self-respect. The parents' acceptance of the necessity for hospitalization is vitally important to its success.

There is no complete correspondence between the degree of parents' disturbance and their adequacy as parents. Some who are irresponsible and unproductive become more mature when they have children, and some who have many personal problems still are able to manage their children and meet their needs. However, the converse is also true. Some people function adequately in society but do not provide good care for their children.

Anthony (1970) has contributed much to our understanding of the reactions of parents to adolescents and to their behavior, underscoring the difficulties that can result from parents' stereotypic views of adolescents as well as transference reactions in which attitudes from earlier relationships are projected onto the adolescent. Stereotypic polarities include seeing the adolescent as dangerous or endangered, as sexually rampant or sexually inadequate, or as emotionally maladjusted or emotionally free. Anthony suggests that therapists who do well with adolescents avoid this kind of stereotypic thinking and empathize with the "in-between" situation as they respond on a person-to-person basis. I think that a good therapist or counselor for the adolescent's parents must have the same qualities in order to help them give up these stereotypes and develop a "good" or "good enough" reaction to their adolescents.

Fortunately, depth psychotherapy is not always needed to modify inappropriate parental reactions. A brief therapeutic and educational intervention can sometimes turn things around, even when parents are struggling with transference of old issues and make stereotypic responses to their adolescents.

Case Example 1

During her childhood, Donna became very close to her father after her mother developed a chronic fatal illness. When she began dating in mid-adolescence, her father became highly critical. He complained that she spent too much time with friends, wore clothes that were too revealing, and did not study enough, despite the fact that she was an honor student. He attempted to enforce a curfew that could be met only if she left school plays and sports events before they were over, and he was furious when she refused to comply. He requested psychiatric evaluation for Donna and was astonished during the feedback session when I commented on his difficulty in giving up his beautiful "little sweetheart" and his reluctance to allow her to grow up with his blessing. I further suggested that he might be picking fights and finding fault with her to keep his loving feelings from getting out of hand. After some discussion, he acknowledged that, since his wife's death, he sometimes had felt "turned on" by his daughter, often while berating her. He said that he thought I might be right because he had not been especially critical of her one-year-younger brother, whose behavior actually merited more negative comment than Donna's. He seemed relieved when I explained normal adolescent development and complimented him on having provided a facilitating environment that had allowed her to cut some of the strong childhood ties to him. I explained that her recent oppositional behavior was a reaction to his strenuous effort to control her at a time when she needed to use her own internal controls. I offered to begin seeing her for therapy and him for counseling.

I was on vacation during the next three weeks. Shortly after my return, Donna's father came in for his session. Things had changed. He and Donna were no longer in a struggle. They had agreed on a mutually acceptable curfew, and he had stopped criticizing her. He added, "You were right about my part in this. I guess I was afraid I would be a 'dirty old man' if I admitted to myself that I sometimes felt excited by Donna. I had been trying to blame her for this—accusing her of dressing improperly instead of accepting responsibility for my own feelings. Even though I want her to become independent and lead her own life, a part of me does want to keep her all to myself and dependent on me. It feels like this is not going to be such a problem anymore. I hope not. It was hard for my mother to let me grow up and perhaps that had something to do with my attitude toward Donna, especially after we lost her mother."

Physical expressions of anger by exasperated parents sometimes increase the intensity of struggles with their adolescent offspring. Violence begets violence. Youngsters who are slapped or beaten are more likely to attack siblings and peers. The message they get is that it is all right to hit when you are angry. Adolescents who have been physically punished since early childhood may finally rebel and refuse to submit passively any longer. An Army captain father was astonished when his well-developed, sixteen-year-old son took from him the belt that he was trying to use on the boy, threatened to call Child Protection, and announced that he would fight back if his father persisted in his efforts to chastise him.

Many parents who were spanked as children assume that they turned out well because they were spanked, not realizing that it could be in spite of this. They feel disloyal to their parents if they do not spank. They insist that physical punishment is necessary and desirable and quote "Spare the rod and spoil the child." Of course, they never quote Ephesians 6:4: "Parents, do not provoke your children to anger." In discussing this practice with parents, I point out the disadvantages, which, in my opinion, far outweigh the advantages. I mention the danger of engendering feelings that their youngster may not be able to handle. I explain that the feelings that are stirred up by physical punishment, which include anger, sadness, fear, and lowering of self-esteem, can lead to despair and that studies of suicide in children indicate that physical punishment is the most common precipitating factor. Also, it is well known that what begins as culturally sanctioned physical punishment can escalate into abuse. As one parent described it, "It's like my drinking—once I start to drink I can't stop and once I start to hit my kid I can't stop. It scares me and it scares my kid.

Afterward I feel ashamed and hope no one will find out what I did." I explain to the parents that physical punishment wipes the slate clean and eliminates guilt, thus interfering with conscience formation in young children and undermining it in adolescents. Having paid the price for their crimes, they feel free to repeat them in vengeful defiance. On the other hand, if parents use firm verbal expressions of their disapproval and disappointment without recourse to physical punishment, youngsters can experience appropriate guilt, which is a more effective deterrent.

Rexford (1969) has called our attention to a split in our thinking regarding children. In America, we give lip service to the proposition that our children are our most precious resource, our hope for the future, our immortality, yet the children's programs are always the last to be funded. In New Orleans, the only public buildings that are not fully air conditioned are the schools. I believe that our attitudes regarding physical punishment are another example of this split. There is abundant evidence that physical punishment can be destructive, yet we jealously defend the myth that it is helpful to children because it is such a fine way to act on repressed, negative feelings for children and then rationalize that the action is motivated by love. I find that many parents who use physical punishment feel somewhat uncomfortable about it and that some can be persuaded to give it up and express their disapproval verbally.

Case Example 2

Tom, a highly intelligent, creative fifteen-year-old was brought for evaluation because he was failing in school. His mother complained that he was a very angry boy, that he made unreasonable demands on her, and that, if she failed to accommodate him, he screamed and cursed her, often calling her a "whore." What she did not tell me, initially, was that she frequently got exasperated by his demands and slapped his face. His verbal attacks on her closely followed her physical attacks on him. He told me that, when she slapped him, he felt humiliated, rageful, and afraid that he would lose control and hit her back. He was a large, physically fit youngster, taller and heavier than his mother. His father's work had caused him to be absent from the home a great deal during Tom's childhood. It was only during the past five years that he had been able to see much of his father. They got on well together for the most part, although his father would become upset on hearing that he had cursed his mother and, on these occasions, would sometimes chase Tom around the house and hit him. Tom's mother had been physically abused during childhood by her alcoholic father. Tom's father did not remember his own father, who died when he was three.

After the evaluation, I explained to the parents that Tom was depressed and unable to apply himself to his schoolwork. I asked them to discontinue physical punishment, pointing out that the slapping and punching lowered his self-esteem, deepened his depression, and provoked oppositional behavior. The parents were surprised and shocked to realize that they had inadvertently contributed to their son's difficulties. They wanted very much to meet his needs and help him mature and were willing to trust my judgment. Tom responded by becoming less demanding and more reasonable. When angry at his mother, he began to use more polite words than those he was thinking. His grades improved, and he joined the school wrestling team. He decided to continue coming for therapy until he proved to himself that he could do well in school. He was terrified that he would not be as successful as his father, a highly respected professional. "My dad is a hard act to follow," he said. "I am very proud of him, and someday I hope I can make him proud of me."

Parents who cling most desperately to destructive patterns are usually those who are conflicted and uneasy about their parenting. We urge parents to acknowledge their children's appropriate behavior—to use positive reinforcement—yet we often neglect to do this with the parents. Even those parents who manage to get most things wrong are doing a few things that are appropriate and helpful to their children. We need to search these things out and let the parents know that these practices benefit their children.

Erikson (1950) and Benedek (1959) regard parenthood as an important stage in the life cycle. Benedek (1959) stated that parents' own developmental crises are revived as their children negotiate these stages and suggested that this gives parents a second chance to work through their conflicts and to achieve a new level of intrapsychic integration. She observed that motherliness becomes more mature with successive babies and that the instinctual wish to survive in one's child and the wish to love the child are somewhat in conflict with the difficult task of child rearing. The survival of humankind in spite of the conflict was seen as attesting to the strength of these tendencies that enable parents to love and care for their children. Benedek (Parens 1973) asserted that the parents' wish to reproduce themselves in their offspring is innate and linked with the instinct of survival. Parens (1973) agreed, suggesting that the proper epigenetic sequence of psychosexual developmental phases might conclude with parenthood rather than adulthood. He pointed out that, in Freud's drive theories, reproduction and preservation of the species are the ultimate aims and stated that, in view of the long period of child care, which is necessary to preserve the species, we may assume that parenting is inherent. Kestenberg (Parens 1973) also agreed that there is evidence to support the concept of a developmental need in humankind to reproduce and rear children. Moore (Parens 1973) disagreed on the grounds that present trends of postponing family formation and turning over of children to the care of others seemed to him incongruous with the concept.

Regardless of whether parenthood is inherent, it is certainly an opportunity for growth and the development of greater maturity. However, it seems arbitrary to label those who do not want children as selfish or immature on these grounds alone. Although giving life to a child and nurturing it may be the most creative thing most of us will ever do, some prefer to express their creativity in other ways.

One's motivations for making a major change in life have considerable bearing on the outcome. This is certainly true of becoming a parent. Jessner, Weigert, and Foy (1970) have explored motivations for having children. They state that a healthy motivation includes strong wishes for a child and equally strong wishes to nurture the child and meet its needs; however, they point out that motives are sometimes less pure. Some individuals who felt unloved as children feel that their own children will have to love them to make up for what they did not get from their parents. These unrealistic expectations lead to feelings of frustration and disappointment. Individuals who are uncertain about their identity may want to have children in order to prove something—that he is truly a man or that she is a real woman.

Even well-motivated parents who want children to love and care for rather than to solve their problems may have some difficulty managing normal, negative feelings about having children. Negative feelings may stem from doubts about one's ability to love a child. Those who are overly conscientious and have excessively high standards are particularly likely to be preoccupied with fears about their ability to be good parents. This is common in individuals who felt that their parents were not able to love them enough. If, as children, they felt jealous of their siblings, they may find it hard to share their mates with a child. Conflicts regarding dependency can lead to reluctance to assume responsibility for meeting the dependency needs of a child.

The ways in which parents manage their negative feelings for their children greatly affect their competence as parents. When the negative feelings predominate and are not sufficiently neutralized by positive feelings, parents develop rejecting attitudes and may neglect or mistreat their children. Even when the negative feelings are not the predominant feelings, they may be acted on and rationalized. Good care may be seen as dangerous spoiling by parents who are unaware of the negative feelings that are evident in their actions. Such parents often defend excessive or inappropriate punishments as "good for the child."

Repression and denial of negative feelings can lead to overly protective attitudes, overindulgence, and inability to be firm or say "no." These attitudes and behaviors serve as compensations for the negative feelings. Unfortunately, rather than making up for anything, they only compound the problem. Having to be excessively protective and helpful interferes with parents' ability to enjoy the child and prolongs the child's dependence on the parent. Children are often resentful of and feel demeaned by parents' excessive solicitude. The children's resentment stirs up still more negative feelings in the parents, which are, in turn, denied and dealt with by still more condescending helpfulness. Thus, a vicious circle is established.

The healthy way to deal with negative feelings is to acknowledge them, accept them as natural human feelings, and put up with them, realizing that some ambivalence is part of the human condition. No one is capable of perfect love. There is nothing shameful about having a few mixed feelings. Our efforts should be directed toward helping parents utilize this healthy way of coping with their negative feelings. To do so before a child is born amounts to primary prevention of mental illness, both for the parents and for the future child. We should endorse and support preventive programs for expectant parents and parents who have not experienced problems severe enough to prompt them to seek our help. Even after difficulties arise, children and adolescents can benefit from our working with parents to enable them to verbalize and master feelings that were previously so unacceptable that they could not be acknowledged.

The GAP (1973) report states that, when individuals are physically mature enough to have children and psychologically mature enough to gratify both the children's needs and their own, they are ready to become parents. As parents care for their children, they reconsider their past and, in learning to be parents, reexperience what happened to them when they were children. They can either take good care of their children and develop into more capable individuals or feel frustrated and unhappy about their deficiencies and regress to a lower level of functioning. Parents as well as children gain self-esteem through good parent-child relationships. Parents tend to fear that their children will have difficulties similar to those that they experienced in their own development. If they were wildly rebellious teenagers with drinking or drug problems, they may dread their child's adolescence and convey negative expectations to them as a self-fulfilling prophecy. Other parents, as they rework what happened to them many years ago, reach a higher level of maturity and contribute to their children's mastery of the same conflicts (Benedek 1970).

Parents' relationships with each other also has a significant effect on their children. Children learn from their parents' example how men and women relate to one another in marriage, how they communicate, negotiate differences, and arrive at compromises. Children worry if their parents do not have a good relationship. Studies of the effects of parental divorce have shown that children often feel that they have lost both parents. One leaves home, and the other is preoccupied and emotionally unavailable. Conflict between the parents before, during, and after the divorce is very disturbing to their children. Weissman and Cohen (1985) have suggested that parents' marital relationship is less important than their ability to form a parenting alliance. They find that divorce does not preclude a good parenting alliance and that intactness of the family does not guarantee it. The parenting alliance is conceptualized as a relationship that sustains parents' self-esteem and enables them to resolve developmental issues that are reactivated in the process of parenting.

Parents have the right and the duty to advocate their values and to try to pass them on to their children while at the same time respecting their children's right to establish differing values. The GAP report gives the example of a college girl who brought her boyfriend home and demanded that they be allowed to sleep together in her bedroom. Because it was within her value system not to be hypocritical, she was being true to herself in taking this position; however, it was contrary to the mother's values to condone this behavior. In order to be true to herself, the mother had to say, "You may sleep with your boyfriend if you wish, but not in my house." Parents must uphold their own values in order to preserve their own self-integrity. Parents must also constantly reexamine their values and be flexible enough to allow them to change.

Similarly, therapists must respect the values of both the adolescent patient and the parents. Cultural and religious values that are not shared by the therapist may be regarded as resistance or as a pathological nuisance when, in reality, they are healthy and useful. Barnhouse (1986) has provided guidelines for distinguishing between pathological and healthy religious ideation. She points out that, although immature uses of religion do not necessarily imply psychopathology, it is usually a reflection of psychopathology when religions ideation is highly idiosyncratic or incompatible with the patient's level of religious development or when religious concerns cause consistent subjective discomfort. She contends that, because "sex and religion are, in some form, universal components of human experience, psychiatrists who know very little about religion would do well to study it" and reminds us that "no psychiatrist would dream of trying to practice without knowing a great deal about sex." She states, "Religious concerns . . . cannot be irrelevant to therapy if they are brought up by the patient. The task is to understand whether they are being used as . . . . (resistance) or whether they are an important component of . . . . healthy functioning" (p. 103).

Conclusions

Research concerning parent education indicates that parents are significantly and desirably changed by participating in parent discussion groups and by individual counseling or therapy. Often what begins as child-centered counseling develops into personal therapy for the parents. We can be confident that people can and do change and that they continue to respond to external influences throughout their lives. Psychotherapists and educators provide something special in the way of an external influence, something that gives parents new information about themselves or about their children, that may help them to alter their attitudes and behavior. Normal parents of normal children sometimes seek parent education or therapy as a preventive measure. Parents of emotionally disturbed children may seek it because they are demoralized by the child's illness, whether they have contributed to it or not. We must bear in mind that some of the disturbance seen in these parents is the effect rather than the cause of the child's illness and that they are very much in need of understanding and support. If we assume that most parents do the best they can with the knowledge and empathy they possess, we will get on with helping rather than blaming them for unfortunate attitudes and actions.

NOTE

This chapter was presented at the Central States Conference of the American Society for Adolescent Psychiatry, "The Troubled Family: Adolescent Abuse and Adolescent Abusers," Nashville, Tennessee, November 13–15, 1987.

REFERENCES

Anthony, E. J. 1970. The reaction of parents to their adolescents and to their behavior. In E. J. Anthony and T. Benedek, eds. *Parenthood: Its Psychology and Psychopathology.* Boston: Little, Brown.

Barnhouse, R. T. 1986. How to evaluate patients' religious ideation. In L. Robinson, ed. *Psychiatry and Religion: Overlapping Concerns.* Washington, D.C.: APA Press.

Benedek, T. 1959. Parenthood as a developmental phase. *Journal of the American Psychoanalytic Association* 7:389–417.

Benedek, T. 1970. The family as a psychologic field. In E. J. Anthony and T. Benedek, eds. *Parenthood: Its Psychology and Psychopathology* Boston: Little, Brown.

Erickson, E. H. 1950. *Childhood and Society.* New York: Norton.

Gilberg, A. L. 1975. The stress of parenting. *Child Psychiatry and Human Development* 6:59–67.

Group for the Advancement of Psychiatry. Committee on Public Education. 1973. *The Joys and Sorrows of Parenthood.* Report no. 84. New York: Group for the Advancement of Psychiatry.

Jessner, L.; Weigert, E.; and Foy, J. L. 1970. The development of parental attitudes during pregnancy. In E. J. Anthony and T.

Benedek, eds. *Parenthood: Its Psychology and Psychopathology.* Boston: Little, Brown.

Kessler, J. W. 1966. *Psychopathology of Childhood.* Englewood Cliffs, N.J.: Prentice-Hall.

Markowitz, I. 1975. Making meaningful advice to parents acceptable. *International Journal of Group Psychotherapy* 25:323–329.

Parens, H. 1975. Parenthood as a developmental phase. *Journal of the American Psychoanalytic Asssociation* 23:154–165.

Peck, M. S. 1983. *People of the Lie.* New York: Simon & Schuster.

Rexford, E. 1969. Children, child psychiatry and our brave new world. *Archives of General Psychiatry* 20:25–37.

Robinson, L. H., and Phillips, C. 1968. A common school problem: when parents become teachers. *GP (Family Physician)* 38:94–99.

Weissman, S., and Cohen, R. S. 1985. The parenting alliance and adolescence. *Adolescent Psychiatry* 12:24–45.

4 REVENGE OR TRAGEDY: DO NERDS SUFFER FROM A MILD PERVASIVE DEVELOPMENTAL DISORDER?

NICHOLAS PUTNAM

There is a clinical syndrome that is easily recognized by both adolescents and the general public but rarely by clinicians. Youngsters identified as "nerds" suffer from a sometimes serious handicap that mental health practitioners generally fail to diagnose and treat, perhaps because no widely accepted clinical label for the syndrome exists. It is important that psychiatrists become better informed about this syndrome and the effect it has on children and adolescents.

This discussion focuses on youngsters commonly described as nerds. More technical terms for the problems that afflict such individuals, such as "mild, nonautistic pervasive developmental disorder," are cumbersome. Nerds can best be understood clinically, however, in the context of the pervasive developmental disorders.

The pervasive developmental disorders (PDDs) are a distinct group of disorders, beginning in childhood, characterized in DSM-III-R (American Psychiatric Association 1987) as involving qualitative impairment in the development of reciprocal social interaction, verbal and nonverbal communication skills, and imaginative activity. Within the category of PDDs, DSM-III (American Psychiatric Association 1980) identified three subtypes, including a residual category labeled "atypical pervasive developmental disorder." DSM-III-R, on the other hand, identifies only two categories: "autistic disorder" and a residual category called "pervasive developmental disorder not otherwise specified." The PDDs actually lie along a continuum. Some forms are quite severe; some forms are less severe or are mitigated in some way by a particular child's cognitive and temperamental strengths. Cantwell and Baker (1988) note that recent research supports a number of subtypes of autistic-like syndromes, ranging from severely retarded autistic children to high-functioning children with so-called atypical personality development.

I maintain that PDDs occur in attenuated forms that are not uncommon. My interest in this topic stems from acquaintance with a number of tragic cases involving bright adolescents with relatively mild, nonautistic, PDDs whose handicap went unrecognized by their treating physicians and who posed continuing diagnostic dilemmas. Those diagnostic difficulties led at times to inappropriate treatment and to a failure to address directly the primary source of the considerable pain that those youngsters experienced. It is my contention that many individuals labeled as "nerds" suffer from a mild or minor PDD.

The mild pervasive developmental disorders (MPDDs) are less obvious than their more severe counterparts but probably much more common. Although children with a mild PDD may not fit easily into the definitional structure of DSM-III-R, the public has never had any question that nerds form a definite subgroup of human beings. Nerds are frequently featured on television, in movies, and in cartoons. In the popular *Far Side* cartoons, Larson illustrates "nerd convoys" and "nerd roundups." In the movie *Revenge of the Nerds,* the protagonists are immediately identified as nerds; their appearance, mannerisms, and speech clearly mark them from the moment they appear on screen. Although nerds generally figure as comic characters, under stress real nerds can decompensate, resulting in significant morbidity and even mortality. For that reason, among others, it is important to describe and classify the syndrome of nerdiness.

Definition

"Nerd" appears in several dictionaries. *The American Heritage Dictionary* (Morris 1985) defines "nerd" as "a socially inept, foolish, or ineffectual person." *Webster's Ninth New Collegiate Dictionary* (Mish 1987) expresses a view of nerds that alludes to the contempt often felt toward these youngsters: "Nerd . . . *slang* (1965): an unpleasant, unattractive, or insignificant person." A more precise clinical definition of the MPDD syndrome from which nerds suffer can be offered:

The syndrome is first apparent in the preschool years, when, in the presence of average or above average intelligence, children exhibit difficulties with reciprocal social relationships, despite a definite desire for companions. These difficulties are manifest in an inability to make and keep friends, in problems understanding and responding to social cues, and in showing little empathy for the feelings of others. The syndrome is accompanied by deficits in pragmatic language skills, often including poorly modulated speech and an inability (rather than an unwillingness) to adopt contemporary jargon successfully. There is, in addition, a difficulty in appreciating the arts, aesthetic pursuits, and other creative, imaginative endeavors. The syndrome is often associated with some degree of clumsiness.

This definition is similar to descriptions of Asperger's syndrome (Wing 1981). Asperger's syndrome, an autistic-like disorder, lies within the spectrum of the atypical PDDs. Because this disorder is "less pervasive" than autism, it is easy to misdiagnose in an adolescent as a personality disorder, such as schizoid or schizotypal (Munro 1987). Individuals with Asperger's syndrome characteristically are socially isolated and display abnormal social interaction (Szatmari 1986). They may be not just shy but also abnormally garrulous or intrusive; their behavior is often not appropriately modified to suit the social situation. There are impairments in nonverbal communication and oddities in the speech of persons with Asperger's syndrome. There is frequently a history of developmental aberration in the preschool years, such as an unwillingness or inability to engage in cooperative or imaginative play.

Perhaps many of the youngsters with MPDD fit the criteria of Asperger's syndrome. Most American psychiatrists are not comfortable with this term, so it is not in common use in this country. The term "MPDD" may be preferable as a clinical designation of nerdiness because it implies that there is a continuum of children with dysfunction in language and social development. Use of the term "MPDD" avoids splitting this group of individuals into specific diagnostic categories, at least until there is more of a basis in clinical research to do so.

MPDD and Adolescence

Adolescence, because of its demands in the areas of social and language functioning, is a period of great risk for individuals with MPDD. With respect to the major PDDs, DSM-III-R notes that, during adolescence, "there is often an exacerbation of aggressive, oppositional, or other troublesome behavior, which may last for many years" (p. 36). Contrary to the stereotype of the bookish nerd, the same is true of the MPDDs as well.

Youngsters with mild pervasive developmental disorders will experience a crisis in adolescence because the skills that are necessary to accomplish adolescent developmental tasks are dependent on rather high-level functioning in the very areas in which these youngsters have deficits. They lack the ability to respond to subtle social cues appropriately and the ability to use language to establish identity and, later, intimacy.

During early adolescence, children display a wide range of social abilities. At one end of the spectrum are the popular, socially facile children, including both delinquent and nondelinquent youngsters proficient in manipulating their social environment. Next in line are the vast majority of children, who are skilled enough to avoid much of the teasing and social pain so common in junior high school. Then come the nerds, who occupy a place in the spectrum well short of the autistic extreme. Whereas autistic individuals, even the high-functioning ones, have trouble from infancy or soon thereafter, the major problems for nerds begin in the older primary grades and intensify in junior high school. Nerds suffer enough limitations in their social awareness and social effectiveness to become the object of rather severe scapegoating, even among adults. They themselves are painfully aware that there is something wrong, yet they and their parents often cannot define the problem.

Secondary psychiatric symptoms often obscure the MPDD, increasing difficulty with clinical recognition. When the coping mechanisms that these children employ fail, as they frequently do during adolescence, they may develop secondary psychiatric problems ranging from aggressive behavior to depression to psychoses. Clinicians tend to focus on these secondary symptoms, ignoring the primary syndrome.

Personal Example

When I began to write this chapter, I decided to do a literature search to find out what had been written lately on related topics. I called a friend I had known well since junior high school. He is a physician in his forties, single, living with his parents. He uses his home computer and modem to do literature searches. I told him that I was interested in the less extreme PDDs and the group of youngsters in school referred to as "nerds."

When my friend sent me a printout of the results of the computer search, he included a note: "Your discussion triggered off a whole flood of memories of mine from junior high school. I can recall how I was accused of being from Mars and of reading the dictionary. I did not read the dictionary and was never conscious of speaking in a different vocabulary than my peers, but I assume my accusers were correct and what were ordinary words for me were peculiar polysyllabic, pedantic nerdisms to them. Occasionally, I would flat-out misuse words or mispronounce them, which you and others called me on on several occasions."

My friend's strongly positive reaction at feeling understood is a reaction that I have had repeatedly from older adolescents and their parents when I discuss this problem of nerdism in developmental terms. I have come to believe that these individuals have felt stigmatized for a long time. Because they are rarely understood, they are relieved and appreciative when someone can say to them, "I think I know what the problem is here, even if we do not have a very good name for it."

My friend's comments brought back some of my own memories of him in junior high school. He was right. He was the object of unrelenting teasing not only for his vocabulary but for his speech, which was mocked for its atonal quality, his mannerisms, his utilitarian way of dressing (with the almost emblematic front-pocket plastic pencil holder), and his lack of athletic skill. He was ridiculed in the cruel manner of which perhaps only seventh and eighth graders are capable. I remember an occasion when a group of boys attempted to push his head through a hole in a concrete wall in front of the school. I remember also how confused and embittered he became, to the point eventually of assisting some of the more antisocial boys in placing homemade explosives down the school toilets, an activity that somewhat broke the ice for him socially. In high school, he was better accepted and even appreciated for his wide range of knowledge, but he never found social situations easy, and the only date he had was arranged by friends. In adult life, he has often been severely depressed.

Holistic versus Sequential Thinking

In order to understand better the particular handicap that plagues youngsters with MPDD, it is necessary to review a number of concepts presented by Tanguay (1984). He pointed out that, among those with PDDs, each child has his own profile of cognitive strengths and liabilities. The more we understand these children and their specific cognitive profiles, the more difficult it is to classify them together, as "autistic," for example.

It appears to be more useful to look at their ability to function along a number of cognitive parameters and to discern patterns in functioning that affect adjustment and clinical outcome for these youngsters. Tanguay suggested that it is important to recognize that neuropsychologists have identified two distinct forms of cognitive processing, the "holistic" and the "sequential" modes of thought. One may imagine that there is a spectrum of social adjustment among adolescents related to social intelligence, which is related to holistic thinking (and perhaps to right-brain functioning). Social intelligence is the ability to read subtle, often nonverbal, social cues, to use social context appropriately in order to modulate behavior, and to use language in socially significant ways. Tanguay (1984, p. 377) writes:

> Holistic thinking is nonverbal, and is presumably carried out using visual, kinesthetic, tactile and auditory images, with multiple parallel information inputs being synthesized and compared. It is particularly well adapted to activities such as facial recognition, spatial manipulation, or processing of the auditory "gestalt" of familiar words and phrases. Holistic processing may play an important role in the manner in which one deals with words in a punning, changing, metaphoric, creative, symbolic fashion, rather than in strict lexical and syntactic terms. . . . sequential processing, in contrast, deals with the coding and decoding of meaning in terms of the relationship of elements within a sequence.

Sequential thinking is logical, both analytic and deductive. Explaining holistic thinking to patients with MPDD and their parents can be difficult. Although facial agnosia is not part of the MPDD syndrome, a discussion of the way in which the brain can recognize faces is often helpful when teaching these adolescents and their parents about holistic thinking. These patients often cannot imagine any mental activity that a computer could not be programmed to accomplish, yet facial recognition, thus far, cannot be simulated in the way that the human brain accomplishes it.

The relation of holistic processing to MPDD is fairly complex. Many youngsters with PDDs have an ability to use simple holistic skills and may even show superior skills in visual-spatial operations, yet they show significant deficits in complex holistic-processing abilities. The latter abilities include the use and understanding of subtle forms of nonverbal communication such as facial expression or gesture.

It is interesting to speculate about why the proportion of nerds among females is so much lower than the proportion among males. It may be that the cognitive pattern associated with MPDD is in some ways an exaggeration of the normal male pattern. Indeed, fathers seem to relate more easily with their children who are nerds, and mothers of nerds often have difficulty in understanding why their sons have such poor social skills. Women with highly developed capacities for holistic, intuitive thinking may have the most difficulty in understanding MPDD children.

It is appealing to think of this in terms of right-brain versus left-brain functioning. Nerds are often capable of superior analytic (left-brained) skills. My friend knew a lot of good words. He just could not understand when or how to use them. Nerds' ability to use the right brain—in the arts or in social situations—is often impaired. They may learn music theory and learn how to operate a musical instrument, but they may find a better niche in the school band by becoming a manager keeping track of equipment and travel arrangements. In fact, nerds gravitate toward such jobs. In the past, it was operating the audiovisual equipment: a special card was issued, lending some prestige, and there was assured involvement with peers who could socialize and perform.

Brothers (1989) recently utilized a broad biological approach in considering the role of empathy in the development of clinical psychopathology. Brothers notes that DSM-III-R "uses a defect of empathy as a primary criterion for diagnosis of autistic disorder" (p. 13) and describes laboratory studies that could someday reveal the neural substrate of empathy—possibly involving the amygdala.

MPDD AND COMPUTERS

For some teenagers, computers provide an escape from challenging social situations and a partial cure for the loneliness of MPDD. The computer itself provides a predictable pseudocompanionship, and computer users can also band together in common-interest clubs. Such teenagers can become involved with computers to the exclusion of almost all other interests. At an early age, they may reach high levels of proficiency with programming and even make contributions to the computer world.

Interaction with computers is satisfying because computers reward analytic thinking with success. This is not true of the adolescent social world. Some of these adolescents may come to identify themselves as "computer people." Since computers are not primarily mechanical devices, such mastery often carries with it a certain mystique and status.

APPEARANCE

The popular youngsters in junior high school have an uncanny ability to negotiate the complex social maze. Appearance, which includes but is not limited to physical attractiveness, is instrumental in attaining social well-being. This involves knowing how to dress and how to dress when. Nerds are easily recognized by their clothes. Front-pocket plastic pen holders are extremely practical, but only a nerd would wear one to junior high school. The same is true for clip-on cases for eyeglasses or eyeglass safety straps (unless they are used for sunglasses).

Early in adolescence, youngsters must learn to make subtle distinctions between what is right to wear and what is wrong. Recently, for example, it was no longer "in" to wear "OP" shorts in Southern California, and there was a switch to a baggier brand of short pants. An entire industry closely watches (and perhaps helps create) such changes in adolescent fashion. Appearance is extremely important in determining one's acceptance among peers, and many youngsters are extremely sensitive to subtle and rapidly changing cues regarding their appearance. Much of this information related to fashion cannot be reduced to logical bits, and the ability to see the whole gestalt must require holistic thinking.

SPEECH AND LANGUAGE

Shapiro (1985) has pointed out that adolescent speech includes endless variations on the theme of establishing group identity, so important to the psychological development of the adolescent. Litowitz (1985) describes three functions of language that are particularly pertinent for adolescents: the use of language to establish one's identity, including gender identity; the use of language to establish closeness of relationships; and the use of language for phatic communication, that is, the socially ritualized and reassuring use of language, as in "Hi, how are you?" or "Have a nice day" for us and "Hey, dude!" for the seventh grader. Litowitz points out that adolescents realize that every utterance embodies two different forces: what one is trying to do with language and what one is trying to get others to do.

These communication tasks, as well as the effective use of language, require the use of both sequential and holistic modes of cognition. Perhaps one part of the brain provides the words and syntax, and another part provides the intonation and emphasis and helps ensure that what is said takes into account the complex social context of the conversation, with emotional tone regulated at still another neuroanatomical site. The individual who experiences difficulties in holistic processing is surely at a disadvantage in both generating utterances and producing appropriate speech acts.

Case Example

Michael was the seventeen-year-old son of two high school teachers. His parents were an attractive, loving couple who set aside a great deal of time for family activities and led an active adult social life. Michael was a high school senior and had for some time been enrolled in special classes as a result of difficulties in school performance, despite his above-average intelligence. His adjustment to school had deteriorated rapidly during his junior year, and, on a number of occasions, he simply refused to attend school. He complained that he was being teased by other students at school and even by a few faculty members. These episodes led to periods of extreme dejection and eventually to crying spells that occurred at school, which exacerbated the scapegoating.

His parents had always been aware of Michael's social problems, but they became increasingly alarmed as his depression progressed and he began to threaten suicide. He would talk with them about having no future. He feared his senior year in high school would "not be anything like it is supposed to be—like it was for my brother." Michael was referring to the high school experience of his more socially facile older brother, who dated, went to the senior prom, and participated in many social clubs.

Michael was seen by a number of physicians, diagnosed as suffering from a major depressive disorder, and treated with antidepressants. When that was not entirely successful, he was treated with thioridazine for anxiety and agitation, and eventually he was placed on lithium. When I first saw him, Michael was on a high dose of imipramine, had a therapeutic serum level of lithium, and had thioridazine prescribed as needed. He had been seen by competent clinicians who had recognized the extreme disturbance in his mood, along with his "odd personality," but who had failed to recognize the underlying PDD that was the root cause of this boy's poor adjustment in school.

When I asked, "How are you?" Michael responded with speech that was classically mechanical and poorly modulated. With a forced smile, he replied, "This has not been a good day for me." Asked to elaborate, he noted that the school had had an end-of-the-year swimming party. He had always admired one of the more popular boys in the class and had approached him at this party, intending to have a conversation. As the boy emerged from the swimming pool, Michael commented, "My! You certainly are wet!" On hearing this, the boy grabbed Michael by the arm and threw him into the pool. Michael, who was not wearing a swimsuit, was acutely embarrassed by this incident and immediately left the party. When I asked him to explain why the boy had thrown him in the pool, he stated, "I guess I just put my foot in my mouth." I asked what he meant by that, and Michael stated that, as he was throwing him into the water, the other boy had said, "Of course I'm wet, I just got out of the pool, Dork. See what I mean?"

Most of the evidence necessary to make a diagnosis of MPDD was apparent to me within the first three minutes of my interview with Michael. His attempt at social contact, both with the psychiatrist and with the boy at the party, required the use of speech for what is known as phatic communication, the establishment of an atmosphere of sociability. At the party, depending on what was "in" at the time, it might have been better for Michael to say, "Hey, dude, how you doin'?" Just saying the proper words, however, would not have saved Michael, as nerds are notorious for saying the words in a mechanical way. The language of teenagers is especially dependent on pitch, tone, and rhythm. In fact, the entertainment industry continuously markets particular speech patterns, such as "rapping," and "Val-speak," as they emerge among adolescents. Michael could not even hope to say "Hey, Dude, how you doin'?" in a way that might have elicited acceptance from his peer.

Youngsters who have poor pragmatic speech skills experience such situations several times a day. The social consequences are disastrous. Michael had a birthday shortly after he began seeing me and invited twenty other teenagers to the party. Such "social optimism" is typical of nerds. Despite the fact that his family was able to offer a nice setting for the party, only two youngsters attended. It is no wonder that Michael was unhappy. Continual rejection can lead to withdrawal or even the symptoms of a major depression, which Michael manifested.

Differential Diagnosis

Psychiatrists frequently mistake MPDD youngsters for schizoid or schizotypal teenagers. Both nerds and schizoid youngsters often have no close friends of a similar age other than a relative or a similarly socially isolated child (the first criterion for diagnosis of schizoid disorder). Schizoid children, however, have no apparent interest in making friends and do not derive pleasure from the usual peer interaction. They generally avoid nonfamiliar social contacts, especially with peers. Nerds, on the other hand, are painfully aware of their difficulties in establishing normal peer relationships. They may have a great deal of interest in making friends and, until their failures become too unbearable, will seek out social contacts. For a nerd, it is better to be at the party, operating the stereo or helping start someone's car, than not to be there at all.

The *Revenge of the Nerds* movies (the original and the sequel) are full of examples of nerds' deep desire for normal social contact. In the first movie, for example, the older adolescent nerds eagerly anticipate an enjoyable college social life, including heterosexual experiences.

61

Both movies demonstrate repeatedly how difficult it is for somebody to escape the social stigma of being a nerd, how easy it is for people to recognize nerds, and how little nerds seem to be able to do about changing their image. Nevertheless, the movies emphasize that, in spite of these obstacles, the nerds have a strong interest in social relationships.

Another part of the differential diagnosis is avoidant disorder. Avoidant teenagers may appear awkward socially as a result of extreme anxiety. This anxiety may make them feel like nerds and even act like nerds. If they can overcome their anxiety, it becomes clear that they have more than adequate social intelligence and normal speech and language development. Nerds do not avoid social situations. They often seek them out, particularly in adolescence, but they misread the social situation miserably.

Thus, the schizoid youngster does not particularly want to go to the prom and asks nobody to go to the prom; the avoidant youngster may want to go to the prom but is too shy to ask. If he finds a partner with whom he is comfortable, then he may well go to the prom. The nerd may ask one of the cheerleaders to go to the prom and is unable to understand why she laughs at him. The avoidant adolescent must learn to overcome the anxiety that surrounds social interactions; the nerd requires specific training in how to understand and negotiate the social maze of adolescence.

Some might argue that nerds are simply extremely intelligent, somewhat eccentric youngsters. For some time now, it has been known (Terman 1925) that bright youngsters are typically healthy and well adjusted. They use both sides of the brain well. While many nerds are blessed with superior analytic skills, particularly those skills important in science and mathematics, they lack social intelligence. The writers of *Head of the Class,* a television situation comedy about a classroom filled with extremely bright youngsters, have recognized the distinction between the nerd and the intelligent young person. They have included one or two boys whose social ineptness provides a great deal of the humor in the series; however, other equally bright adolescents in the class are socially quite adept. Woody Allen is able to identify with the bright but socially inept nerd and can humorously portray a nerd, yet he obviously is an extremely skilled observer of relationships and subtle social cues and could not himself be called a nerd.

MPDD and the Media

Many of the situation comedies on television include a nerd, usually as a friend of the family. Nerds provide a constant source of humor, but, when this form of dysfunction happens to teenagers in real life, it is not at all funny. One reason for the heavy use of nerds in television and movies is that many people identify in some way with nerds. We all can feel nerdy at times. We all have taken things a little too literally, have misread social cues, or have stuck our foot in our mouth. It reassures us to see someone on television who behaves inappropriately in the extreme—when we know that it is not real. Perhaps because of feelings of discomfort over our occasional social miscues, we also enjoy seeing socially inept persons reap revenge, as they do in the *Revenge of the Nerds* movies.

Another television sitcom, *Small Wonder,* is about a little girl who is actually a robot created by her parents and programmed to perform all the functions of an ideal child. She also provides humor in the show by misreading social situations. Tact is something that is difficult to teach. In all these television sitcoms, the person who plays the role of the nerd will frequently be too candid in situations that cause embarrassment to others and eventually to himself. Another television show employs an extraterrestrial, Alf, who is quite engaging and has the potential to learn appropriate earth social behavior, but he has many of the difficulties that nerds have with understanding family life. He is constantly "in the doghouse," so to speak, with his adopted, earth family.

Adjustment to New Family Situations

There are special problems for kids with MPDD whose lives lead them into complicated family situations, as occurs so frequently today with the high rate of divorce and remarriage. It is extremely difficult for a healthy adolescent to deal with all the complex social problems that arise following a divorce, but it is even harder for an adolescent who is a nerd. Two teenagers whom I saw recently had parents who had remarried; both boys were living with their fathers, stepmothers, and stepsiblings. In each case, not only were the new stepsiblings embarrassed to be associated with these youngsters at school, but both boys found it almost impossible to develop relationships with their new step-mother and stepsiblings. They each quickly became the family scapegoat, blamed for nearly all the tension inevitable in blended families. These youngsters had special difficulties with stepsisters, and, interestingly, both went through periods of hostile acting out toward these girls.

Nerds in School

Although the social problems of nerds with peers are obvious, they may also have significant problems in the classroom, which is usually seen as their "home turf." Educators are well aware that, beginning in preadolescence, students are expected to practice various levels of higher-order thinking. Rather than merely decode information, the fourth grader is expected to put information together in interesting and informative packages. This involves the ability to encode information already learned and produce an original product. It also involves the ability to identify with a potential reader of one's work, to evaluate the work of others critically but sympathetically, and to develop skills such as persuasion.

In adolescents with MPDD, teachers may notice either undue formality or familiarity with adults in the school. The teen may continue to raise his hand with the answers when it is clear to all that he has already had his fair share. He may not know when to stop with his answers, exploring every aspect of the question to the exasperation of all. He may direct poorly tempered criticism at the creative projects of other youngsters.

From a diagnostic standpoint, written material may not reveal the problem, as it might with a thought disorder or a language disability. One needs to know the nature of the assignment in order to judge the writing of a child with MPDD. For example, in English class, the assignment might have been to write about an experience that the child had over the summer. Expecting a personal reply, the teacher may receive, instead, a science article on the recent heat wave and changes in climate caused by a hole in the ozone layer.

Treatment

In the movie *Back to the Future,* the protagonist, played by Michael J. Fox, is an adolescent cursed with a socially inept father.

While the father sits glued to reruns of situation comedies, laughing periodically in the same bizarre way that the nerds in *Revenge of the Nerds* do, the mother has turned to drinking. When this teenager is able to travel back in time, he meets his parents as they were as adolescents. He discovers, to his dismay, but not his surprise, that his father was a nerd. He spends much of the movie teaching his teenage nerd father social skills in order to make him attractive to his mother and thereby ensure his own eventual birth. When he returns to the present, he finds that the social skills he taught his adolescent father have resulted in a radical change in his adult father's new present life: an improved marriage and participation in sports and social activities.

In theatrical presentations, there is often the implication that beneath the exterior of a nerd is a warm, empathic individual. The male nerd need only remove his eyeglasses; the female nerd need only let down her hair (as Marian the librarian does in *The Music Man*). Although social skills training with real adolescents is rarely as successful as it is in the movies, when these children and their families begin to understand their handicap better, rather than becoming discouraged or hopeless, they begin to feel as though there are things that they might do to make the problem better. One can tell people that this kind of a problem is not so much an illness as it is a handicap, and, as with other handicapping conditions, one can work to minimize its effect and hope for improved functioning over time.

Many schools are beginning to recognize that there are children whose adjustment to school and to life will be enhanced by specific training programs. Some schools offer groups that specifically assist youngsters with pragmatic language skills, such as asking someone to join you at the movies. Some colleges actually offer special programs for young adults with PDDs. As a part of these programs, a big-brother-type relationship is developed for the impaired freshman to provide him with an adviser about college social life. Such advisers teach these young adults how to avoid scapegoating (which, sadly, does continue into college) and how to develop appropriate friendships with the opposite sex.

The treatment of this disorder begins with treatment of any secondary psychiatric disorder that is present. This could include psychiatric hospitalization and medication when severe psychiatric complications are present. Next, it is important to provide speech and language therapy in pragmatic speech skills. Social skills effectiveness training includes a number of topics: how to begin a conversation, how to maintain good eye contact, how to request something from a peer, how to listen carefully to others, and many more skills that can be analyzed and taught. My patient, Michael, whom I have described, once said to me, "Notice how I'm making good eye contact?" (His rhetorical question suggests that he has learned social skills mechanically, in much the same way that autistic youngsters learn social skills.)

Finally, it is necessary to manipulate the home environment to enhance social success. Although there is often more than one nerd in a family, particularly a father/son combination, it has been my experience that many MPDD children have parents and siblings who are quite adept socially. Reframing the patient's problem for other family members can decrease scapegoating within the family so that siblings may become more sympathetic and less isolating or hostile toward the MPDD youngster. Family members can engage in role-playing with the adolescent, teaching him how to deal with typical social snags that occur in the course of daily living. The child can be encouraged to join special interest groups that provide for social contact around a particular, well-defined activity. Stamp, chess, train, and computer clubs are all examples. Some of these youngsters do well in scouting because the merit-badge system is structured to enhance self-esteem in highly defined ways. Sports activities that involve clear, simple goals, such as body building or blocking on the offensive football line, and minimize teamwork and instinctive sports skills, such as anticipating an opponent's behavior, can enhance self-esteem. The more accepting and adult supervised the group is, the better, and church youth groups are often ideal, with minimal scapegoating of unusual youngsters.

Conclusions

I am suggesting that nerds suffer from a syndrome with defining characteristics of its own. For a number of reasons, the syndrome can be classified as a mild form of PDD. The problems with social communication and imagination typical of nerds indicate a type of PDD. In particular, nerds' notorious difficulties in holistic thinking appear to involve inadequate information integration, possibly involving a minor neurospsychological handicap. The core problems in these youngsters are often missed by clinicians. The diagnosis of a nerd as suffering from an MPDD does more than give him yet another label. It suggests possible interventions, and it can change the way the patient and his family perceive the way he functions.

Do nerds ever get revenge, as in the movies? Perhaps when we read about computer viruses, we are seeing the product of a bright MPDD youngster who harbors enormous anger at society. In fact, the cost to society of not providing help and sympathetic understanding to these youngsters may be bigger than we realize. Most nerds never do get revenge, nor do they seek it. Our goal as clinicians should be to avert the tragedy of emotional pain, loneliness, and secondary psychiatric disorders that have gone unnoticed in the past. I believe that this goal is worthwhile and that it can be accomplished with early recognition and appropriate management of the syndrome.

REFERENCES

American Psychiatric Association. 1980. *Diagnostic and Statistical Manual of Mental Disorders*. 3d ed. Washington, D.C.: American Psychiatric Association.

American Psychiatric Association. 1987. *Diagnostic and Statistical Manual of Mental Disorders*. 3d ed., rev. Washington, D.C.: American Psychiatric Association.

Brothers, L. 1989. A biological perspective on empathy. *American Journal of Psychiatry* 146:10–19.

Cantwell, D., and Baker, L. 1988. Issues in the classification of child and adolescent psychopathology. *Journal of the American Academy of Child Psychiatry* 27(5): 521–533.

Litowitz, B. 1985. The speaking subject in adolescence: response to Theodore Shapiro's essay. *Adolescent Psychiatry* 12:312–326.

Mish, F., ed. 1987. *Webster's Ninth New Collegiate Dictionary*. Springfield: Merriam.

Morris, W., ed. 1985. *The American Heritage Dictionary*. 2d college ed. Boston: Houghton-Mifflin.

Munro, A. 1987. A possible case of Asperger's syndrome. *Canadian Journal of Psychiatry* 32:465–466.

Shapiro, T. 1985. Adolescent language: its use for diagnosis, group identity, values, and treatment. *Adolescent Psychiatry* 12:297–311.

Szatmari, P. 1986. Nonautistic pervasive developmental disorders. Symposium presented at the thirty-third annual meeting of the

American Academy of Child and Adolescent Psychiatry, Los Angeles, October 17.

Tanguay, P. 1984. Toward a new classification of serious psychopathology in children. *Journal of the American Academy of Child Psychiatry* 23(4): 373–384.

Terman, L. 1925. *Mental and Physical Traits of a Thousand Gifted Children*. Stanford, Calif.: Stanford University Press.

Wing, L. 1981. Asperger's syndrome: a clinical account. *Psychological Medicine* 11:115–129.

5 THE FIRST FEW MINUTES: THE ENGAGEMENT OF THE DIFFICULT ADOLESCENT

PHILIP KATZ

A number of opportunities to engage or repel the adolescent patient may occur during the first few minutes of the first interview. Those opening moments, the dynamics involved, and the tactics available require special attention. I first became aware of the importance of those first few minutes after an experience as a fellow in child and adolescent psychiatry.

Case Example 1

Johnny was thirteen when we discussed the opening minute of our first contact, which had occurred when he was only ten. He had been described in the referral material as a precocious, bright youngster, severely neurotic, with high levels of anxiety and some depression. He was seated on a bench in the waiting room of the hospital's outpatient department. I walked up to him and addressed him in the way that I had been taught.

"Hi, Johnny. I'm Dr. Katz. I will be working with you. Would you like to come to my office with me?" Johnny stood up, took my hand, and we walked down the hospital corridor to my office.

About three years later, when we were terminating therapy and agreeing that things had gone very well between us, he commented that he never would have expected it after the opening greeting from me. I was surprised and asked what was wrong with the opening greeting. He asked if I remembered it. I said that I did remember it and repeated the above introduction.

He said, "Yeah, and it took me six months to get over it!"

I was jarred because for six months he had done nothing in treatment despite major efforts on my part to get the relationship rolling. I asked, "What was so wrong with that introduction?"

"You were so damn patronizing! You put me in my place. You were the doctor, I was the patient."

Rather defensively, I said, "If it was so bad, how come you took my hand?"

"I was desperate, and I needed a friend."

I said to the now thirteen-year-old, "But the waiting room was absolutely no place to talk; it was crowded and noisy. What would you have liked me to have said?"

"Just that! Hi Johnny, I am Dr. Katz. This is no place to talk. Would you like to come to my office with me?"

My colleagues and I, in discussing this afterward, felt that Johnny was quite right, that the statement "I am going to be working with you" did preempt the field and did imply that the power of decision was taken away from the youngster. For this bright, sensitive boy, who had already been steamrolled by several events in his life, being presented with a fait accompli was not going to encourage his engagement in therapy. It took six months to convince him that we could work together.

While the first few minutes of an interview are significant with all patients, they are particularly significant with adolescents, as many of them are struggling for independence, trying to establish an identity, and choosing their place in the world. They are particularly sensitive to any signals from the therapist that their powers of decision, their intelligence, and their perceptions will be ignored. As Barish (1971) wrote, "The critical time for engagement is often in the first session, sometimes in the first few minutes, and almost invariably within the first few sessions. An adolescent who is not engaged early is likely to be off and running or, perhaps worse, to remain in body only" (p. 530). This is particularly true when the adolescent has been compelled to come or has been tricked into coming.

In over twenty-five years of practice and teaching, I have seen many adolescents who could benefit from therapy lost to treatment in the first couple of minutes of the first meeting with the therapist. It is, therefore, important that the therapist be oriented to the issues involved and be prepared for this first encounter. Even before they meet, the therapist must know and understand what emotions he and the patient will be experiencing, he must know what his goals will be, and he must have an armamentarium of responses ready for the difficult adolescent.

The Preinterview Emotional Environment

The emotions that are at play within all therapists and all patients in those last few minutes before the interview reflect that they come to this appointment in the hope of getting satisfaction for their individual needs—the patient for relief from his troubles, the therapist for success and reward in his chosen profession.

They each come with fear. The patient fears loss of control over his personal destiny; the therapist fears helplessness and loss of control over the case. The patient fears punishment for not fulfilling the requirements; the therapist fears legal action for not fulfilling the requirements. The patient fears a failure to get the help that is needed; the therapist fears being unable to enlist the needed cooperation of the patient. They each come with anger. The patient is angry at having to face the risk of humiliation in surrendering privacy. The therapist is angry at the risk of humiliation should he fail to help the patient, yet, in those first few minutes of the initial interview, he has to try to allay the patient's fear and anger.

Frieda Fromm-Reichmann (1952) wrote, "The psychiatrists should remember that intensive psychotherapy is a mutual enterprise, if not a mutual adventure, between two people who are strangers and who are likely to be as different from each other as are the average personalities in this culture. Yet, at the same time, there is much more likeness between themselves and their mental patients than some psychiatrists may wish to see. As Harry Stack Sullivan (1940) put it, 'We are all much more simply human than otherwise' " (p. 45).

It is essential that therapists be aware of their own fears, fears that they will be unsuccessful, that they will be embarrassed, that they will be challenged, that they will be frightened. They must be aware that they are angry that they have to walk into that room and face the patient. The therapists must try to deal with their own fear and anger by establishing a therapeutic process that will give them the hope of a chance for success. The therapists must keep in mind that the patients

71

are fearful that they will be humiliated and that they will not be helped and that the patients are angry that they must surrender their privacy and seek help from someone else, a stranger. They need the hope of receiving help to start to reduce the fear and anger.

It is helpful for the therapist to remember that there are circumstances that greatly increase the chances of being successful with adolescent patients. One does not need to be so fearful of failure or so angry at the risk. All adolescents, particularly difficult delinquent adolescents, are hungry for adult relationships, that is, for relationships with adults who are open and emotionally available, who are accepting and approving of them as human beings, who will be nonjudgmental about what they have done, and who, on looking at them, do see neither the "crazy" adolescents that their parents or parent figures see nor the "disturbed" adolescents that the charts portray; instead, therapists see their potential, what they can be in the future. If a psychiatrist, in the course of working with a difficult adolescent, develops a negative reaction to the patient, he should look down the line, study the patient's potential, and try to see what he can be in the future. It makes it much easier, then, to give him the acceptance and approval that he so desperately needs. Adolescents hunger for such a relationship, and that kind of relationship is therapeutically potent. In general, the odds heavily favor the success of psychiatrists with their adolescent patients. The awareness of that potential should strengthen a therapist's confidence in his ability to work successfully with the difficult patient, thereby enabling him to quell the anger that rises owing to the fear of frustration and failure.

Hilde Bruch (1974 , p. 2) wrote:

> Whatever he has heard about his patient-to-be, or read in the sometimes voluminous case history, when the first interview finally takes place [the psychiatrist] does well to remember that this is an occasion where two strangers meet, with both having to take the first tentative steps to learn to know one another. It is a time of mutual assessment, though there may be only limited awareness of the interplay of many subtle emotional factors. How the initial interview turns out depends not only on the patient and his problems, how he presents himself, how he perceives or misperceives the situation, but also on the therapist's openmindedness, his awareness of himself and his feelings and reactions, his

confidence in what he is doing, and his sensitivity to the patient's need for help and understanding.

It is helpful in working with difficult patients to remember that the patient who comes into a psychiatrist's office only occasionally resembles the description given by parents, referring doctors, social workers, and so on. I had the experience of being on a child welfare board of review that consisted of three mental health professionals, two other professionals, and two lay members. We assessed over 400 adolescents who had all been committed to a reform school. Almost invariably, it was our finding on interviewing the adolescents that they bore very little resemblance to the hardened, callous youngsters portrayed in the charts.

Case Example 2

I particularly remember Dale, a sixteen-year-old Indian youngster who was described as being one of the most vicious, violent, and uncooperative youngsters ever encountered by the probation service and the residential treatment center in which he was placed. He had been charged with an assault, and the judge requested a psychiatric assessment. I was asked if I would do the examination quickly and was told that it would take only a few minutes because he would not talk to me anyway. Fortunately, I booked the standard hour. Dale wheeled into the office, asked for a cup of coffee, put his feet up on a stool, and talked for an hour and a half, during which time he gave me a mass of information about himself and contracted to come for psychotherapy. Months later, when we discussed what had lead to that unexpected first interview, he told me that, the night before he came to see me, he had decided that he was on the road to jail and that he did not want to follow that path to its end. He decided that he had to let somebody get to know him and help him with his problems and that he would take a chance on the interview with me the next day.

Case Example 3

Another illustrative case was that of Bill. The boy's father had phoned me saying that the seventeen-year-old youngster was heavily into drugs, dangerously suicidal, and that it was an emergency. The father was a very overbearing, angry man whom I had known for many years. I expected to see a very hostile and resistant young man, only to discover that he had been trying to figure out for a year how he could trick his father into telling him to go for therapy. He wanted therapy but thought that if he asked for it his father would say no.

Adolescents often have their own agendas when they come to see a psychiatrist. In the majority of cases, the adolescent comes willingly, knowing what he wants help with and hoping that the psychiatrist will be helpful, will make him comfortable and not embarrass him, and, in the end, will become a special kind of friend. The challenge is with those who could also benefit from therapy but who either do not see the need for treatment, have had previous unpleasant experiences with therapy, or, for a variety of reasons, are too fearful of the psychiatrist-patient situation. It is with this group that the psychiatrist must hone his skills, be aware of his own reactions, be sensitive to the patient's fears, and be ready to respond immediately. His initial questions and his reactions will tell the patient about himself and will either encourage the patient to engage with him or scare the patient off.

The First Few Minutes with the Difficult Adolescent Patient

The engagement of the very difficult adolescent, who comes in hostile and resistive right from the opening moment, tests the psychiatrist's skills, creativity, empathy, and tenacity. I believe that one should have available a thought-out array of approaches, an armamentarium, to use in such situations.

It is helpful to have information about the patient to assist in planning an approach. A good history, particularly from the parents, is invaluable, but one must keep in mind the earlier caution that the patient who comes to see a psychiatrist may have his own agenda and, therefore, may not resemble the description.

The first basic strategy in planning an approach is, *Clarify your role as a stranger.* When there is an immediate flash of distrust, I respond to that with a ready acceptance of the distrust, pointing out to the patient that I know that I am a stranger to him, that he does not know what I am like, that he has no reason to trust me, and, indeed, that there would be something wrong if he did immediately trust a stranger.

I invite him to test me out, see what I am like, and find out if I am the kind of person with whom he would like to work.

The verbalizing of the thoughts that are already uppermost in the patient's mind shows the patient that the psychiatrist has possibilities for understanding him. The psychiatrist's acceptance of the fact that he has to prove himself to the patient protects the psychiatrist, a bit, from the powerful negative reactions that the patient has already built up against authority figures. It recognizes the patient's position of control. There is an implicit acceptance of the patient's intelligence and ability to make good decisions.

Case Example 4

Peter was thirteen, delinquent, depressed, and hostile to psychiatrists after a couple of unsuccessful attempts at therapy with other psychiatrists. He walked into my office after being ordered to come see me by his treatment center staff, stood just inside the doorway, and said, "I don't like psychiatrists!"

I said I knew that but that I was a stranger to him, that he did not know what I was like, and that he should try me out and see whether he could work with me.

He said, "Okay, then I will ask the questions."

I said, "Shoot!"

He asked what I liked to do when I was not being a psychiatrist. I thought for a moment and said, "Many things, but I particularly like to travel." He sat down and asked where I had been. I listed a number of places. When I mentioned Russia, he lit up and asked if I had really been to Russia. We spent the entire session discussing my trip to Moscow and Leningrad. When the staff came to take him back to the treatment center, I looked at him questioningly, and he said, "That's okay Doc, I'll come back again."

We moved easily into a therapeutic relationship. When some months later I discussed with him his reactions to that opening session, he said that what he liked was the feeling that I respected his mind, that he was genuinely interested in my experiences in Russia, and that he could see that it was important to me that he was interested in them. He felt that he was not there just for my purposes; I was interested in him.

A second strategy is, *Analyze the situation to the patient*. One of the more useful tactics that I have used when in a jam with a patient is to analyze the situation to the patient and enlist his assistance. Many times, the patient has information that can be helpful, and usually he will not react negatively to the situation but will work together with you on it.

Case Example 5

Perry was a sixteen-year-old very bright foster child who had recently become severely depressed. He had broken up with his girlfriend, was making a mess of his schooling, had become very difficult to live with in the foster home, and was engaging in some delinquent activities. The agency had been unable to work with him, and he was refusing to see any therapist. I suggested that they order him to see me once, telling him that he had to come one time but that they would not make him come more than that.

Perry slipped past the secretary and booted open the door to my agency office. He slammed into a chair and glared at me. I said, "You think you have it so bad! How would you like to be me, facing you? What would you do, Perry, if you were a psychiatrist and a social worker came to you saying that she had this very bright sixteen-year-old who is going to hell, who is screwing up his school, who is screwing up at the foster home, who has broken up with a real nice girlfriend, who is doing delinquent things, and is getting more and more depressed, but he is refusing to see a psychiatrist. You feel that you would like to try to help him, but you do not know how to get him to give you a try. He does not know you, and he does not know what you are like. If you were me, Perry, how would you get you to give me a try?"

He looked at me with a faint smile, was thoughtful for a few moments, and then said, "I don't know, but I'll give you a try."

In planning this approach, I had thought that, from the description I had been given of the youngster as someone who was bright, thoughtful, and sensitive, he would be intrigued by my approach. We went on from that beginning to a successful course of treatment.

A third useful strategy is, *Seek opportunities to empathize with the patient.* The therapist should try to demonstrate as quickly as possible his powers as a therapist, the power to see things from the patient's point of view and in a way that the average adult does not and the power of understanding what is going on in the patient, especially what the patient himself does not understand. One often has very little time in which to do this, so one looks for quick openings.

Case Example 6

Elaine was thirteen and well developed physically for her years. The product of a broken marriage, she was described by her mother as a terrible child who would not obey either parent. Currently, she was using drugs and alcohol heavily, quite promiscuous, and had been expelled from school. Her parents were not sure that they could get her to come. She stalked angrily into the office and announced that she would not sit down. I said that that was okay, that it was obvious that she was very angry at being forced to come see me. I said to her that it was also obvious from the description that her mother had given me that she was in a lot of pain, was very unhappy, and did not know what to do with it. I said that her parents seemed to be confused also and were reacting with anger to her. She then strung out a list of belligerent episodes with her parents. I asked what made them react so angrily to her. She said that she did not know. I then asked if she understood why her parents reacted so negatively to her on so many issues. She said that she could never figure them out, that she did not know what to expect from them. I said that that was something that needed to be worked on, that she had to understand them if she was going to have some control over what happened between her and them.

She then said, "Okay if I sit down?"

I said, "Please do, and can I offer you a drink?"

She raised an eyebrow and said, "Vodka?"

I laughed and said, "Nope. Sorry about that. Soft drinks only, or coffee."

She laughed and said, "Thought I would try. A Coke will be okay." From there it was an easy move into the therapeutic work.

The offer of a way of looking at things (that one could understand the causes of her parents' anger and thereby control it), in effect the offer of power, as well as the support of a sympathetic, understanding, accepting adult, moved her quickly out of her defensive hostile position into a friendly age-appropriate relationship.

Case Example 7

Don was thirteen. An appointment had been made for him two weeks prior to the first interview. I had seen his mother one week before. She was quite intelligent and troubled because this youngster seemed to be traveling down a delinquent path, whereas the other children in the family did not seem to be on that road at all. Don walked sullenly into the office. I asked when he found out about the appointment with a psychiatrist. He angrily replied, "Fifteen minutes ago! On the way down here! And she said I was going for a doctor's appointment!" I asked, "Does your mother usually play games like that with you?" That opened the flood-gates to a torrent of examples about how she manipulates and outmaneuvers him and his fury and anger about it. We were off and running into a working relationship.

My calling his mother's handling of the appointment "a game" signified to him that I was not going to be protective of the adult establishment but that I would have an open mind in looking at his relationship with his parents. I felt that I needed to make a quick move to ally with this angry patient, who felt apart from his family. There are other adolescents who would resent the implied criticism of their parents.

Don's parents were very helpful because, after the interview, in the car on the way home, Donald unloaded on his mother, telling her what he had learned in the session about her manipulation of him. She phoned me that evening to thank me for opening up the communication that she had not had with him for years, saying that she had not realized the way she had been manipulating him.

Case Example 8

In contrast, I misread the parents involved in another case. Mark was fourteen, an angry child of a doctor father; he was doing miserably in school, getting involved with drugs, and totally uncooperative at home. Father forced him to come to the first session. Mark walked into the office, sat down in the chair, and pulled his large turtle-neck sweater up over his face. He sat there for the entire fifty minutes, silent, with the turtle-neck covering his face. I monologued off and on throughout the session, analyzing the situation to him, trying to be empathic, trying to make a connection one way or another. Nothing worked. As the fifty minutes ended, I told him that our time was up but that there was one thing I wanted to say to him, which was that I admired his guts for being able to sit there for fifty minutes silent like that. As he pulled the turtle-neck down, back around his neck, he grinned at me rather delight-edly and walked out. As his father met him in the hallway, I prevented any communication in front of Mark by saying to the father that I would phone him. When I called the next day, the father said that the boy had said simply that the session had gone okay, that there had been no indication that he would not go again, so we set up another appointment.

Mark came and this time talked fairly freely on a variety of topics. We had two more sessions, and I felt that everything was going well, but I failed to move quickly enough with the parents. Mark did not want to come to the next appointment because it conflicted with something else that came up, but his father was insistent. Mark absolutely refused to come to that appointment and would not come to any others after that. He would not talk to me on the phone either.

If the parents had called me, I would have either moved or canceled the appointment in order not to conflict because Mark was not yet sufficiently engaged. I would not have tested his commitment to therapy against his other pleasures. I had hoped that we were on the road to something.

Looking back at this case afterward, I felt that to some extent the parents had sabotaged my work with the youngster, perhaps because they did not see any change occurring in him with respect to his behavior with them. I had not properly prepared them for Mark's course of treatment. Obviously, one has to try to make the environ-ment as cooperative with the therapeutic goals as possible.

A fourth strategy is, *Offer immediate help to the patient.* Each youngster who comes unwillingly to the office is being faced with the evidence of his helplessness. One seeks to offer power in the form of knowledge, and help, if appropriate, by interventions in patients' situations. This offer of help comes from someone who is considered potent, from someone whom society endows with a certain mystique, and from someone to whom the parents or guardian agency have turned for help. It can counteract a youngster's fears of being involved with an unknown authority figure.

Case Example 9

This bizarre example begins when I was late for a meeting of a child welfare board of review and walked in to find Danny on the floor, with three guards sitting on top of him and my colleagues on the board sitting white faced and stunned. There was some disarray in the room; obviously, Danny, a sixteen-year-old Indian boy who had been in the reform school for over a year, had blown up at the board. I had read the advance material and knew that Danny had suddenly and inexplicably asked the board to discharge him from the reform school. The situation suggested that they had refused and that he had exploded.

I went and sat down, crosslegged, on the floor, at Danny's head, and said "That's not going to work. You are not going to get what you want that way."

He yelled, "Well how the ———— am I going to get out of there?"

I said, "You have got to do it by talking, Danny. Obviously you are very desperate. There must be something terrible about being there for you to get this desperate and blow up like this. You have got to talk about it. You have got to get across, in words, to the board, why you are so desperate. Only, this time, I will help you. I will help you get those feelings out, and I will help you explain to them why it is so terrible."

He said that he could not talk with three guys sitting on him. I asked if he would sit and talk with me if they let him up. He said "Sure." I signaled the three guards to let him up. They did so, warily. As Danny got up, he was startled to see me in suit and tie and all the conservative attire, but then sat down, crosslegged, facing me on the floor, and talked with me while the board listened.

Gradually, Danny got out a description of the incredible situation that he was in. He was being used as a guinea pig in an operant-conditioning unit, where he was being kept in a large cage until he earned a certain number of points. It would be months before he earned the necessary points to get out of the cage, as he was so far behind in penalties. He felt he could not take it any longer and that he was going to crack up. He was terrified of some of the hallucinatory experiences that he was having. The board agreed to get him out of that situation, but we just could not release him onto the street. He agreed to wait a week, saying that he could handle it if he knew he would be out in a week and that would give us time to have arrangements made for him for his discharge. The institution, knowing that he would be discharged, placed him in a special holding situation away from the operant-conditioning unit. At the conference with the review board a week later, at the end of his meeting, after we had formalized his discharge, Danny came over to me and asked if he could see me for treatment. His treatment course was erratic, due to continuing difficulties with the law and with drug abuse, but the positive relationship with me that began that day at the review board has continued to this day.

By using these four strategies of acknowledging one's role as a stranger, analyzing the situation to the patient, seeking opportunities to empathize, and seeking opportunities to offer help, one can develop an array of approaches that will be available for use when a hostile, resistant adolescent comes into one's office. I have used these strategies many times in the twenty-five years that I have been in practice with the over 2,000 patients that I have seen during that time.

Conclusion

In trying to engage the very difficult adolescent, the work begins inside the psychiatrist's head prior to the time that the patient arrives. The psychiatrist has to deal with the fears and anger that well up in him before the interview and has to be prepared to deal with the fear and anger that the patient brings to the interview. It is often necessary to prepare a strategic plan for those opening moments or have a number of them available, depending on what the psychiatrist is confronted with. He has to prepare to present himself for study and exploration, to enable the patient to decide whether the psychiatrist is the kind of person with whom he would like to work and whether the psychiatrist has something to offer. The psychiatrist has to have confidence in what he has to offer: understanding, knowledge, empathy, and a warm and positive view of what the adolescent can become. They are the essentials that will meet the adolescent's need for control of his chaotic life, for self-esteem, for hope of a better life. The proper preparation of oneself will enable the psychiatrist to engage the difficult adolescent in a therapeutic journey.

REFERENCES

Barish, J. 1971. Engaging the adolescent in psychotherapy. *Adolescent Psychiatry* 1:530–536.
Bruch, H. 1974. *Learning Psychotherapy.* Cambridge, Mass.: Harvard University Press.
Fromm-Reichmann, F. 1950. *Principles of Intensive Psychotherapy.* Chicago: University of Chicago Press.
Sullivan, H. S. 1940. Conceptions of modern psychiatry. *Psychiatry* 3:1–117.

6 THE TERMINATION OF TREATMENT IN ADOLESCENTS

DEREK MILLER

The initial stages of treatment in all adolescent care imply diagnosis, the setting of therapeutic goals, and planning for termination. The therapeutic goals that are set by the psychiatrist are, however, not necessarily those of the patient or of the family. Between the adolescent and his or her parents, a conflict of interest and of goals almost certainly exists, whatever the developmental stage of adolescence, early, middle, or late (Miller 1984). The therapist's goal should be the cessation of the symptomatic behavior that is developmentally and perhaps realistically destructive, along with the resolution of those etiological issues that are significant precipitants of such behavior.

Adolescents in the early and middle stages of this psychosocial developmental period generally do not enter treatment with the overt acceptance that this is something they need or want. Such a statement would imply an abandonment of the struggle for autonomy. Usually, such adolescents enter treatment at the behest of their parents or other authority figures. Late adolescents are more likely to see the necessity for treatment but often, particularly university students, guiltily feel that they are not "sick enough." Those who are not initially motivated because of a legalistic preoccupation with their civil rights often do not get any assistance. This is particularly likely to occur in those with bipolar illness and those who abuse alcohol or drugs.

An initial goal of treatment is the creation of a therapeutic alliance so that projection is abandoned. The end of treatment implies the dissolution of this alliance without the destruction of the internalized attitudes and feelings that it has helped create.

The indications for treatment determine both the goals of therapy and its likely termination. When an adolescent, as a response to perceived frustration, behaves in a symptomatic way that is developmentally destructive and/or dangerous to the self or others and that cannot be contained by interpersonal relationships within the family and the social system of society, therapeutic intervention is indicated. Developmentally destructive behavior may include school failure and refusal, drug abuse, alcoholism, and sexual promiscuity. Alternatively, the patient may be suffering from psychic pain of such intensity that it precludes age-appropriate functioning. Finally, the environment may be so psychonoxious that healthy personality development is impossible. If the relationship that is established with a therapist in an outpatient setting cannot contain such situations, there is then a clear indication for more intensive care in a hospital setting.

The Timing of Termination

The timing of termination may not be a function simply of the adolescent's needs. Constraints, which inevitably modify what can be done, are placed on therapy by a variety of factors, some of which are constructive. These may be a function of growth and development; a youngster who appears for treatment in the last year of high school may be leaving for college. Not uncommonly, termination may occur when the patient develops a wish for autonomy and insists that therapy is no longer needed. The rather abstract issue for the adolescent, as to whether problems remain, may not be considered. It is generally better on such occasions not to try to keep the patient in treatment but rather to indicate availability should the attempt at autonomy fail. More destructively, at the present time, there is current social and economic pressure on parents and therapists to limit the provision of care. The general goal of society seems to be at best to pay for limited therapeutic intervention irrespective of what may be optimally indicated. Sometimes only a stated amount of time, money, or number of therapeutic sessions may be spent, a particular quality of health maintenance organizations, government agencies, and insurance carriers. Designated physicians are sometimes offered regardless of their expertise.

The belief that interventions can be time limited is often one that is unwittingly colluded in by therapists. If the reality implies an inappropriate time constraint, the therapist should refuse to intervene at all if the severity of the disability is such that no positive gains can be made: for example, a demand that a potentially suicidal patient be inappropriately discharged from the hospital. Sometimes, however, gains can be made, although these are far short of optimal, and this should be clearly stated both to parents and to the regulatory agencies. Termination may be unplanned when the parents cannot tolerate the growth to autonomy of the patient and exercise their power over their child, who is then withdrawn from treatment. The adolescent may revert to behavior—drug abuse, for example—that makes psychotherapy impossible. If other theraputic parameters cannot be introduced, the therapist should terminate treatment. Termination may also occur because the therapist's countertransference is such that, in inappropriate ways, the patient is encouraged to leave.

Ideally, termination occurs when the family no longer defines their offspring's behavior or attitudes as pathological, when the adolescent can deal with stress without inappropriate psychological and behavioral responses, and when personality development can proceed "independently of the therapist's direct presence" (Group for the Advancement of Psychiatry 1982, p. 57). Optimally, at the termination of therapy, the adolescent should reject the therapeutic situation but not the therapist. The therapist, in turn, should not reject the adolescent by telling him or her that treatment is no longer needed.

In seriously disturbed adolescents, who require high-intensity care in a hospital, the nature of termination is also determined by the treatment philosophy of the therapeutic setting and the availability of resources. If genuine continuity of care from inpatient to partial hospital to outpatient status is available, the patient terminates with a whole social system in which he or she is developmentally involved as well as withdrawing from psychotherapy. It is clear that object cathexis in such settings may vary and that involvement with parts of the setting may continue even when psychotherapy has terminated. This is particularly likely if a biological intervention—the long-term use of mood changing drugs, for example—is necessary. Medication may have to be monitored after psychotherapy has terminated. Families too may continue their involvement with parental groups, if these are available, long after their offspring has terminated.

Termination and the Developmental
Phase of Adolescence

The developmental age of the patient affects both the type of therapy recommended and the nature of its outcome. Some patients may be chronologically in their teens but not yet be able to be adolescent. They may show the psychological responses to puberty, but there is no indication that development of secondary autonomy is occurring (Miller 1986). In the course of successful treatment, these patients will become adolescent. In that the therapist and the therapeutic situation will inevitably have been "transitional objects" (Winnicott 1953) to make this possible, therapeutic termination will differ from that in those who have become adolescent prior to the onset of treatment.

Early adolescents, struggling with the turbulence of puberty and the initial steps toward autonomy, remain an integrally dependent member of their family unit until this developmental phase is over. Termination then is related not only to the cessation of symptomatic behavior and a return to a healthy developmental track but also to the level of homeostatic interaction between the patient and the family. Paradoxically, rebellious and difficult behavior that may initiate the parents' wish to have the child go into treatment may continue with a different developmental mode. The behavior may be a function of the child's mixing rebellion and independence as part of the wish to become autonomous rather than of the child attacking internal objects that have been projected onto the world outside the self.

Those in the middle stage of adolescence may continue autonomous growth away from the family. This is likely to create parental conflict with their awareness that successful therapy implies the loss of a dependent child. Parents of this age group are likely to be much more conflicted about the need for therapy than are those with excessively turbulent children in the early stage of adolescence. In that case, a healthy child is returned to the family, and the loss of childhood has not yet occurred. In late adolescence, the termination of therapy is much more related to the capacity of the patient to handle the real world because the nature of external parental support inevitably has changed. A young adult now relates to adult parents.

The situation may be complicated by several issues, one of which is the etiology of the adolescent's difficulties. If neuroendocrine pathol-

85

ogy is evident, or if the capacity to make trusting relationships has been seriously and irrevocably impaired, this must affect both the outcome and the nature of the termination.

If the patient is the offspring of a broken nuclear family or one that functions in relative social isolation, the therapist may occupy two significant roles in the adolescent's life. Apart from being a purveyor of the designated psychotherapy—expressive, supportive, or behavioral—the therapist is likely to be a developmentally significant extraparental adult. Personality development does not just depend on the resolution of internal conflict; it requires emotional involvement with parents, peers, extraparental adults, and stable social systems (Miller 1984). In an increasingly fragmented society in which large numbers of adolescents are being brought up by single parents or in which the quality of parenting is affected by both parents working, it is inevitable that a therapist becomes a significant developmental object, a significant other adult as well as a psychotherapist. This may well mean that with the partial resolution of conflict, which makes trusting relationships possible, the adolescent may appear to improve rapidly. Identification with the perceived qualities of the therapist, and the therapeutic interaction with all its ramifications is made. If the nurturing environment is deficient, it is believed that this must be accepted: a "cure by identification" is better than no cure at all.

The Nature of Termination

Termination in psychoanalysis occurs when a patient has relived much of the primary infantile situation and has begun to resolve infantile conflicts. Old conflicts are successfully reworked with more adaptive results. The goals for analysis have been thought to have been reached if the patient is free enough to develop in his or her own way, although such development may not be apparent until long after the analysis is completed. [Stewart 1980, p. 2126]

The analytic patient who successfully terminates treatment is able to confront reality, and the transference neurosis has been resolved. The final resolution of transference bonds is said to differentiate the termination of analysis from the termination of other types of treatment. However, even in analysis, it can be argued that the patient identifies with a process that has gone on within the analytic situation and also identifies with the perceived qualities of the analyst, although this identification, in an adult, is not a bar to conflict resolution.

Termination in adolescent therapy is successful if the patient is becoming autonomous and is able to return to, or become involved in, a developmental track that will produce mature adulthood. This latter concept implies the ability to be empathic, to test reality, to be loving and productive, to love and work, to play, and to trust. Termination, however, is not graduation (Yalom 1970). Successful termination in adolescents does not imply that the patient has to feel resentful of the therapist (Stekel 1950), although, in order to part from a significant extraparental adult, the adolescent needs to deal with the anger that makes rejection possible.

Ideally, termination depends on the child and the family's acceptance of a "mutually satisfactory balance of mastery over problems" (Group for the Advancement of Psychiatry 1982), and the process of secondary individuation continues in a satisfactory manner (Ekstein 1983).

Successful Termination

Successful termination will depend on the therapist's ability to mobilize his or her concern for the patient, to get inside the youngster's head and imagination, and to think and feel developmentally with the adolescent at his or her own level. Such termination results partly from the therapist's expectation of success, which is related partly to the therapeutic process and to the therapist's personality. At termination, the family no longer defines their offspring as pathological. The patient no longer projects all difficulties onto the family and attempts to function on the basis of this projection (Miland 1987).

There is no indication for the therapist to indicate the end of treatment. As soon as the adolescent is no longer functioning in destructive ways and no longer needs to have tension "held" by the therapist (Winnicott 1957), the adolescent can decide when to leave treatment.

Termination in Hospitalized Adolescents

Seriously disturbed adolescents who have to be admitted to a high-intensity-care hospital setting have often felt repeatedly rejected and betrayed by adults, including parents and psychiatrists. Thus, they constantly test the strength and stability of those involved in their treatment. The psychotherapist has to be perceived as a person of strength and integrity who does not reject the patient. The adolescent has to respect the therapist and the therapeutic process (Easson 1969). The therapeutic situation has to be perceived as enriching, not just in terms of cognitive understanding, but also in terms of creative and imaginative stimulation.

In all adolescent patients, relationships are used to help contain symptomatic behavior. Initially, adolescents who are behaving in symptomatically destructive ways will abandon this behavior, not because conflicts have been resolved, but because they feel sufficiently supported by the therapeutic situation.

Hospital care implies the need for external controls because of profound deficits in ego functions and the lack of ability to make trusting relationships. Hospital care should include the provision of planned growth-promoting experiences (Knesper and Miller 1976). The adolescent who leaves hospital care is in a different situation than the adolescent who is being treated solely as an outpatient with individual and perhaps family therapy. On the one hand, the therapist has been seen as a facilitator of growth and an individual who helps resolve problems and contain tension and anxiety. On the other, the therapist has become significant in the development of the adolescent's autonomous sense of self. When the adolescent leaves therapy, he or she has to retain the new identity that has been developed and allow this to grow.

Termination in adults includes separation, mourning, and giving up a love object (Freud 1913). Termination in adolescence does not necessarily include all this. The adolescent patient may continue to retain the internal image of the therapist. Thus, the adolescent who leaves therapy may not mourn and may not genuinely be giving up a love object. The issue is whether the therapeutic imago has been internalized as an introject or whether it has been incorporated into the adolescent's personality. If the perception of the therapist is only as an introject, the likelihood that the therapeutic intervention will continue to contain developmentally destructive behavior after termination is less unlikely.

Conclusions

A particular problem in termination for adolescents requiring hospital care is that traditional treatment repeats the developmental trauma of the premature separation that led to disturbances in ego functioning in childhood and adolescence. Hospital care may show little regard for the importance of continuous and emotionally meaningful relationships, including that with the psychotherapist. Within the setting of a hospital ward, interpersonal relationships between staff and patient are often attenuated. Staff may spend many hours in treatment team meetings, but it may be that, without considerable emotional support, inpatient staff cannot tolerate the affective distress projected into them by emotionally disturbed adolescents. This may explain why techniques of isolation from adults with a variety of rationalizations are used, even though this has no developmental rationale.

When adolescents improve, the reward in moving to a less restrictive setting may be the loss of contact previously made with adults and peers. In some hospitals, even the therapist changes, and this is particularly likely to be the situation when an adolescent is ready to move back into the community. If, through high- and low-intensity care (Miller 1986), a genuine continuity of relationships exists, this reinforces their value so that at termination the adolescent is more able to deal with their loss. If relationships are not therapeutically valued, the loss of a therapist merely confirms that adults have little to offer. Frequent therapeutic separations may repeat the child's experience of that early separation from parents, which was developmentally destructive. Such premature separations are highly significant in the development of personality disturbances and deprivation depressive syndromes. Inappropriate separation from therapists and therapeutic systems may replay the loss of a mother who was either not available or not able to contain instinctual tension and possibly the loss of a father through separation, divorce, or noninvolvement. In treatment, emotional maturation is impeded, and the process of psychotherapy is made more difficult.

REFERENCES

Easson, W. M. 1969. *The Seriously Disturbed Adolescent*. New York: International Universities Press.

Ekstein, R. 1983. The adolescent self during the process of termination of treatment and termination, interruption, or intermission. *Adolescent Psychiatry* 11:125–146.

Freud, S. 1913. On beginning the treatment: further recommendations on the technique of psycho-analysis. I. *Standard Edition* 12:121–144. London: Hogarth, 1958.

Group for the Advancement of Psychiatry. 1982. *The Process of Child Therapy.* New York: Brunner/Mazel.

Knesper, D., and Miller, D. 1976. Treatment plans for mental health care. *American Journal of Psychiatry* 133(1): 65–80.

Miland, O. 1987. *Systemic Family Therapy.* New York: Basic.

Miller, D. 1984. *The Age Between.* Northfield, N.J.: Aronson.

Miller, D. 1986. *Attack on the Self.* Northfield, N.J.: Aronson.

Stekel, W. 1950. *Technique of Analytic Psychotherapy.* London: Bodley Head.

Stewart, R. L. 1980. Psychoanalysis and psychoanalytic psychotherapy. In *Comprehensive Textbook of Psychiatry,* vol. 4. Baltimore: Williams & Wilkins.

Winnicott, D. 1953. Transitional objects and transitional phenomena. *International Journal of Psycho-Analysis* 34:59–97.

Winnicott, D. 1957. *Mother and Child.* New York: Basic.

Yalom, D. 1970. *The Theory and Practice of Group Psychotherapy.* New York: Basic.

PART II

THE CHESTNUT LODGE ADOLESCENT EXPERIENCE

EDITOR'S INTRODUCTION

We need . . . an experimental hostel or boarding school for half a dozen children to be located in the area where psychoanalysts live and work. Only in this way can a beginning be made to the problem of the treatment of these children of any age who need treatment of two kinds at once, treatment of specialized management and treatment by intensive personal therapy. [D. W. Winnicott]

For more than a decade, there has been a psychiatric center at Chestnut Lodge near which psychoanalysts and psychoanalysts in training live and work with adolescent children needing two kinds of treatment at once.

What this special section attempts to show, as clearly, as candidly, and as comprehensively as possible, is just how a long-term psychiatric hospital for adolescents goes about its regular daily business of helping patients think, feel, and behave better and more in keeping with average age expectations that allow for a certain amount of turbulence, rebelliousness, withdrawal, and, in common parlance, discombobulation. When patients apply for admission to the Lodge, the careful evaluation addresses three basic and crucial concerns: the likely responsiveness to the long-term dynamic approach, the level of management needed to hold and contain the patient, and the intensity of the psychotherapeutic process to which the patient is open. When things are going relatively smoothly within the total milieu, the boundaries between the interpersonal and intrapersonal domains are more or less lost and less contended. The aim is to establish a seamless continuum within the therapeutic program. At moments of crisis, to which all psychiatric settings are prone, the parts of the treatment transitively become more visible than the whole. This becomes evident in all the clinical contributions in this section, particularly at times of major change linked with the arrival or departure of more charismatic staff or patients.

The importance of management needs some explanation. Even before Donald Winnicott wrote so inspiringly about this aspect of treatment and had been criticized by some "depth" psychotherapists for contaminating the purity of psychoanalysis, Chestnut Lodge had decided to split the functions of the therapists and administrators since the combined function seemed too complex and too complicating to be left entirely to one individual. This arrangement ensured that psychotherapy could be carried out privately and confidentially with a primary focus on the intrapersonal and that the "other twenty three hours" spent in the group, the family, the unit, the school, and the general community could be free to activate their own powerful therapeutic potentials. Keeping an objective appraising eye on this rich tapestry of treatment is the research team whose functioning is described in the second half of the section.

The Chestnut Lodge experience underscored Winnicott's (1961) conclusion that the managerial activities represented the professionalized aspect of the caregivers responsible for "holding" the patient "while growth tendencies are given a chance" (p. 237). The goal in all such situations is to correct earlier failures in the environment. What parents do when this occurs is to "exaggerate some parental function and keep it up for a length of time, in fact until the child has used it up and is ready to be released from special care" (D. W. Winnicott 1963, p. 227). This is what therapeutic management implies, and Winnicott goes on to itemize its details: applying oneself to the case; getting to know what it feels like to be the patient; becoming reliable to the limits of one's professional responsibility; behaving oneself professionally; concerning oneself with the patient's problems; accepting an internal subjective position inside the patient while at the same time dealing with him objectively; accepting his love and hate confidently without acting on it erotically or revengefully; tolerating the patient's illogicality, unreliability, suspiciousness, muddle-headedness, fecklessness, meanness, and recognizing these as symptoms of distress; and not being scared or overcome with guilt feelings when the patient goes haywire, disorganizes, or tries to kill himself or others but able to take appropriate and needed action; recognizing that although you are a person deeply involved in feeling that you are not responsible for the patient's illness and that your powers are limited to alter a crisis but that if you are able to hold the situation together, it is possible that it will resolve itself, and that this would be because you have held fast (p. 229). In the milieu, the administrator and his or her staff are to a large extent real people dealing with external events and other figures in the patient's life while, at the same time, attempting to bridge the gap between the external world and the feeling about it (see C. Winnicott 1963, p. 45). The psychotherapist, on the other hand, means largely a subjective figure who can thus play a major transference role but can be deployed systematically in the service of the psychotherapy. The administrative group are therefore important as bridging people who actually live through significant life events with the patient, including transitions between the family and the inpatient milieu.

In the first chapter of the section, I have attempted to convey something of the atmosphere of the "dynamic long-termness" shared by patients and personnel, comprising the qualities of an Eriksonian moratorium, but with sufficient "oxygen" (Redl 1968). In this unique setting, one can observe the gradual progression, complete with setbacks, from chaos to coherence along various diagnostic pathways as fundamental transformations help to convert action into words.

The second contribution by Douglas Chavis is focused on the intensive personal therapy of a typical Chestnut Lodge case with a predominance of narcissism that renders the treatment situation often difficult and disappointing for the therapist until his persistence and reliability gradually makes the therapy more acceptable to the patient and more successful. Years of outpatient treatment had failed to do so and the therapist is the first to admit that it is only because of the specialized management by the milieu staff that made it possible for him to continue his work in spite of the severe ups and downs. The patient is now attending college.

The family approach practiced at the Lodge is delineated in the next chapter by Boots, Goodman, Loughman, and Anthony, demonstrating often through vivid case material the work done in improving parent-child relationships, parental understanding of what is taking place in the hospital, the philosophy of treatment, and the capacity to contain the anxieties and aggression involved in the therapeutic process. The work done in family therapy complements the parallel efforts in individual and group treatment as well as adding a crucial aspect to the total clinical portrayal of the patient.

The next chapter by Fort, McAfee, King, Hoppe, Fenton, Abramowitz, Woodbury, and Anthony is devoted to the intensive long-term group psychotherapy carried out in small weekly groups that, because of their composition, have a somewhat chaotic, incohesive quality about them that is shed almost automatically as the patients return to the daily school program. As one patient remarked, "Without the group, I would have to keep my scream inside me." Over many years, the groups have shown a remarkable capacity to contain the overwhelming disturbances brought to them at different times. The treatment is conducted within a largely maternal type of ambiance with regressive phenomena to the forefront and the group activity largely consisting of holding, facilitating, mirroring, and sharing. The patients use the opportunity provided by the group to test the tolerance of "nuisance" behavior; when this is satisfied, the "work" of therapy can then proceed. As might be expected, the communication patterns vary from session to session and from group to group, revealing shifting levels of insight and coherence.

At the Lodge, treatment, management, and research go hand in hand in ways that are mutually helpful: the managers make the treatment of very difficult patients possible and the investigators enable the psychotherapists to understand more objectively what is taking place in the patient and in the patient-therapist relationship over time. The chapter by Fritsch, Holmstrom, Goodrich, and Rieger brings together unlikely bed fellows—research methodology (cluster analysis) and a psychodynamic model based on object relations theory to investigate adjustment of borderline patients. What emerges from the study is the interaction between gender, object relations, and management problems that, in turn, bring up crucial questions about the efficacy of analytic psychotherapy, at least in the early phase of hospitalization.

The chapter by Fritsch and Goodrich scrutinizes the role of attachment as a workable, dependable alliance to major milieu figures and concludes that it is an important treatment variable albeit functioning differently with different diagnostic groupings. The resistance offered to the attachment process may be characteristic and expectable for the severely disturbed adolescent, while in the more psychotic patient it may constitute a sign of health. In the chapter by Rieger, the attachment process is viewed from a different angle: the capacity of some organically impaired adolescents with severe psychiatric symptoms to make the initial attachment to both the therapist and the milieu, reinforcing earlier observations by Mahler and Goldfarb.

Fullerton, Yates, and Goodrich examine the therapeutic improvements with adolescent patients from the viewpoint of the therapist's experience and gender during the initial phase in hospital and come up with findings that suggest an interaction between the two variables. This is clearly an important area for further research on the determining influences at work in helpfully evolving therapists-patient dyads.

The chapter by Wells Goodrich brings together a summary of knowledge derived from the Chestnut Lodge research experience of the adolescent program taken as a whole over time and manifesting different characteristics at different phases of treatment depending on the diagnostic grouping of the patients. The treatment model provided at the Lodge appears to be highly ameliorative for certain disorders of the patient and permits the family to grow and change within the framework provided, but, at the other end of the scale, there is a small group of adolescents whose pathology defeats the system. Goodrich concludes that perhaps newer and more focused interventions are required for this resistant type. Until such measures are available, it might be more effective for both the program and the patient to screen them out of the program.

Berman and Goodrich investigate still another aspect of treatment—adolescents who run away from it and adolescents who run away from it and return to it. Factors of age, sex, diagnosis, and adoption are all seen to play a part in this particular symptomatic behavior. The study throws still further light on the phenomenon of attachment that runs like a red thread through all these therapeutic considerations.

Bullard's reflections on the ever evolving program on the Adolescent Unit covers not only its history but the rationale behind the various developments and points a finger at the relatively neglected role of maturational factors in long-term treatment. The future is already with us at Chestnut Lodge as a new admissions unit and a new transitional unit make their appearance on the campus to be gradually incorporated into the total Chestnut Lodge experience.

If this section seems like a shining one, I must acknowledge the editorial gifts of Linda Berman, who took the whole work under her careful and professional editorial eye and enabled it to flow as smoothly as it does. I and the other contributors thereby express our gratitude for her diligent efforts.

REFERENCES

Redl, F. 1968. In G. Caplan and S. Lebovici, eds. *Adolescence*. New York: Basic.

Winnicott, C. 1963. Face-to-face with children. In *Child Care and Social Work*. London: Codicote.

Winnicott, D. W. 1961. Varieties of psychotherapy. In *Delinquency and Deprivation*. London: Tavistock.

Winnicott, D. W. 1963. The mentally ill in your caseload. In *Maturational Process and the Facilitating Environment*. New York: International Universities Press.

E. JAMES ANTHONY

In my previous professional career (which I now refer to as "b.c.," or "before Chestnut Lodge"), I worked with adolescent patients who were, for the most part, neurotically conflicted, prone to depression, confused about their developing selves, and underachieving at school. With their background of a good-enough environment, a strong-enough constitution, and a smooth-enough development, they were often a therapeutic joy to treat since the course ran predictably through well-defined stages and the alliance, once established, held together under the most taxing vicissitudes of the transference.

At the Lodge, I found the circumstances to be somewhat different. In mythological terms, Oedipus was here approaching the crossroads but had not yet encountered his father and dispatched him or continued on his way to the consummation of his desires with his mother in Thebes. At this point, he was still a preoedipal youngster, still suffering from infantile abandonment and the trauma of a cruel exposure that was far from healed by adoption.

At this hospital, I found adolescents who fell short of "classical," were fixated somewhere in the pre-Oedipus with little or no latency development, and were still traversing an infantile path that had made them into even more monstrous babies than they once were—more hungry, more greedy, more cruel, more dirty, more curious, more boastful, and more egocentric. Not only had they pursued their development with sticky feet, but they had also emerged at the far end of childhood with a heavy burden of traumata. They appeared to be inextricably bound up in endless love-hate struggles, merging relationships, and blurred identities. Their sexuality and aggression floundered unpredictably

99

and awkwardly all over the place and were generally confluent with an enormous neediness. The critical question was whether they could be held long enough to initiate treatment before they or their families took flight. Yet the facility was talking, with much experience behind it, about two to four years of uninterrupted therapeutic care with no promise of a rose garden.

Coming from an over-crowded academic department, I was surprised at the spaciousness of this well-put-together and charming campus, comprising self-contained cottages along a little street, lying within easy walking distance from the school, the treatment offices, the recreational and rehabilitative facilities, and, surprisingly, the Research Institute. Here, I found an intriguing interest in the investigation of the therapeutic processes and their efficacy. In my academically trained mind, I was wedded to the idea that there should be no treatment without research and no research without treatment, and this conjunction was therefore highly congenial to me.

The campus was insulated from the everyday competitive life on the outside and had a life of its own that eliminated much of the stressfulness but still maintained the normal challenges to living in the manner of remote villages and townships that preserve their traditions and live by standards that grow naturally out of their particular needs. Time did not dominate the campus as it did in the majority of psychiatric facilities. Treatment was not expected to end at some artificially dictated point and at a stage when treatment could hardly have begun. The long-term philosophy permeated the air and gave it that quality of interminableness that Freud discovered, by trial and error, to be the very quintessence of psychoanalytic treatment. To work comfortably on this campus, one needed a long-term perspective coupled with the long-term dedication of a long-term staff, all of which must appear to the outside as "dodoesque." In today's psychiatric world, the treatment tends to be short, mindless in the sense that the brain is the target of therapeutic endeavor, and chemical. Here, it was different; here, the mind, especially the unconscious mind, was in the ascendant.

As I thought about this uniqueness, I began to see it as an actualization of an Eriksonian moratorium (Erikson 1968), lasting years but not haphazardly since a sequence of therapeutic stages could be discerned in the progression and regression of the patients that dealt with the technical problems of forming an alliance and testing it out, working through with the help of transference, and terminating.

Moratorium Activities

The need for a long-term, fairly structured, therapeutic moratorium has become imperative since the increase in severe adolescent disorders (excluding the psychoses) in the latter half of the century. Every moratorium generates its own particular set of phenomena (Anthony 1982), such as the emergence of a pseudo species with its own "tribal" creations, its own folklore, and its own group identity. Within this setting, there is a gradual delineation of a personal identity, but a delineation put in abeyance in the milieu while the adolescent tries on different "masks" with much relished exhibitionism, such as the outrageousness of the "punk," the vulgarity of the street urchin, the aloofness of the alienated, and the craziness of the psychotic. There is also much experimentation with gender through autosexual, homosexual, bisexual, and heterosexual trials. Then, with the help of an encouraging learning environment and the undoing of learning inhibitions, cognitions begin to thrive, allowing for reflective "stock taking" and the construction of loosely or tightly put together "metatheory" in which deviances from the norm find an understandable place. Finally, the moratorium offers a "second chance" to undo and redo the dynamic complications of earlier and later life, long covered over by massive and somewhat primitive defenses. In this "second chance," a gradual attempt is made to establish the workable complementarity between the synthesizing functions of the adolescent ego and the treatment environment. These moratorium activities gradually lead to the development of new emotional and cognitive competences with the help of "tools" provided by an intensely therapeutic environment in which each mode of treatment sets out to engage a particular aspect of personality.

It is my expectation that developmental research findings will support the view that the moratorium has found a significant niche in the human life cycle and that cognitive, linguistic, and symbolic functioning all stand to gain considerably from this psychological incubation. I would expect the same from the therapeutic moratorium. Although the gains in question have not been too closely examined as of yet, studies of "representational competence" (Anthony 1974) offer some evidence of gain following a total therapeutic approach. This involves an assessment of the degree of coherence in the patient's narrative account of his disorder that is much more clearly, comprehensively, and succinctly articulated by the end of his stay on the campus. All this in response to the simple request, "Tell me about yourself."

The moratorium works within a milieu, and the creation of a therapeutic milieu represents one of the most exacting challenges of hospital treatment, especially in the long-term mode. The staff, like the patients, become better at handling their own feelings and frustrations, with and without treatment, the longer they are steeped in the therapeutic milieu, and there is a careful regard for their psychic equilibrium. "Burnout" is a problem when the setting is emotionally opaque and the staff lack opportunity to air their concerns through regular meetings in groups while these are still uppermost in their minds.

The emphasis at the Lodge is on flexibility: both structure and control are used in the service of growth and maturation and not for the purpose of surpressing such phenomena, as "acting out," that are the norm for the average teenager. It may also be the only form of communication available in the initial phase of treatment to the primitive ego of patients, deficient in thinking, coping, and reality testing. For many of them, it has been their customary way to obtain attention and is readily understood by the staff as such. The house-parents, with supervisory help, become empathically sensitive to their charges and learn, on the job, to recognize their own strong departures of feeling in both positive and negative directions. They seem like natural "containers" of the excesses on their units: supporters for those who feel despairingly helpless and hopeless and tolerant acceptors of periodic regressions. Most of all, they become deeply involved in the sad predicaments that the patients bring to them and sometimes suffer along with them, but on the right side of humanness. I have often been surprised in my meetings with the staff at how skillful they are at decoding the mixed messages directed at them, even in very abstruse nonverbal forms.

In this setting, which is so much an interpreted one, intuitions also play a vital part and help to regulate staff-patient interactions. This is not to say that the long-term staff does not sometimes feel impotent, inadequate, and suffused with self-doubt in response to certain very difficult patients who specialize in the mechanisms of splitting and projective identification, but they seem to sense when their counter-transferences develop irrational aspects and to pull out when weekly supervision points out that they are falling into the adaptive pattern already perfected by the patient in his home environment. It takes time to tolerate being treated as an object, "not related to but dictated to" and not loved but clung to in the manner of hungry babies.

One should stress that the path to long-term patienthood is strewn with expectable and often inexplicable resistances and reactions. On initial exposure to the multiple therapies, the sense of vulnerability is often elevated so that a phase of helplessness may ensue. There is also a concomitant burden of shame attached to the prospect of becoming a long-term case, a sense of stigma that seems never to be completely resolved in certain patients. In the same context, the adolescents may sometimes complain of condescension when the reaction is actually rooted in the inevitable tiltedness of the therapeutic relationship. As the patients perceive it, the staff's mental health is enviably beyond question: every day they go home to their normally functioning families and are free to go where they please. Why was life so unfair? Why did they have to end up in a mental hospital? One can work with guilt in psychotherapy, but adolescent shame is hard to eradicate even within the benevolent, nonjudgmental milieu of the Lodge.

The Setting as a World of Testable Theory

The long-term psychodynamic setting provides an excellent field for researching the vicissitudes of therapeutic process as they ramify within the milieu.

First of all, there is the evaluation of psychoanalytic theory as it deals with severely disturbed pathologies. One likes to think of the models that have grown up as noncompeting. The classical model provides understanding of the individual process such as attaching, relating, transferring, defending, repairing, and recovering. Nonclassical psychoanalytic theory tends to focus on primitive object relations, envy and greed, persecutory anxieties, and intense feelings of annihilation or abandonment and is largely preoedipal in its perspective. The question still under consideration is whether at the Lodge one is dealing predominantly with a deprivational, traumatic, or conflictual psychopathology or whether elements of all three are present with any one predominant depending on the diagnostic category of the patient in question. It is not easy to pinpoint a "basic fault" or assess the accumulations of multiple traumata or the savagery of conflicts when these are tainted by severe character disorders. In dealing with disturbed adolescents, one is often more conscious of the self in operation chiefly because of the obtrusive narcissism. The emergence of a "nuclear self" is still impeded by the many selves that struggle for expression in these disordered individuals. As with the Eriksonian identity (Erikson 1968), the nuclear self gives the therapist something to focus on as an important dimension of the individual's life, and he can set up "nuclear programs" designed to enhance the ideals, skills, orientations, and autonomy (all aspects of milieu activity) away from the constant intrusions of the grandiose, exhibitionistic self.

The long-term setting also provides ample opportunity for exploring the ideas of a "second individuation" resulting from a loosening of infantile ties, the integration of childhood traumata, the development of "signal" responses as part of the security system, and the genesis of a historical sense of continuity associated with wholeness and a stable gender identity. All these integrative functions are mirrored in the daily operations of the milieu and can be checked independently by the researchers as treatment continues.

One can observe, in patients from chaotic and disorganized homes, a gradual internalization of the protective environment so that a sense of safety and poise is recovered and the world no longer impinges on them as a constant source of danger. It is only when the patients feel less threatened, less persecuted, and less overwhelmed that milieu enhancements (controls, competences, consistencies, continuities, coherences, containments, and copings) add a positive overlay to the recuperative processes.

When patients have undergone a disorganization of thought and speech, it becomes the prime aim of the treatment to restore and sustain coherence and reestablish meaningfulness. This is effected by furthering the process of internalization interpretatively against the persistent tendency of the adolescent patient to externalize inner conflicts and concerns and to help him replace his primitive defense system with a more mature set of mechanisms. Furthermore, the empathic response of the milieu presents the patient with a more articulate and integrated core of being, thus making up for the central failure of the developmental environment. By the time the patient is discharged, there is an expectation that he will be able to construct a life narrative that will include significant participants; significant facts, episodes, and states of mind; stages of beginnings, middles, and endings; sequences and causes; and, finally, some sense of purpose. Such a whole amounts to an experiential Gestalt, and, through this, the patient tries to give shape and coherency to his life (Lakoff and Johnson 1980).

Bion's (1977) notion of containment (of a container and the contained) is based on the early mother-infant relationship but can easily be extended to portray the happenings within the long-term milieu. The staff become the containers of psychic events and processes of exchange that take place constantly between the patient and the milieu and help to contain and transform primitive states of being and hand them back to the patient at a higher level of process and integration. In this way, or in some way related to this, the patient acquires the capacity to do for himself what the environment does for him, and so structural and maturational development take place. These holding and containing functions are the invariants of the therapeutic process and emerge from the reliability and sensitivity of the setting.

An observer, such as Fairbairn (1941), might examine the relationships existent on our adolescent campus and pronounce them all schizoid, that is, showing at the same time extreme dependency and denial of dependency, a sense of self-desolation experienced simultaneously with merging, and what Anna Freud (1958) described as a state of primary identification. The three main features of these schizoid relationships—the attitude of omnipotence, of isolation and detachment, and of preoccupation with inner reality—are used to exercise control of therapeutic relationships, to prevent actual relationships, and to affirm the primacy of internal life. In individuals with those propensities, any act of giving leads to inner impoverishment, and, therefore, there is a predominance of taking in all relationships, a feature that elicits special countertransference from the milieu staff. This may very well represent the nuclear psychopathology of the patients that we admit, although I am aware of much more variability than this would suggest.

The cases that present themselves seem on the whole to be a curious admixture of developmental stages from the most primitive to the episodically mature. They are not as doomed to pregenitality as they appear on first impression. Once they develop the therapeutic habit of "putting (their feelings) into words," it is surprising how more advanced they seem to be.

Transformations

The different therapies at work in the milieu form a complex interactional pattern and, for the most part, carry on in concordance, but they can become antagonistic at times and generate therapeutic discord. This, in turn, may produce a crisis unless the supervision of the system is both careful and constant. Competitiveness among therapists evokes its own special kind of countertransference that seeks to downplay the rivals in many subtle and almost undiscernible ways. Each treatment modality, however, brings about its own specific transformations so that there should actually be no contest. The individual responds to the therapist, to the family, to the group, to the cottage unit, to the classroom, and to the milieu as a whole in different ways since his resistances, defenses, and interpersonal skills vary with each therapeutic situation, as do the gains and losses, the advances and regressions. Bion's (1977) concept of invariance recognizes the fact that some parts of the original pathology may remain relatively unchanged, even though reduced considerably in significance, and that the effect on change of different therapeutic modalities may differ a lot. The processes of transformation, it must be remembered, are carried out in the patient's mind, and, with the different techniques in use, different patterns of transformation are induced. Sometimes the same situation can be transformed in different ways at different times, by different parts of the personality and by different therapies. To what extent the patterns of transformation begin to look good or bad depends on the concomitant elements involved. There can, for example, be large transformations associated with poor adjustment or relatively small transformations with striking progression in adaptation. Whether one could ever develop a grid system, similar to Bion's, to particularize these developments in the long-term milieu is something for the future, but a development of this nature, in a more comprehensible form than Bion's, would represent an advance in our total grasp of the therapeutic environment.

Adolescent Agonistes

The adolescent at Chestnut Lodge is struggling with himself, with his developmental phase, with his family, and with his immediate environment. There is always meaning in the perpetual struggle, but this is not always conscious. The unconscious meaning of the milieu lies in the interweaving of treatment that carries the patient sequentially to different places, where he reenacts different individual, family, group, and community struggles of the past in the present and begins to find meaningful connections between his contribution to the various interactions and those of the participants who also figure in them. The patient may also carry an unconscious meaning for staff members who may respond to him out of their past. Soon after admission, he sets up transferences within the institution and receives countertransferences in return. Sometimes the staff replicates in an almost uncanny way the family configurations of the patient and may then be sucked into the drama currently playing in the home. The polarization of family members into good and evil, through splitting, generates a similar dichotomy in the staff, who, in supervision, can be made aware of their logical role in these unconscious operations.

What sustains the therapists that treat those adolescents, live daily with them, talk about them, argue about them, dream about them, and even daydream, aggressively and erotically, about them is that the adolescents represent perhaps the most appealing type of patients one can treat, delightful in their spontaneity, in their creativity, and in what Winnicott (1974) referred to as their most precious commodity of immaturity. These, in greater or lesser amounts, act as a spur to the therapists' long-term endeavors in spite of the acting out, the unpredictability, the negativism, the arrogance, the narcissism, and the feelings of entitlement.

The more explicit goals are shared by every part of the milieu and involve a variety of transformations: acting out into self-reflection and verbalization; outer controls into inner controls; low self-esteem into normal degrees of narcissism; isolation into mutual relationships; primitive defenses into more mature ones; the sense of despair into some degree of hopefulness; and spilling over anxieties and aggressions into a capacity for containment on the part of both patient and family.

At the end of his therapeutic moratorium at Chestnut Lodge, the adolescent Oedipus is, it is hoped, on his way once again, having resolved at best some of the infantile impediments that had held up his progress and ready to tackle the developmental problems lying ahead of him in Thebes.

REFERENCES

Anthony, E. J. 1974. The syndrome of the psychologically invulnerable child. In *The Child and His Family*, vol. 3. New York: Wiley.

Anthony, E. J. 1982. Normal adolescent development from a cognitive viewpoint. *Journal of the American Academy of Child Psychiatry* 21:318–327.

Bion, W. 1977. *Seven Servants*. New York: Aronson.

Erikson, E. H. 1968. *Identity, Youth and Crisis*. New York: Norton.

Fairbairn, W. R. D. 1941. A revised psychopathology of the psychoses and psychoneuroses. *International Journal of Psycho-Analysis* 22:64–80.

Freud, A. 1958. Adolescence. *Psychoanalytic Study of the Child* 13:255–278.

Lakoff, G., and Johnson, M. 1980. *Metaphors We Live By*. Chicago: University of Chicago Press.

Winnicott, D. W. 1971. *Playing and Reality*. London: Tavistock.

8   THE INTENSIVE PSYCHOANALYTIC
PSYCHOTHERAPY OF A SEVERE
NARCISSISTIC PERSONALITY DISORDER
IN ADOLESCENCE

DOUGLAS A. CHAVIS

It is not unusual for many of the adolescents in long-term residential treatment to have been in therapy, sometimes even intensive long-term therapy, prior to their admission. Yet these past treatments were unsuccessful. Frequently, our adolescents have started out in outpatient psychotherapy, gone on to brief hospitalizations and the use of neuroleptics, and then arrive at the end of the road and are admitted to hospitals like Chestnut Lodge.

This chapter will examine the therapeutic process enveloping one such "untreatable" adolescent here at Chestnut Lodge and attempt to illustrate this process with a special focus on the four-times-per-week individual psychotherapy. An additional theme will be to illustrate the opening to early middle phase of the treatment of a severe narcissistic personality disorder in adolescence. It is noteworthy that, while adolescents with narcissistic personality disorders have been described in the literature and technical and countertransference problems have been explored, there is no real description of the actual treatment process with these extremely difficult patients (Bleiberg 1984, 1987, 1988; Egan and Kernberg 1984; Frankel 1977; Kernberg 1984; Rinsley 1980a, 1980b; Spruiell 1975; Tylim 1978).

Background to the Disorder

Tom was admitted to Chestnut Lodge when he was fifteen years old. He had been in psychotherapy from two to four times per week, with three different therapists, almost continuously since he was seven years old. Something clearly was not working for Tom in his family of origin. His father was an extremely successful businessman, and his mother was a housewife. Tom was the second youngest of seven siblings. The family system was characterized by a depressed, over-whelmed mother with too many children and an absent father. While Tom's developmental milestones were all normal, there were difficulties at every stage of development. As a toddler, he was described as clinging and needy of affection. He was enuretic until age ten. At three years old, he attended preschool. No separation problems were noted by his mother, but Tom was overly aggressive with teachers and peers. He liked to wear nail polish at ages four and five, possibly suggesting a feminine identification. It was noted that he was irritating, provoking, annoying, and constantly trying to draw attention to himself. At age seven, when he was first seen by a therapist, he was described as disruptive in school, a know-it-all, entitled, irritating, angry, resentful, and occasionally assaultive toward teachers and peers. His superior intelligence was recognized as being enlisted in the service of his psychopathology.

Tom's first therapist was a female, who, after one and one-half years of treatment, referred him to a male child analyst because of Tom's problems around his sexual identification: she thought a male might work better with him. The child analyst observed that Tom had inordinate degrees of dependency, anxiety, inferiority, oppositionality, shame, and humiliation that made him intractable to analysis. After two years of attempted analysis, the analyst shifted to an intensive, psychotherapeutic approach for the next several years. This phase of the treatment stopped when Tom was twelve because the parents, the therapist, and the patient himself were dissatisfied with the results. The male analyst was now of the opinion that Tom might work better with a female therapist, and such a referral was made.

By this time, Tom was aged fourteen and becoming increasingly maladapted. He was unable to perform academically, showed no motivation to work, was constantly provocative with peers and teachers, and, during one period of crisis, attempted to attack one of his sisters with a knife. His low self-esteem made him vulnerable to severe depression, and this, together with his impulsivity, was thought to put him at risk for suicide and homicide. In more reactive ways, Tom was counterphobic and hyperactive and manifested extreme fluctuations in ego functioning. He was treated with lithium carbonate in conjunction with an antidepressant and was seen thrice weekly in individual psychotherapy. His parents were seen for counseling by a family therapist. All these measures proved ineffectual. Indeed, Tom became actively suicidal within one year. He was hospitalized briefly and medicated with trifluxoperazine and lithium. The diagnoses considered on that admission were bipolar affective disorder, variant syndrome; a combined bipolar affective disorder with ADD; or a prodrome of paranoid schizoaffective disorder. He was referred to Chestnut Lodge for long-term residential care. The referring female therapist advised us that she thought Tom might work better with a male therapist.

It has been noted that Tom was one of seven siblings. There were twins aged twenty-four, a brother and sister; a sister twenty-two, a brother twenty-one, a sister eighteen, the patient fifteen, and a brother five years old. Since none of them appeared as disturbed as Tom, it is interesting to speculate why he seemed most afflicted. There is certainly a phenotypic spectrum of genetic expression that would vary with an individual child's endowment and his particular familial experience. This would include variations in resistance and vulnerability. Second, there are fluctuations in a mother's maternal drive and availability for mothering. Tom's mother apparently became more depressed with each additional child she bore. Moreover, there was the fact of Tom's prepartum rejection by his mother: he was an unwanted child. When her next child was born eleven years after Tom, she was again refreshed and more available. Also, there is the factor of a father's availability. Tom's father was traveling and largely unavailable for most of his early years. Around the time of the birth of the last sibling, the father was home more often.˙ A factor related to this concerns the father's attitude toward each child's personality. It was clear that the father viewed Tom's particular style of attention seeking with contempt. This leads to another element, that of the presentation of symptomatology. This can range from provocative to passive, belligerent to reticent. It is possible that some siblings might be as disturbed as Tom. However, their pathology might be expressed more passively, not demanding the notice that Tom attracted. Another consideration is the ordinal position and gender of the siblings in the family. As the youngest sibling for so many years, Tom was abused by the older male siblings and mothered by the older female siblings. He was thus in a unique position. Finally, there is the element of the relative deprivation experienced by each sibling in a crowded family situation. Tom expressed this in his complaint that there were no more bedrooms left for him. There are consequently a range of factors that might have coalesced to form Tom's distinctive set of difficulties.

This is not an atypical admission for Chestnut Lodge. Our usual adolescent is characterized as a difficult case, a failed case, or an over-treated case. What they all have in common is the need for long-term, intensive, psychoanalytic psychotherapy in a therapeutic milieu. Tom specifically had been unsuccessfully treated since age seven. The pharmacological treatments were not effective, and they were all discontinued on his admission. The many psychological treatments seemed to have been of a probing, uncovering style. Tom was resistant to this mode to begin with. His history of treatment only made further work more difficult since it heightened his sensitivity to therapeutic intrusion. This problem is even more important when there is severe narcissistic pathology because the pathological style expresses itself in a wish to avoid depth. Tom, for instance, stated that he was not interested in history or philosophy. He wanted to "stay on the surface of things." He feared that, if he "paid attention to the thoughts of great men, a seed might be planted in my head and then my thoughts really wouldn't be mine."

The Initial Phase

When I first saw Tom nineteen months ago, he seemed to be in a state of extreme disequilibrium, franticly clutching out for a hand to stabilize him. He was short and well-groomed in a "preppy" manner. His speech was rapid, and opposing trains of thought appeared to fight for expression. His motor activity was constant. He let me know that he was in the hospital voluntarily and that he was depressed and hopeless. After so many years of psychotherapy, he was no better. He felt like a circus act with a sign saying "freak" because he had no friends. If he lost a game, he said, he would stop playing it. He described himself as intelligent, but he could never concentrate in school and thus did poorly. He would constantly interrupt classes with joking, talking, burping, and farting. He reported that he did best in the fifth grade, when a male teacher showed an interest in him and thought that Tom had promise. Tom liked to draw, but he drew the same thing over and over again. That is because, he explained, he will draw something only if he can do it perfectly. One of the pictures he had perfected was what he called a "snail's angel." It was a picture of a small snail with bruises all over its body, a long tail, and very big antennae. He said that he yearned to be like the "snail's angel." The picture seemed to represent a small but tough and resilient character, not afraid of fighting and getting injured, and coming through with body and integrity intact. On the other hand, it also conveyed the image of a vulnerable, hypersensitive person who could withdraw from traumatizing experiences that made it difficult for him to adapt to the outside world.

Tom was fearful to go outside by himself. The fears seemed to be of bodily injury and homosexual attack. He said he was small and feared having a gang jump him or people make fun of him. The concerns about his body were legion. He talked of his toe size, of corns, of fears that his body would become covered with spots, and of wishes to have a perfect body. He complained constantly of pain in his body, blisters, burns, fears that his fingers would be chopped off, and fantasies of bodies bursting. He was troubled with fantasies of nuclear war and radioactivity burning his limbs, melting them, or causing them to fall off or to disintegrate. He was constantly on the verge of disintegrating panic. In our hospital setting, this anxiety could be contained without medication. He seemed to feel protected in his therapy hours with me, and outside the hours he could feel constantly protected and taken care of by the milieu.

Varying attitudes toward me were expressed initially. For instance, if I did not quite grasp his rapid speech, he would impatiently and impulsively yell at me, calling me "thick." He was constantly farting without regard for me. But, then, he seemed anxious to identify with me, to try on my glasses, and to buy a plant for his room like the one in my office. He was always on time for our sessions.

I think that, because Tom was so panic stricken, frightened, and fragmented when he arrived at Chestnut Lodge, he was able to reveal a great deal about himself in his quest for some measure of security and stability. He said he was terribly upset because he had no friends and that it was humiliating and shameful for him to have to rely entirely on his parents. He felt only barely tolerated by his peers or hated for being spoiled, needing to have everything his way, and thinking of himself as special. He felt sad and different from others. He was also preoccupied with tortures, such as skinning people with razors and cutting off their limbs, but he never linked these fantasies to any specific person. He was greatly interested in bombs and liked to see them explode. He once called in a bomb scare in a public facility and then called his schoolmates to watch it make the news on television. He said, "I felt great, scaring people the way I go around [being] scared all the time." Even though he showed it sparingly, I was impressed with his psychological mindedness.

Tom initially presented his father as being like a "drill sergeant." Even such a mild criticism tended to arouse guilt. Tom was unable to talk to his father because he felt that his father treated him as a business associate. Nevertheless, he would like to feel closer to his father. He would read about his father's business and eavesdrop on his business conversations. Tom saw his father as a superstar, at the peak of his achievement, and was proud of him. Nevertheless, his father had a severe temper that could embarrass the family, and Tom was scared of him. There were times when the father would get physically violent with Tom, and this was extremely frightening. In general, Tom felt guilty about his angry feelings toward his family and displaced these onto authority figures outside the home. In this regard, he liked to test nonfamilial authority, always picking the most vulnerable and marginal rule to challenge and persisting until he had won his way. He would try to mobilize his peers to rally around his cause and help him obtain his objective.

During this time, there was little reference to his mother. He acknowledged feeling disappointed in her, especially when she sided with his father. He could not be angry with her, though, because he loved her.

The period of fragmentation and panic gradually subsided over the first three months Tom was at Chestnut Lodge. As he felt less desperate, he became less and less communicative. I believe this had to do with the fact that the lessened anxiety allowed the consolidation of a grandiose identity with which he could deny his needs. During the therapy hours, Tom started doing crossword puzzles and reading the sports section of the newspaper. I would greet him in the waiting room, and he would walk past me as if I were not there and sit in my office reading his magazine as if he were alone. Occasionally, he would ask my help with a crossword puzzle. It was obvious to him that, while I could do the puzzles better than he could, I was still not very good at them. I told him I was glad at least to help him with his crosswords. It seemed to me that this type of interaction was important at this stage, in that it allowed Tom to experience me as someone not needing to be in control, someone interested in what Tom found interesting, and someone willing to acknowledge that he was not perfect and always right, like a superstar. (There was no conscious attempt on my part to manipulate the developing transference and afford Tom a "corrective emotional experience." But it did feel right at that time and still does in retrospect.) At the end of the sessions, even though I scarcely appeared to exist for him, he was reluctant to leave, suggesting that he was finding some value in simply being there with me. He often would arrive early but stressed that this had nothing to do with his feelings toward me; he just wanted to use his sessions to miss as much school as possible. Frequently, he would fall asleep during the sessions, covering himself up with various articles from around my office, as if to create a safe place. At this time, he felt rejected and picked on by his peers at the Lodge School, and I had the feeling that he found the therapeutic situation a maternal haven from these abuses. He did not want me to know too much of these outside difficulties and was angry if I pressed him for details. What he seemed to want more was a reliable friend, a secure refuge, and an accepting and nurturing parent who did not think badly of him and did not focus on the things he felt badly about.

Interestingly, Tom's apparent self-sufficiency and noncommunicativeness flowered concurrently with a covert and unacknowledged increase in dependency on me. Before a four-day holiday weekend, he expressed fears of being alone in a small car and getting crushed in an accident. He said he needed a larger car. I tried to connect his fears and wishes for more protection to our not meeting for four days, but Tom denied this and then asked if he could have a book of mine to take with him over the weekend.

Homosexual themes also made their appearance during this period. His conversation became liberally sprinkled with the phrase "buttfucking." Frequently, he would bend over and exhibit his rear to me or widen his legs, seemingly to show his genitals. Once, he wondered why he had had "all kinds of sexual thoughts, especially involving anal sex," since he was seven years old. I told him that I thought he was very confused about who and what he really was and that the sexual thoughts probably contributed to his anxiety and restlessness. Tom said that, when he was in the third grade (about eight years old), he was troubled by questions of who and what he was, whether male or female, and that he then started to get bad grades. He was generally regarded as lazy, even by himself. I told him that, with questions like that on his mind, he must have been very anxious and that perhaps it was this anxiety that made him tired or lazy. He insisted, however, that he was lazy and, as if to confirm this, went to sleep in the session. I continued to talk to him, saying that I could imagine him thinking that I also considered him lazy but that in fact what I really thought was how very hard it was for him to talk of things that disturbed him so much. It could surely drive him to sleep. On another occasion, he sat down next to me and touched my leg. He made a reference to something "gay." He explained he did not mean anything homosexual by this but rather something queer or strange. He started getting upset and went to the window and said, "Look's like a storm is coming." This was followed by his wondering how people saw him, his belief being that he was seen as "short and a pretty boy."

After being at Chestnut Lodge for about eight months, Tom found his first girlfriend, a tomboy. The anxieties he experienced in this relationship, which remained nonsexual, gradually threw him into a panic. The extreme anxiety seemed central to his identity concerns over who or what he was, a male or a female, and to his fear of being challenged and ridiculed by other males. He began to build up his body, constantly exercising. The sessions were now filled with push-ups and exhibitions of his musculature. He either ignored me or hoped that I would admire his physical development. I told him that I was glad that he could use the sessions for body building because I was all for his building himself up. It was important for him to know that there were other ways to build himself up, though, and therapy could be a tool for that. He replied that body building made him feel masculine and that he wanted to make sure he was not a baby (like a newly admitted patient on his unit) or a girl (like his girlfriend). While not acknowledging any reference to me, he often sang the song "Stand By Me" during this period.

His overt stance, however, remained one of not needing me and treating me contemptuously. He appeared to fear that, if he talked more, I would demean and belittle him and treat him contemptuously. He felt "dicked over" everywhere and seemed to fear that, if he let down his guard, that might happen in his therapy also. There was very little that he could talk about, and frequently the sessions were filled with more flatulence (actual) than words. Once, when we were walking into the office together, he feigned throwing a stick and said "fetch" to me. I told him that I thought he was fearful of being my puppy, chasing after me, and needing desperately to have my protection and that yet he acted as if I were a nothing whom he could control and for whom he had no need. I also said his fear was that, if he trusted me more and talked with me, I would end up humiliating him. These interpretations elicited several kinds of responses—silences, farts, curses, and abuses. He ranted at me, "You should keep the psychiatry shit to yourself— I've heard it for years and it's shit. No one's ever helped me before, why should you help me now?"

Toward the end of the first year of therapy, enough trust had developed that Tom could let me know more of his feelings at times. Compared with his six siblings, he felt that his parents had deprived him. He said that his needs would always come last. However, he felt that he could not cry or complain about this or anything else with his parents because he would then be a shamed and humiliated crybaby. Additionally, he revealed his concerns about father's drinking. Once, his father came to Chestnut Lodge to pick him up and was drunk. This showed, Tom felt, that father did not have his interests at heart, would risk his son's life, and really could not take care of him. Nor could he trust his mother to remember his needs and take care of him. She had too many other things on her mind. He said he felt "fucked over" by his parents in the past but could not be angry about it. In fact, he felt compelled to make excuses for these perceived shortcomings.

In the transference, at this time, there was still predominantly Tom as the self-contained grandiose self, with space for no one else in the room. One person was dominant, and the other was a nothing. I suggested that one of the reasons he did not like to listen to me was because, if he felt he was not in total control, he would be a nothing. He stated that the person with no control, "the nothing," would be filled with envy and jealousy of the dominant person and would make efforts to belittle and sabotage that person. His wishes enviously to destroy the ascendent other have only rarely become explicit since. They would arise in those situations in which he would try to confuse me with his rapid speech and tangential thoughts in order to throw me off the track that I would take.

117

We were now in the middle of football season, and Tom had a keen interest in football as well as an encyclopedic knowledge of the subject. Most of our sessions were filled with his reading silently, or at times out loud, about various happenings in football. I made it clear that I respected his vast knowledge of football, indeed, that I was interested in it, and that he had much to offer me concerning football. He eventually said, "I feel you are the only person in the world who listens to me about the thing I love most—football—and I love it because I feel I have your attention in the palm of my hand." He therefore let me know that, while he might have been treating me as if I did not exist, my existence was quite important in the sense that I am there to admire, appreciate, and listen to him. Nonetheless, if it were not for the fact that I genuinely enjoyed football, it would have been extremely hard for me to endure this period.

It was virtually impossible for Tom and me to talk about this because he could not tolerate me as a person with an expertise of my own. To confront him with this via my "psychiatric" comments would only provoke rage. I acknowledged with him how I felt he was using me, but I felt that he needed me in that way to consolidate an identity and maintain a tolerable self-esteem. I hoped that he would eventually trust me more and feel secure enough with who he was to acknowledge me more as a separate person. I realized, of course, that this approach was problematic in that I was also being treated contemptuously. When this became extreme, I would confront him. He at times would reply, "That is what psychiatrists are for, to take shit." I told him that I would not tolerate that and that I was not there to be abused by him. While he argued, he seemed to enjoy hearing this, and, at times, it would provoke a transient, overtly idealizing transference. I would be no longer identified, for the moment, with the devalued expelled parts of himself. It is noteworthy also that hateful countertransference feelings were greatly alleviated by the realization that his grandiose responses were for the most part defensive. When he was at his most rejecting, it was usually obvious to me that I was enormously important to him, even though he rarely acknowledged this fact.

In another session around this time, Tom came in and read silently for half an hour. I once again pointed out his contradictory feelings for me: either I was nonexistent, or I was treated with so much importance that he wanted to reschedule his sessions so as not to miss them. He responded that he wanted to reschedule only in order to miss math. He felt that I just wanted the satisfaction of knowing that he wanted therapy and was getting something out of it. I told him that he liked to think that we just exploited each other and that it was easier for him to think that way rather than think that he might miss our meetings. He did not respond. However, several days later, he talked of how people at Chestnut Lodge just liked to lord over him and did not really care about him. I said it seemed to me that he wanted people to care about him very much and that he got upset when they did not appear to do so. Later, Tom said that he felt I was trying to get him to say something. That was not my intention, and I indicated so. Minutes later, he exclaimed, "Ha! I've got you cornered." I reflected aloud my thought that for him therapy was a power game, a struggle between doctor and patient, with one trying to get the better of the other. This made it hard for him to talk because it led him to feel that I was trying to dominate him rather than feeling that he and I were working together. When he agreed to this, I was surprised that he could even acknowledge what I had said.

Toward the end of the first year, another aspect of transference began developing. Tom revealed the feeling that he and I were alike and that I was chosen to treat him because we were similar. Moreover, I had things that he needed. He perceived me as calm and unflappable and felt that he might learn these traits from me. Our similarities seemed to involve his feeling that we were both "come-from-behinders." I was a contemptible and abused person—a Jew—and I had managed to succeed; perhaps he would succeed too. But there was also ambivalence in this. A part of him believed, as he said that his father did, that the only respectable thing was complete and total domination from the beginning. Furthermore, the "come-from-behinders" would be character flawed, as opposed to admirable. He occasionally revealed a wish that we would become like Batman and Robin, engrossed in mutual admiration for each other and helping each other achieve greatness. He wanted me to accompany him to his unit or to the recreation center so that others could see us together and know that I was his doctor. He would bask in my light; we would be a glory-filled pair. It must be noted, though, that most transference manifestations left me nonexistent, with his narcissism filling the room.

Tom frequently tested me to see if I would forget about him like his parents did. He would be late for sessions (forgetting about me), and it seemed very important to him that I call the school asking for him. He suggested that I see a movie that he felt was very significant—Pink Floyd's *The Wall*. A week later, he asked if I had seen it, and I had. We were able to discuss the story of an unloved young man who built a wall around himself to prevent pain, further disintegration, and hurt. The important thing seemed to be that he had asked me to do something for him, to test whether I was interested in understanding him. I told him that he was concerned whether I would forget about him in the way he felt that his parents did.

After the first year of treatment, I was assigned a new patient in the adolescent division. Tom came in shortly after this in an abusive frame of mind and said, "Let's talk straight—I am nothing to you and you nothing to me. Therapy is useless and you are just a slot in my day." I told him I thought he was worried that I thought so little of him that I could cast him aside as a "nothing" slot in my day in favor of my new patient. Because of this, it became easier for him to reverse the situation, cast me aside, and tell me I was nothing. I wondered if this might not have been the way he felt when his brother was born and displaced him as the "baby." (At that time Tom, aged eleven, had overdosed and had tried to hang himself.) I said that maybe he was frightened of how important I had become to him and (smiling) how much safer it was to have me for garbage. He would wish to be closer to me but could not quite, as yet, trust me. His big fear was getting dependent on me. As a reaction to this, he continued to devalue me and to do everything by himself. While there was no verbal assent to these interpretations, he quieted down, and the abuse subsided.

The Early Middle Phase

Over the following month, Tom did allow himself to become a little closer to me. He talked of wanting to be the center of attention and wanting to be recognized as special. In relation to this, he revealed that, just prior to his first hospitalization, he learned from a sister (who heard from their mother) that Tom was an unwanted child. He began to express anger and disappointment that his mother had not valued him or given him the time he needed. Themes of murderousness emerged, and the anxiety associated with this seemed barely containable in the sessions. It was also becoming clearer to me that Tom projected the devalued and despised parts of himself onto me and would treat me accordingly. To see these feelings and behaviors as part of himself was humiliating and unacceptable. Ordering people to do things or brusquely telling them what he wanted from them made him feel a lot less needy and dependent than asking for his wants to be met did. He had always intruded into my desk and taken things like pencils and paper that he wanted to use. We were able to talk about these acts more easily, especially as he became more open about his feelings of inadequacy. But narcissistic injury was ever just around the corner. Tom complained constantly that he felt cheated and shortchanged by others, did not acquire the friends he chose, and lacked the social skills he needed to get friends and keep them. In fact, he did not have the cathectic power to survive in the world.

Shortly after this, a new theme was introduced. Tom felt that people should be stricter with him, not let him get away with too much, and applied this to home as well as to the Lodge. I wondered aloud about whether the setting of limits would seem to indicate to him that he was cared for and valued and that he needed more of that. He talked of how on his unit in Chestnut Lodge he felt entitled to be rude and demanding because he thought he was being cheated of the attention he needed and that his family was paying for. He had to be rude because to let people know how hurt he was would be humiliating and they would think he was a crybaby. Following this, for several weeks he treated me as if I meant nothing to him and he had no use for me. I told him again that he felt humiliated by his neediness and that he had to act as if he was totally self-sufficient and needed no one. This, I said, was very sad for him because it left him alone and frustrated.

Tom began to acknowledge that there were two sides to him—a hurt, vulnerable, needy, and dependent side and another that proclaimed that he needed and cared for no one. He also let me know an aspect of himself that he had kept hidden: he sometimes ran himself ragged to please an admired friend whom he wanted to respect and admire him and for whom he felt loyalty and devotion, albeit ambivalently. Tom was not sure he could trust this man and suspected that he was being taken advantage of and used. The more he pursued this theme, the more it became clear how enraged he was at this individual who left him feeling unappreciated, cheated, and unloved. In his treatment, at least overtly, the opposite relationship prevailed. With Tom's stance of grandiose aloofness, I had felt at times as if I were running myself ragged trying to make contact with him. In a sense, I was also proving my loyalty to Tom by doing this and by putting up with him and his arrogant attitudes. I again brought up the mixed messages that he sent me: on the one side, he had no need for me; on the other side, he wanted to be with me and not leave me. To my surprise, he replied that he liked the sessions because they were the only place in the world where he did not feel put down. He added that he refrained from talking about his problems because it made him feel as if he was "talking up" to me, and he felt "scummy" talking to me like that. His preference was to speak to me "adult to adult."

It appeared, then, that there were two main levels of relatedness in the transference. The first involved Tom as "grand" and me as the container of his despised and shameful feelings and behaviors. When he talked of "adult to adult," what he really meant was that one person was in control and the other was compliant. "Control" in this sense was to be understood as one person's grandness suffusing the room in the way that an odor from one person might obliterate the odor of another. The second level was less conscious and seemed to involve me as an ideal with whom he could merge and thereby share my power and luminosity. For this to be thought of consciously would be too threatening to Tom's autonomy and would necessitate his running himself ragged to please me. I then would become a person of overwhelming importance to whom he was homosexually linked and whom he would need in order to stabilize his self-esteem.

A third level of relatedness was slowly developing. For instance, Tom's comment "I feel I'm talking up to you" indicated a capacity to examine what went on in the room between us. This could occur only when trust became sufficient so that constant security operations to maintain the integrity and stability of the self did not dominate our interactions. Recently, Tom has told me that he would like to take me out to lunch because "I realize that you have put up with a lot of shit and you continue working with me, and I want you to continue . . . after I leave the Lodge." He was now able to make reference, at times, to his grand attitudes and ideas as a defense against object loss and has been able to acknowledge his need for admiring people and material objects to maintain his self-esteem. At this third level of relatedness, there is the beginning of a reliable therapeutic alliance.

I want to expand on the scattered references to countertransference that I have made. In a sense, the therapy consisted of my efforts to help Tom recognize my psychological existence vis-à-vis him, to make contact with him, and to rescue him from his narcissistic insulation.

Insofar as I was not present for Tom in the room as a person with my own psychological existence, the defense of projective identification played a major role in our communications (Kernberg 1975). The helplessness, impotence, and anger that I would feel at times in struggling with my allocated nonexistence, or with being the object of so much narcissistic rage and contempt, were all informative "signal" affects that allow me to be more empathic with Tom's experience. More troubling was a tendency to counter his narcissistic stance with my own narcissistic withdrawal. I had to examine my silences at times, wondering whether I was saying to him, "You don't recognize me, well, who needs you? I won't pay attention to you." At other times, the countertransference fantasies took a different turn: I would be struggling ineffectively to make contact with him and not withdraw into my own reverie and feel as if I was an insect, a mosquito or a fly, buzzing around a giant animal. I would become overactive, darting up, down, left, right, striving to get his attention. It seemed to me that the insect fantasy was an identification with those early experiences of Tom's in which he must have struggled desperately to get the attention of the "sleeping giants" in his life. At other times, I felt I had the same degree of reality and separateness in his experience as a thought in his head might have. Recently, he came into my office for a session, did not acknowledge my presence, sat down, read, and was unresponsive when I talked to him. Finally, when I got his attention and asked him why he had not called me to tell me he would not be in for the previous two sessions, he replied, "What sessions?" I was surprised when I started to think that what I had believed was a growing relatedness with Tom was really a thought, a fantasy, in my head. It made me feel foolish. I wondered whether I had created a fantasy relationship to ward off feelings of narcissistic isolation and rage. To continue to see him, did I have to deny the extent of his nonrelatedness? On reflection, I realize that these thoughts and the feelings of insecurity and foolishness that accompanied them were also identifications with Tom. This was certainly an aspect of his concerns, doubts, and distrust when he was "running himself ragged" out of loyalty to an idealized friend.

I have already alluded to my strategy of balancing an empathic understanding of Tom and what his plight might be at any given moment with the need to confront him with the reality of my feelings and the way he treated me. When I was struggling toward an empathic approach to him at such times as I felt that he needed this most, I would wonder to myself whether I might not inadvertently be engaged in a masochistic countertransference enactment. Likewise, while there might have been an empathic element involved in confrontation, it most often was not experienced in that way. When I chose to confront him, therefore, I would question myself about possibly being sadistic and revengefully provoking narcissistic rage or further nonrelatedness.

It is interesting to note in this context the problem of Tom's sleeping. While this could be viewed as the ultimate narcissistic withdrawal, I found it paradoxically to be a time when he could also get something from me and allow me to affect him. Historically, he has always had problems falling asleep. In latency to preadolescence, he would take a blanket and curl up outside his parents' bedroom or attempt to get in bed with a sister. He was too anxious to fall asleep and was therefore chronically tired. At Chestnut Lodge, he would stay awake ruminating and reading, struggling with feelings of disintegration and castration anxiety. After a year of therapy, with much relief, he was finally able to get to sleep regularly before midnight. I gradually sensed that sleeping in the sessions largely represented the safety reunion within a maternal envelope. The couch, at least, could physically contain him and hold him, even if at that time I was unable to do so. He slept in a position in the room that was much closer to me and that involved a shift from his chair to the couch. There was no hostility, or positive feelings, involved in the move. I was simply not a presence in the room to be concerned about—he acted as if he were alone, and on becoming tired or anxious he would simply resort to sleep. In a sense, the couch and I were one, and my presence would appear to suffuse the room. When he would awaken, he would announce that he was finally able to sleep and felt refreshed and replenished. I got the sense that the couch and I had shared in his internal maternal representation.

As Tom's anxiety subsided, the character of the sleep changed somewhat. My office was now valued by him in part as a place where he could relax and not be bothered or demeaned, a place where he could rest his tired self and wake up refreshed. When I would talk, he would sometimes escape my intrusion through sleep, but, on other occasions, he would let me know that he was just feigning sleep. While this withdrawal warded off impingement, he would let me know later how replenished he was after his nap and how positively he felt that I was respecting his needs and integrity in not disturbing him. Most of the time, if I said anything to him after he awoke, it was, "I am glad you can feel renewed," or "I am glad you can find something of value in our meetings."

Recently, I have been confronting him more since I have felt that he was more trusting and secure and more able to allow himself to recognize my presence. For example, after coming into my office, he would scarcely acknowledge my presence for about twenty minutes, after which he would yawn and move to the couch to sleep. At this point, when I started talking to him, he would get angry with me for bothering him, calling me rude. He would then go to sleep. I would wake him up toward the end of the session, and he would say: "Could I spend a few more minutes in here, just waking up slowly? You know how much I like that." I would reply that I was indeed aware how very important it was to him that I recognize his needs, but I added that, when it came to my needs to have him listen to me and to acknowledge me, he seemed to think that my feelings were not important. He replied that he just forgot and left.

I thus experience a dilemma with Tom. I feel he is a boy who has never experienced an adequate response to his feelings and needs. Further, his self-esteem is extremely labile, and he needs a secure, containing, therapeutic environment to foster a sense of security and cohesiveness. The hope would be that, as Tom feels less anxious and threatened, his capacity to recognize the existence of significant others would broaden. He would also be more able to integrate my confrontations (regarding his abuse of me, for instance) and make use of them without feeling demeaned and catapulted into narcissistic rage or withdrawal. In my mind, this process requires a careful intuitive titration of empathy with confrontation, along with a constant wariness of any masochistic and sadistic trends in myself.

It is apparent to me that there is something therapeutic happening between Tom and me at the early middle phase of his treatment here at Chestnut Lodge. While the therapeutic alliance is still not fully established and he remains vulnerable to regression, and even while the major therapeutic work remains to be done, many gains have been made. There is a diminished reliance on hypomanic defense, and the transference is becoming the critical focus of his treatment.

In the Lodge School, on his unit, with his peers, and with his family, dramatic changes in his behavior have been noted. He is much less anxious, grandiose, contemptuous, obnoxious, and disruptive. For the first time in his life, he has made some male friends whom he respects and has recently dated a girl who is respected by her peers and managed himself well. His grades are improving in school, and he has recently taken the SAT. He does a good job, outside school hours, landscaping. His goal is to become an architect.

He was recently retested by a Lodge psychologist. A shift from the initial testing was noticed, in that now there is a focus on personal loss rather than an uncontrolled picture of total violent devastation. The theme of fraudulent authority has shifted to a perception of a magical benevolent figure who restores hope. There is the emergence of some early benevolent object representations, along with evidence of a growing attachment and drop in cynicism about psychotherapy.

Discussion

I have attempted to demonstrate how an adolescent with severe narcissistic pathology has become engaged in a treatment process at Chestnut Lodge that holds high hope of being helpful to him in the restoration to normal life. Prior to his admission at age fifteen, he had been in almost continuous outpatient therapy since age seven with three different therapists, with little success. At the time of admission, he was suicidal, hopeless, and in near-psychotic fragmentation. Why were we able to help him? Why would he be untreatable as an outpatient and become treatable in Chestnut Lodge? It is possible that for the first time he has been treated by a therapist with whom he is well matched. Certainly, a patient like this who is demeaning, devaluing, contemptuous, rejecting, and silent presents huge technical and countertransference problems. My own approach, which I conceive of as an empathic acceptance balanced by a gently confrontative realism, seems to be useful. I have become a benign, potentially helpful figure. I have felt that too much emphasis on empathic understanding might lead to a sadomasochistic enactment, while too much confrontation might lead toward chronic narcissistic rage to such an extent that it would not be possible for Tom to be treated.

This approach borrows from the valuable contributions of both Kernberg (1975, 1984) and Kohut (1971, 1977). It is similar also to the approach evolved by Bleiberg (1987) in his treatment of a latency-aged child.

However, more must be involved. I personally know Tom's past therapists, and they are well-trained, competent people. It could be argued that Tom is simply older, more capable of reflection, and, therefore, more available to treatment. But this belies the fact that, when he was admitted, he had reached the end of the psychotherapy road, was being turned in the direction of the pharmacologists, and being labeled within the schizophrenic spectrum. He was fragmented, hopeless, and saw psychotherapy as just another fraud.

To account for the changes that we have seen in Tom in his nineteen months in treatment, the Chestnut Lodge milieu must be considered. The milieu was significant in helping Tom develop and put into practice new social skills as well as in providing for many therapeutic opportunities. In addition to the intensive individual psychotherapy, weekly family therapy meetings have been especially important. Tom also participated in group psychotherapy. However, the hospital was most crucial in simply providing a setting within which therapy was possible. It must be noted that the therapeutic alliance is still not firmly established. If Tom were to become my private patient, I am uncertain whether he would continue his therapy, at least with an effective frequency of sessions. His narcissism has still not sufficiently been worked through so that he can acknowledge consistently his need for treatment as well as my importance to him in helping him resolve his problems. Under these circumstances, the milieu was necessary to keep him engaged in intensive treatment. His parents, overburdened as they are with the events of their own lives and with their own narcissistic issues, cannot ensure their son's attendance at his therapy hours. That would entail a recognition of his needs and a taking care of him that they have never been able to do. Therefore, in the early stages of treatment, which might be quite lengthy, hospitalization is necessary to allow for the establishment of a true therapeutic alliance.

It is apparent, then, that Tom was simply not able to be treated as an outpatient because there was never enough containment to allow him to feel taken care of and cared for. In the outside world, the narcissistic rage and depression were too great to allow him to engage in a treatment process in which he could begin to allow himself to be helped and become aware of his vulnerability and needfulness. Skilled intensive psychotherapy was crucial, but it was not enough. The family milieu was never able to contain Tom and to give him a secure feeling that he would be taken care of and protected. The ambivalence and anxiety around family members was too great to allow for any relinquishing of defenses. Too much energy had to be spent on defense for a therapeutic encounter to emerge. For such adolescents as Tom, treatment is possible only when they are provided a milieu in which they can feel taken care of and secure. Then individual psychotherapy can be useful, and the untreatable can become treatable.

REFERENCES

Bleiberg, E. 1984. Narcissistic disorders in children: a developmental approach to diagnosis. *Bulletin of the Menninger Clinic* 48:501–517.

Bleiberg, E. 1987. Stages in the treatment of narcissistic children and adolescents. *Bulletin of the Menninger Clinic* 51(3): 296–313.

Bleiberg, E. 1988. Developmental pathogenesis of narcissistic disorders in children. *Bulletin of the Menninger Clinic* 52(1): 3–15.

Egan, J., and Kernberg, P. F. 1984. Pathological narcissism in childhood. *Journal of the American Psychoanalytic Association* 32:39–62.

Frankel, S. A. 1977. The treatment of a narcissistic disturbance in childhood. *International Journal of Psychoanalytic Psychotherapy* 6:165–186.

Kernberg, O. F. 1975. *Borderline Conditions and Pathological Narcissism.* New York: Aronson.

Kernberg, O. F. 1984. *Severe Personality Disorders: Psychotherapeutic Strategies.* New Haven, Conn.: Yale University Press.

Kohut, H. 1971. *The Analysis of the Self.* New York: International Universities Press.

Kohut, H. 1977. *The Restoration of the Self.* New York: International Universities Press.

Rinsley, D. F. 1980a. The developmental etiology of borderline and narcissistic disorders. *Bulletin of the Menninger Clinic* 44:127–134.

Rinsley, D. F. 1980b. Diagnosis and treatment of borderline and narcissistic children and adolescents. *Bulletin of the Menninger Clinic* 44:147–170.

Spruiell, V. 1975. Narcissistic transformations in adolescence. *International Journal of Psychoanalytic Psychotherapy* 4:518–536.

Tylim, I. 1978. Narcissistic transference and countertransference in adolescent treatment. *Psychoanalytic Study of the Child* 33:279–292.

9 THE FAMILY IN TREATMENT DURING THE LONG-TERM INPATIENT CARE OF THE ADOLESCENT

SANDRA BOOTS, DAVID GOODMAN, SUSAN LOUGHMAN,
AND E. JAMES ANTHONY

In the adolescent division of Chestnut Lodge, the clinical social workers have several roles to play—manager, mediator, and therapist. It is as family therapists that the social workers bring their specialized knowledge and skills to bear on patients and their families, not all of whom, however, are taken into family therapy. For some, the geographic distance is too great; for some, it is clinically contraindicated; and for some, the prospect of dealing with a family psychopathology that includes their own contribution can lead to implacable resistances. In their role of family therapists, the social workers must, first of all, create and maintain a working therapeutic alliance that in time grows into a high degree of dependency and closeness that helps to foster the other therapies in which the patient is involved.

The arrangements of treatment may vary with the nature and stage of the therapeutic process. The family may be seen as a whole, as a triad of parents and patient, as a dyad of one parent and patient, and as a dyad of two parents. Grandparents, stepparents, siblings, and other relatives may be included as the case requires. Such flexibility in the treatment of the family is an advantage that this approach has over other treatments at work in the milieu. It also seems, at times, that a dynamic upsurge in the family therapy appears to energize developments in other treatment modalities, especially in bringing buried preoedipal and oedipal material into the realm of consciousness for the patient's individual therapist. Such therapeutic gifts may not always be appreciated. While the manifest aspects may be in phase in the family work, the latent material may still be under heavy resistance in the individual psychotherapy. Such asynchronisms are inevitable in any cluster of ongoing treatments and require correction within the context of the team meetings.

For family therapy to function smoothly in a psychoanalytic milieu, the theories governing its practice must be concordant with the general philosophy of the treatment center. This is equally true for all other therapies that operate within the milieu.

The multiple roles and relationships of the social workers activate enactments and reenactments by the family so that both current and past family predicaments manifest themselves in the therapeutic situation. In identifying these occurrences and demonstrating them to the family members, the therapist can help to control compulsive repetitions. Multiple roles, however, may also render the therapist more vulnerable in various ways. Since every role has its own appropriate arena for action, the therapist may sometimes play the right role in the wrong setting, or vice versa. The manager's role may clash with the mediator's role and both with the family therapist's role, generating perplexity and incoherence. The family, in turn, must learn to respond appropriately to the different "hats" worn by the social worker.

The theory of containment can be well applied to family work. The family therapist must hold, contain, and understand the intense feelings of hatred, despair, and sadness that inundate the interactions of parents and their adolescent children without retaliating, abandoning, neglecting, or avoiding responses. However, to contain is not enough; one must also be attuned to, identify with, and understand what is occuring within the family group. When parents observe the rage and demandingness with which the adolescent approaches the family therapist, they can come to realize how understanding comes from direct experience and empathize with that. It is a challenge to the family therapist, functioning as a container, to identify and to deal with the primitive mechanisms of splitting, projective identification, and denial that press for containment.

Family therapy in a long-term, adolescent psychiatric hospital requires an understanding of the phases of inpatient treatment in their interaction with family functioning. To understand the vicissitudes in these parallel processes, the therapist to the family needs a theory to work with that is in keeping with the theoretical orientation of the hospital—psychoanalytic object relations theory. It captures and conceptualizes both the interpersonal and intrapsychic elements and helps account for both manifest and latent aspects of parent-child interactions, the core self of each family member, and the representations they have of one another.

Crucial to this type of family work as carried out at Chestnut Lodge are theories of understanding the phases of hospital treatment for severely disturbed adolescents (Rinsley 1980); projective identification (Klein 1964), as elaborated and refined by Boszormenyi-Nagy (1965), Fairbairn (1952), and Framo (1970); concepts of environmental holding and facilitating, mirroring, recognition of true and false selves, object usage and the failure to retaliate in the face of object usage, and the emergence of quiet space (Winnicott 1965); the understanding of family defenses, fantasies, and assumptions, the uncovering of repressed needs and fantasies in family treatment, and delineations describing parental verbal and nonverbal behaviors that convey to the children how the parents see them and that are based not on what the children are like realistically but on the defensive needs of the parents (Shapiro 1979); the importance of engaging the fathers to help in the resolution of pathological mother-child relationships (Abelin 1975; Balint 1968); and the preparation of the family for the patient's return home (Anderson, Riess, and Hogarty 1986).

In the first case to be described, one could observe from the early stages of treatment the symbiotic attachment between the mother and her hospitalized daughter, the isolation and disengagement of the father, and the patient's lack of any differentiated identity and sense of self. Mother's capacity to differentiate the others was limited; she saw her daughter as "beautiful and sweet" and father as the "bad guy."

The therapist's initial strategy with the family was to engage the parents in a secure relationship while their daughter began to attach herself to her individual therapist and to others in her unit. The therapist's next task was to persuade both parents how important the father's involvement with the family was to the family and to the daughter's recovery. Once this had been accomplished, the therapist could begin to identify and reveal to the parents their strengths and disordered interactions at a pace and in a manner that would be in tune with what they were already aware of preconsciously. The parents had to be helped to come to terms with their own internal selves so as to make them aware of their unconscious efforts to perpetuate old conflicts. Mother especially would have to identify her anxiety over separating from her daughter, contain it, and become aware of the projective identifications that were interfering with the daughter's emergence as her own person. The unconscious assumptions of all three family members required uncovering in the relationship with the therapist.

Case Illustration 1[1]

Julia was thirteen when she was admitted to the adolescent and child division of Chestnut Lodge with the diagnoses of schizophreniform psychosis in remission or major depressive disorder and borderline personality disorder. She revealed that she had auditory command hallucinations, the gift of clairvoyance, and a concern about being poisoned. Her illness had started about eighteen months earlier, when she was eleven. The recommendation for long-term hospitalization came after six months of short-term hospitalization as her thought disorder, suicidal preoccupation, and vulnerability persisted. The patient and her parents agreed to discontinue her medication when she was admitted to Chestnut Lodge in order to evaluate her condition and her responsiveness to the new treatment environment.

The parents were from an upper-middle-class background and lived in an upper-middle-class neighborhood. Both had college degrees. Father lived in another town Monday through Friday and commuted home on weekends. There were two other children, a girl and a boy, two and four years older than Julia, respectively.

Julia was not a planned child, but was welcomed by mother, although not by father. She was born, said mother, "healthy, gorgeous, and dainty as a doll." Her mother had a considerable investment in Julia's beauty from the beginning. "If there is anything that I have done to make Julia neurotic, it is to be too interested in her beauty." The maternal grandmother was described by the mother as "beautiful, I adored her," until mother realized that her mother had no interest in her feelings but only in her being good, nice, pretty, and successful. Her father was concerned perfectionistically with high standards and preoccupied with hypochondriacal concerns. Julia's maternal grandmother was also taken with her daugher's prettiness and spent many hours beautifying her. The paternal grandfather was "a workaholic, not a communicator, and never played with the children." He remained remote from his family, and, not surprisingly, Julia's father reported being lonely and friendless as a child. Julia's parents' marriage was never a success. Mother was unhappy with it and experienced great loneliness. Father was less critical about the relationship but recognized his wife's need for closeness and his own wish to withdraw and avoid any stress or conflict. With the help of alcohol, exercise, and a commuter existence he managed to keep his distance, yet his wife saw in him the wish to be mothered and to control. He was filled with anxieties that hindered him from offering his wife any support. With her background of emotional deprivation, mother tried hard to be interested in Julia's feelings but instead often projected all her own anxieties and needs onto this very accepting child. When Julia was first hospitalized, mother went weekly for individual treatment with a psychoanalyst.

THE TREATMENT OF THE FAMILY

During the two and a half years of Julia's hospitalization, mother was seen individually by the family therapist once weekly. Mother and father were seen jointly in therapy biweekly for thirteen months until father moved away and then jointly about once every six to eight weeks. There were also biweekly telephone sessions with father and the family therapist and then weekly phone sessions when he moved to the Midwest. After the first six weeks of hospitalization, Julia joined the parents for their sessions except during her one period of psychotic regression. There were also joint phone sessions with Julia and her father when he moved away. The family therapist also met with Julia individually when this was clinically indicated to deal with family issues and to keep in touch with the patient's feelings. The two siblings joined the family sessions on six occasions. After mother moved to the Midwest to be with father (about three months before Julia's discharge), she came back twice for family therapy sessions and had a telephone session once a week.

THE FIRST PHASE OF FAMILY TREATMENT
(SEPARATION, RESISTANCE, THERAPEUTIC ENGAGEMENT)

The six-week separation of parents and patient (except for a weekly phone call) was used to orient the parents to the therapist, to obtain an in-depth history of the family, and at the same time to allow Julia to begin attaching herself to her individual therapist and the unit staff.

In the individual sessions, mother could be pressuring and demanding, then compliant, clinging, dependent, and idealizing, all the while defending against the considerable anxiety and hostility with which she was still not in touch. The lack of information about Julia's illness was to a large extent based on mother's denial and avoidance. When mother spoke of reincarnation, clairvoyance, vitamin deficiencies, and chemical imbalances, the therapist listened without comment because her opinion was not being elicited and because mother needed to be heard. Mother wanted details of Julia's weight, menses, bowel movements, and eating patterns, conveying an intrusive and obsessively controlling interest in her daughter's body. She accepted the therapist's understanding that these concerns had to do with her worry about separation from Julia and about whether she was being taken care of properly. It was also related to her feelings of guilty responsibility for Julia's problems and her helplessness in dealing with them and yet at the same time to a wish to be able to control them. The therapist acknowledged how difficult it was for mother to hand over her child to others for them to do for the child what she could not do. This was the anxiety underlying mother's questions that she needed to understand. At this point, it became increasingly clear to the therapist, by virtue of the feelings that the mother was evoking in her, that Julia may well have been engulfed by the flood of mother's anxieties and projections.

Mother began to ask the therapist for advice as to what to do and what not to do to affect Julia's treatment positively. The spate of questions presented an interesting appeal to the therapist's narcissism: what did she want the mother to be? The therapist bore in mind that being good and successful had been what mother's mother valued most and that this had set a standard toward which mother constantly strove. Sensing the inquisitiveness behind the questioning, the therapist commented on mother's curiosity. Mother then revealed that her mother had considered it impolite to ask questions and so in childhood her curiosity could not be indulged. The therapist reflected that there was much to be curious about regarding the way that treatment worked at the hospital, particularly Julia's treatment and mother's ideas and feelings about it. This position permitted mother's questions to come, and sometimes the therapist would answer, sometimes the therapist and mother would look for the answers together, and sometimes the therapist would expect mother to look inside herself and find the answers there. At times, when the questions were unanswered, the mother would be reminded of her mother, and, in the context of transference, the answer would accrue a new level of significance and depth.

In this first phase of treatment, the therapist also worked to engage the father, and then the couple, on the issues of the marital relationship. Father, at first, committed himself to attending sessions only once a month, and the therapist would spend two hours in session with him and then two hours with him and his wife. He was quite agreeable to work with, but there was a puzzling absence of distress and involvement on his part as to what was happening to Julia. The therapist felt in herself the urge to drag information out of him. In an individual session, father shared the thought that commuting home on weekends served to cut down on the stress in the marriage. As the therapist carefully explored this, he said, "I don't like talking about myself," but nonetheless proceeded to do so. In phone sessions with him, the therapist pointed out how important he and his ideas were in helping both Julia and her mother, and she reminded him that his own father had been so remote that perhaps he had had no model of helpfulness to identify with. Furthermore, the constant arguments between his parents had left him without any knowledge of how marital partners could resolve their differences. Julia's mother had reported to the therapist that her husband did not like women therapists, so the mother was understandably shocked when he asked to be seen every other week.

One of the issues to be dealt with in therapy with father was a crisis at work involving a possible job change in addition to a relocation. That situation generated the anxious conflict between his own needs and the family's needs to have him around. In the past, father had upset them by these relocations. As we examined the conflict in therapy, he felt himself drawn into the family work as an aid to himself. The conflict was too deep and too longstanding to be easily or quickly resolved, and all the subsequent family work was periodically haunted by this specter of father's job dilemma and by mother's parallel dilemma between following him and staying near to Julia. The patient's needs were always in danger of being caught in the middle of this conflict. It was decided not to tell Julia about father's possible move until the middle phase of her treatment.

135

The marriage was characterized by distance and the fulfillment of traditional roles, with the husband devoted to earning a living and the wife to caring for the house, the children, and all the social arrangements. There was very little evidence of intimacy, of sharing concerns, of cherishing, or of respecting the other person. Mother expressed interest in closeness and mutuality and saw herself as the good and loving one and her husband as the bad guy who avoided and devalued her. The father, rational at times and at times remote, did have a sense of humor that he used to defend against direct and open communication and to cut through his wife's earnestness. Both parents feared conflict, anger, disappointment, and the intolerable pain of sadness, both their own and Julia's. Each parent was in need of comfort and help, but unable to comfort and help the other, and unable to bear the other's pain. Both had felt needy and unheard as children with parents whom they could recall idealizing. Mother felt needy and unheard now as well, helpless to control and direct her own life, and very much at the mercy of father's decisions to move. After three months of treatment, they both agreed that the marriage needed serious work. Father felt the necessity to become more responsive and less frightened by his wife's needs for a closer relationship and more support in handling the children. Mother felt that she should work on being less pressuring, less controlling, and less projecting of her anxieties and frustrations onto her husband. They seemed at times to be at two different poles, with the mother determined to have changes made, especially in the direction of becoming closer, and the father fearful of changes and closeness. This central issue was recognized by both.

The joint work with mother and Julia began six weeks after admission. The patient sat quiet, rigid, and withdrawn, wearing a masklike expression reminiscent of a puppet. She had no idea why she was in the hospital and why she was sitting in the office with the therapist and her mother. The therapist reminded Julia that she had been very unhappy since the seventh grade, so unhappy that she was finally unable to attend school. Asked if that was how she saw it, Julia nodded, and the therapist then said that they were all in the office together to get to know and understand the family and to discover ways of helping and understanding one another in the same sort of way that Julia was learning about herself in her individual therapy. It was obvious that the manner in which the mother and Julia interacted made it difficult for her to make choices or obtain some sense of herself. Mother would fill the void with talk, questions, answers, and guesses at Julia's feelings. The therapist spoke of what she was observing in the therapy sessions and suggested that a few statements of interest on mother's part coupled with a "quiet space" for Julia to respond would be what they needed now.

After each joint session, mother and therapist would process the time spent with Julia and deal with mother's sadness at having Julia remain so mute. Mother was pleased, however, to learn that Julia could be more spontaneous at times on her unit. The therapist stated that she understood how much mother wanted to be able to make her daughter happy and that together they would have to bear first this quiet period and then the sadness, anger, and even hateful feelings that would emerge as the patient got better.

Mother identified her need for a smothering closeness with Julia and asked her daughter if this was how she experienced it. Julia confirmed this but then began to vacillate in the joint sessions between three states—a distancing of herself, a compliant symbiosis, and an occasional venture into self-differentiation. Julia's attachment to her individual therapist, a woman, and to the unit staff had become much closer. When father joined the sessions, Julia, perhaps coincidently with the parents commitment to work as a couple on their relationship, asked mother to divorce her father so that she could live alone with her, indirectly expressing an alienation from him.

In one of the sessions at this time, Julia blurted out that "bullshit" had been going on in the family for years, with people not saying what they felt. The therapist agreed with her that both she and her parents had been afraid of strong feelings such as anger, disappointment, and sadness but that they were now all beginning to work on this. Mother was also able to validate what Julia had said and added that she herself planned to try and work on these issues with Julia's father. She would not divorce him but would continue to work on their problems in therapy. The therapist wondered to herself if the members of this family shared a common fear that, if certain feelings were expressed, something catastrophic would happen.

THE MIDDLE PHASE OF TREATMENT
(REGRESSION, DEPRESSION, AND WORKING THROUGH)

Julia entered a period of regression, lasting about one month, during which she became floridly psychotic and was stabilized on a low dose of trifluoperazine. During this time she did not attend the family sessions. The regression initiated the middle phase of treatment. During it, she was flooded with angry feelings, intensely erotic urges, wishes to merge with various members of the treatment team, and delusional ideas of being royalty. The therapist worked with the parents on their own issues and also shared with them some of the content of Julia's psychotic thinking, incorporating some psychoeducational work on how to understand what was happening to their daughter and how Julia's present condition affected the goals that they had set for her and the family. As Julia came out of the regression, she entered a bulimic phase in which she began to induce vomiting after eating in conjunction with an obsessive interest in counting calories and weighing foods, an effort on her part to establish control over herself. Her behavior toward the unit staff became increasingly demanding. It was as if she were asking her environment to react to and verify her existence.

When Julia finally stabilized, it was suggested to father (who now showed an active investment in being helpful) that he call his daughter weekly and write her occasional notes. He followed this recommendation faithfully. At the start, their talks were brief, but gradually, over a period of several months, Julia was able to engage in a lively outpouring of news and feelings with her father.

In the individual sessions with mother, an exploration about what lay behind her extraordinary emphasis on looks began. She would always make complimentary valuative comments about how pretty Julia looked at the expense of expressing interest in many other aspects of her daughter. Mother recognized that it was her way of greeting her child in an attempt to make her feel good and decided that she could just say that she was glad to see her or show it. She recalled her own growing up and the way in which her family constantly discussed and valued looks. She identified projections of her own needs and anxieties about attractiveness.

With the therapist's support, mother also began to desist from falsely reassuring Julia and thus denying the validity of her feelings. Initially, mother felt safer discussing these issues with the therapist alone, feeling narcissistically vulnerable, but subsequently she was able to work on them in sessions with Julia present. She brought in material about her other children who were also struggling, to a lesser degree, with issues of separation. It was clear that she overfunctioned with all the family members and was unable to absorb their tensions and anxieties. She would try to solve their problems rather than set limits that might incur their anger, feeling unable to live with the tension until a solution was reached. As mother made progress in understanding these dynamics and worked to contain her behavior, she became more depressed and cried frequently.

In the work with the couple, as mother and father started to share their differences, the therapist remarked that they each had characteristic ways of dealing with things and of seeing the other's way as bad. She wondered what good they saw in each other. Mother commented on father's humor and ability to stay calm, while father reflected on mother's attractiveness, her intense capacity to care, and her interest in many different things. With these positives in the forefront, the therapist wondered what prevented them from being able to resolve their conflicts. Father actively explored how avoidance and denial had become a pattern of defense for him. He described his powerful and overbearing mother, who toilet trained him far too early and who scrubbed him vigorously in nightly baths, and his father, who was so dominant. Father could see how much he missed out by not having a father who played with him or by not playing with peers. He accepted complete responsibility for his drinking and other past problematic behaviors. As time went on, he became increasingly self-revealing, and the couple were able to share memories of not listening to each other because it made them anxious or sad. The therapist linked this with what mother and Julia were currently working on.

The problem of father's relocation again tormented the parents and panicked the mother. She wondered whether she should move with her husband and take the children with her until their oldest daughter finished high school the following year, at which time the situation could be reevaluated. She decided to accompany her husband on a visit to the new location and to set up his apartment with him. With this separation imminent, both Julia and mother became highly anxious, the anxiety taking the form of concerns about the patient's health: her temperature and heart rate, her sore throats, and her fainting attacks. The mother began to bombard the unit staff with directives, and it was clear to the therapist that her state of mind needed to be contained. The therapist arranged a weekend session where mother angrily complained that the Lodge staff did not do what she wanted them to do. The therapist redirected the anger, pointing out that she was the real target for this ragefulness and that the better thing to do was to explore the way in which mother and daughter were infusing each other with hypochondriacal concerns rather than talking about their feelings about being separated. This interpretation at first drew some of the displaced anger from the mother, but she then remembered her father's hypochondriasis. The family tendency to worry about bodily health and functioning had originated with him and transmitted through her mother, thereby covering over other fears and feelings. In their following session, mother portrayed all this information as a "breakthrough." "I discovered that I could be very mad at you and that you could still like me."

In the family session with Julia and mother, the therapist brought up the fact that Julia developed physical problems whenever mother went away and wondered what thoughts Julia had about this. The patient spoke of two feelings that she had: being angry when her mother left and then feeling "kind of paranoid that I might get into trouble." Soon after this meeting, father made his decision to take the job, following which he reported to his wife a nightmare in which Julia was dead and in her grave, her ghost beckoning to him.

For the next three months, mother and the therapist struggled with the decision that now included mother's determination to stay and not move with father. The therapist pointed out the issues of overcontrol, the projection of blame, and the refusal to take responsibility for decisions. The parents became angry with the therapist when she insisted that it was within their power to shoulder their own responsibilities and collaborate with each other in the crucial months ahead. Both rose to the challenge and developed an elaborate travel schedule in which they would alternate visits with each other every four to six weeks after father moved. The therapist encouraged father to begin his own treatment after he moved, and he chose a minister in his new church who had been psychoanalyzed.

When Julia joined her parents in the sessions, and when the therapist went with her on a home visit, she noted that there were times when the patient let her parents treat her like a mindless and much younger child. When Julia was asked how she felt about this, she was able to recognize what was being talked about and mentioned several recent occasions when it had happened. The therapist then asked her how she would feel about letting her parents know when this was happening, adding that sometimes parents needed help with this because they had mixed feelings about children growing up and she was their youngest child. In the sessions with the parents, it was suggested that they look for cues that their daughter gave and that they might need to take the lead in this matter. At a subsequent family meeting, Julia turned angrily on the therapist when she wondered why Julia had asked her mother to pluck her eyebrows rather than do it for herself. This was the first occasion on which Julia was able to express her anger at the therapist, although, on the unit, she had become much more outspoken and assertive.

Mother, as in the past, was overdoing some of her reactions to Julia's progress. She greeted every sign of advance as the most wonderful thing in the world, once again not helping with her daughter's reality testing. Inevitably, her enthusiasm would reduce the patient to silence. When this was pointed out to mother, she agreed to stay alert to this behavior, realizing that her fear was that Julia would develop no sense of herself without mother's affirmation. In the joint session, Julia looked uncomfortable about what her mother said in this context, and the therapist then reminded her of how she herself had spoken of the years of "bullshit" in the family. The therapist shared with mother and daughter her knowledge that Julia was now able to tell people on the unit when she did not like something and that recently she had told the family therapist when she did not like something the therapist had said. Could Julia now begin to tell her mother this in the same way, and could mother bear it if she did? Mother responded with a willing yes.

On mother's return from a visit to father, Julia said to her, "You tried to make me the person you wanted me to be—not what I wanted to be—at other times all you wanted to do is please me—sometimes I like this." In a subsequent session, the patient was again able to become extremely angry with the therapist and to carry some of her feelings into a lengthy, very typical, heated adolescent daughter-mother debate about what was an appropriate bathing suit for Julia. The therapist acknowledged the patient's standing up for what was important to her as well as her mother's efforts to help her understand what was age appropriate. Julia then said to her mother, "I'm afraid if I get angry, I'll kill you."

Before the therapist went on her vacation, mother spoke to her of the hospital not taking adequate care of Julia, and the therapist wondered if mother felt this because the therapist would not be around to take care of her.

141

Prior to mother's next trip to visit father, Julia tried to pressure mother to allow Julia to go with her out of the hospital. The therapist told Julia that they had learned that she did not like her mother or her individual therapist to leave and asked if Julia could say something about this. Julia reported thinking that something would happen to her when her mother was gone, but would not say what. She sustained her anger with her mother for several days, calling her father and telling him, "You have a special place in my heart and I feel better when mother goes to be with you." Mother, herself, showed little anxiety before this departure, and, on her return, she told the therapist that she was beginning to think that she could let Julia have her feelings of anger and sadness without feeling the same or trying to fix them. As the parents dealt repetitively with departures, separations, and reunions, father began to regard Julia's treatment as an obstacle to his wife and children being with him. Sensing his frustration, the therapist kept him closely informed about Julia's progress, reiterated the important phase she was undergoing in her treatment, and stressed how crucial his support was at this time. The therapist said that she could understand how much he wanted to have his family all together now that he and his wife were feeling so much better about their marriage.

Mother then entered a period when she began to grieve actively over her daughter's illness and about not having the perfect child. In the phone calls and office sessions with father, the therapist worked on his learning to do with his wife what she had been learning to do with Julia, that is, to listen to the sadness, accept it, and try not to fix it. Mother told her husband that she felt he was really changing, and he admitted to having been very self-centered and insensitive to her and to taking out his work frustrations on her. As they continued to feel better about their relationship, the mother became increasingly interested in being with her husband. Every now and then, her need to deny Julia's complaints or engulf Julia's ideas with an inappropriate fervor resurrected itself, but we continued to work on this. Julia would now smile at her mother's excessive enthusiasms, and, when asked about this, she said that her mother was "pretty funny" sometimes when she got excited.

As mother became clearer about saying no to Julia, not needing to make her happy, Julia began to get increasingly angry. When she slapped a female staff member, the family therapist made the connection between this incident and her anger at her mother. In a mother-daughter session, Julia spoke of how she had been afraid of her mother in the past and afraid to show her anger, and she recalled that her mother had once slapped her. Mother, when meeting alone with the therapist, had a recollection of being afraid of Julia's strength and anger when she was only three years old and found herself unable to contain and modify the little girl's aggressive feelings. She had never felt that strength and anger in herself. The therapist suggested that she might have been cut off from her own expressions of anger and strength because she had felt that her parents expected her to be good and beautiful. The therapist also mentioned that she had experienced mother's anger and strength and knew them to exist. Mother said that she had never been afraid of her son.

The ambivalence about joining her husband still preoccupied mother. The therapist wondered whether mother was stuck on this problem and needed to work much more on her mixed feelings. There was a danger that Julia and her treatment might provide the everlasting excuse for not rejoining her husband. This made mother very angry, and she returned to the next session to say that she had been very troubled by what had been said and had worked with her individual therapist on this and would continue to do so. In time, she ruled out a divorce and made a decision to move to be with her husband when her other daughter graduated from school. Once again she would use a consultant to make the decision about Julia's treatment. The parents worked for several weeks on their thoughts and feelings about mother moving and leaving Julia in the hospital. Mother was very anxious about telling Julia about this and was irate with the father when he revealed it to Julia and then left town.

The administrative psychiatrist reviewed Julia's treatment and affirmed the need for the patient to continue to consolidate her gains and understand her problems further. Julia then asked mother if she could go with her when she moved. Mother replied that Julia's hospital treatment was not finished, that mother would visit her every four to six weeks, and that Julia could visit them until it was time for her to rejoin the family. Julia was angry and accused her mother, "You don't trust me, you don't have a mind of your own, you always do what the hospital says." Mother tearfully took a firm stand but conveyed that she understood that Julia would be upset and that it was a difficult decision to make.

When father joined the next session, he took responsibility for making the decision to move away and gave Julia permission to be angry at him. He wanted her to stay in the hospital until she was able to join them. Julia's siblings also attended the session and supported their father but then aligned themselves with Julia against the parental coalition of authority that had decided to keep her in the hospital. The older brother was attending college near the hospital and offered to visit or talk on the phone. Julia felt supported in her anger.

The next time that father left, mother became faint in the therapist's office, revealing that she was upset about leaving and was trying prematurely to terminate her individual therapy. The family therapist suggested that this was her way to avoid painful feelings about ending her work and that it was very important for her to return to her therapist and do the essential work of expressing and understanding these feelings. Mother then ventilated her anger at the administrative psychiatrist who was "too busy to give her precious time." The therapist reflected that time was indeed precious and that there was not much left. She explored with mother what this feeling about time was about, pointing out that, while the administrative psychiatrist's time was in fact precious, she was willing to give as much as the parents needed to help them at this time. Mother concluded that her anxiety about what was happening and her guilt about leaving Julia had fueled this angry outburst. She realized that she would need considerable support during the time she was leaving.

TERMINATION (LETTING GO)

Mother planned to move to be with her husband in four months, and there were about seven to eight months of inpatient treatment left for Julia.

In joint sessions with Julia and mother, the daughter showed an increasing separateness from mother, laughing at her idiosyncracies, seeing her more realistically, and trying "to get her goat"—all very early to middle adolescent ways of dealing with psychological separation from mother. Julia was now also able to share ideas, feelings, opinions, and analyses of people and experiences. She began to talk directly about what she felt like when she was psychotic, describing it as though she had mastered and understood the experience.

As mother planned her next trip to visit father, planning was begun for Julia to have her first trip with mother to the new home. The parents were given the name of a psychiatrist in a day-treatment program for

Julia to consult when she went out for the visit. The parents were also alerted to Julia possibly acting out during this time because of mother's impending departure and Julia's own mixed feelings about being left behind. Julia had been talking with the unit staff about staying and getting more help for herself. The parents were surprised to learn from her that there was a part of her that did not feel ready to leave treatment and would have a difficult time leaving the Lodge.

Through a combination of individual sessions with mother until she moved and family sessions with father every six weeks, a review of the family therapy work and an outline of the areas of particular importance in "saying goodbye" began. An attempt was made to understand what atmosphere in the household would enable the patient to maintain her gains when she returned home to live with her parents. Julia was tearful in sessions about leaving, as was mother in individual sessions. Mother expressed anxiety about the psychiatrist who would be doing the family work. "He seems so serious," she said, and that prompted a reminiscence by the therapist and mother about how anxious she had felt about trusting the present family therapist initially. Father admitted that he felt anxious also about being in family therapy with someone new and that he never thought about the work as therapy but "just sessions with you."

Mother called just before she was to leave for the visit. She said that she felt "stung" by the therapist in the last session (but had been unable to mention it in the session) when the suggestion had been made that she could handle something in another way. She had felt very angry and had never wanted to come back because the therapist was so insensitive. This had been a session in which Julia had made fun of her mother and revealed things that she and her siblings had gotten away with in mother's absence. Mother had turned to the therapist to ask her opinion about something and, rather than ask mother her ideas about it, the therapist had answered. The therapist then told mother that she was glad that she had called and that what had happened in the session had made mother feel like a bad parent and that what had transpired was not good for mother, especially at a time when she was gathering confidence in herself in preparation for leaving her treatment here. Mother experienced relief and said that she would be coming back for sessions after her trip. While she was away, she became overwhelmed and called on the therapist to get support and understanding about all that lay ahead of her in moving, getting used to living with her husband again, and making a place for Julia. On her return, she reminisced about difficult sessions in the therapy and moments when she had been very angry with the therapist.

When the family met next, they wanted permission from the family therapist and the administrative psychiatrist for Julia to leave the hospital soon. Instead, a strong recommendation was made for her to continue in her treatment. The school system funding the educational program had done their own psychological testing and had recommended continued treatment. A discussion ensued about how it would not be long before Julia would be joining them, that this was a very crucial time for her to deal with her feelings about ending her treatment, and that endings are often painful and hard to bear. Parents agreed to support her continuing in treatment for a while longer before terminating. Mother had begun her own therapy with an analyst in the new town, and the couple had established the treatment program that Julia and the family would begin when she was discharged from the hospital in four months.

When the parents terminated the family therapy, they had reinternalized much of their own formally projected neediness, showing a potential for empathic understanding of each other and a higher threshold for difference of opinion. A month after discharge, mother sent a letter and multipage summary of notes she had taken for herself after some of the sessions. The following is a quotation from mother's notes:

> I learned to allow Julia to feel what she is feeling, step out of our space, give her the faith that she can experience the feeling and get through it. I allowed her to talk about her feelings, express them into tears if she wished, and see that she could get through the sadness and be okay again. The last time this happened, we had dropped her sister off to go to a party. She said how sad she felt to miss out on being a normal teenager and going to parties like her sister and her friends. I sat with her while she cried. I acknowledged her feelings without fear that I would not be able to handle those tears and deep feelings of hers or that I would feel the same deep feelings and not be able to handle my own. . . . It was a momentous occasion.

This case illustration provides a vivid picture of the intensive and dynamic family treatment provided by Chestnut Lodge. Rinsley's three phases of treatment have been more or less validated by Goodrich (1987) and Masterson (1972), and this presentation bears out the characteristics of the three phases. The family pathology is clearly delineated, and the therapist steers her way carefully and cautiously through a clinical mine field within which, at times, inordinate detection mechanisms are required. The parents came to learn empathically from their therapist how to handle each other, their family, and their sick daughter in ways that left them comfortable and communicative.

The two other clinical illustrations will be brief and will address specific therapeutic issues that therapists working with the family in everyday life can encounter.

Case Illustration 2[2]

The interdisciplinary, psychoanalytically oriented, long-term treatment approach is unique and special in what it endeavors to accomplish with adolescents and their families. The overall therapeutic experience certainly exceeds the sum of the separate therapeutic parts, and there is a synergistic interplay between the different members of the treatment team that lies at the heart of what happens in the total effort. Integrating the various therapies and making the families not only conscious of all that is being done on their behalf but also aware of the processes involved are challenging tasks for the family therapist. Chestnut Lodge has endeavored to create an environment insulated from the pressures and demands for magical, superficial, and immediate cure. There is a vital recognition that meaningful and lasting change and growth take both time and patience. This attitude provides the foundation for the containing and holding environment that is a critical aspect of the Lodge experience. In this safe environment, adolescents can play out and work through the many and serious conflicts that have impeded their growth and development prior to admission.

The highly disturbed families being treated in this setting have often had many unsuccessful and frustrating encounters with therapists and therapeutic centers and consequently arrive loaded with mistrust, hopelessness, and resentment. Faced with a new therapeutic alliance, they are understandably guarded and somewhat skeptical. The therapist who treats these families, therefore, has to be prepared for massive resistances that seem tailor-made for failure. The major strength of the approach lies in the capacity of the sustaining environment to provide a highly individualized and flexible range of treatments geared to the needs and circumstances of each adolescent and his family. Both strengths and weaknesses of the family group are incorporated into the treatment process. There are, however, some family situations that do not belong to the mainstream of admissions, and, in such cases, the therapeutic flexibility becomes critical.

Vincent, a fourteen-year-old boy, was admitted to the Lodge after three unsuccessful hospitalizations, characterized by threatening and assaultive behavior toward staff, self-destructiveness that included mutilation, and frequent AWOLs. The family situation was unique in that neither mother nor father were immediately available to participate in the treatment. Vincent was the oldest of two children and the only son of divorced parents. He had been living in New York with his father under primitive circumstances that included Vincent's being sexually abused by his father. His life was without structure or supervision, and he drifted inevitably toward alcohol and drugs and toward becoming increasingly out of control. The paternal grandparents had been approached several times to assume responsibility for Vincent, but, being in their sixties, they were hesitant to do so. However, after a brief visit, during which they witnessed what they considered to be life-threatening conditions, they felt compelled to intervene. After much soul searching and ambivalence, they decided to bring Vincent home with them and to assume legal custody. They had not anticipated the extent of the disturbance to which they would then be exposed. Vincent moved in with his grandparents and was enrolled in the local public school system. His unsocialized, primitive, and aggressive behavior led to a rapid deterioration, both at home and at school. His grandparents rapidly realized that they did not have the resources to contain or to cope with Vincent's overwhelming needs, for which the only answer appeared to be hospital treatment. In each of the three hospitalizations previous to Chestnut Lodge, there was a failure in containment. Vincent was admitted to the Lodge with a disorder of conduct, substance abuse, a borderline personality disorder, and a diagnosis of seizure disorder from the history.

Vincent was estranged from both parents. His mother was living in Ohio with her daughter and harbored a great deal of resentment toward her son, who she felt was responsible for much of her unhappiness. His father was living in New York under marginal circumstances and was essentially unavailable. It seemed that the grandparents not only were the most constant and reliable figures in his life but also the only parental figures open to participate directly in his treatment. A family treatment plan was developed that included establishing and maintaining contact with the mother and father, but the major focus lay in involving Vincent and his grandparents in family therapy.

His first year in the hospital proved to be extraordinarily trying for staff as well as for patients as Vincent tested the capacity of the milieu to contain him while he engaged unrelentingly in acting out that included fire setting, self-mutilation, AWOL, and explosive verbal abuse. The abuse frequently spilled over into the family sessions with the grandparents and necessitated containment and limit setting. A psychoeducational approach was used to guide the grandparents through this extremely difficult phase and to help them understand the defensive underpinnings of much of his behavior. Vincent gradually began to feel safer and more trusting of the therapeutic environment and, after the first year, began to move slowly into the second phase of treatment. His acting out diminished, and he became more reflective and available to engage in the therapeutic effort.

Vincent began to explore and to challenge the parameters of his relationship with his grandparents, initially rejecting their authority and role as surrogate parents. He sought a reconciliation with his mother and began actively to reach out to her. Eventually, she came for a brief visit, and Vincent used the family session to work through a great deal of unfinished business with her. As a result, his relationship with the grandparents improved, and they began to spend increasing amounts of positive time together outside the family sessions. These also began to take on a different flavor as Vincent's curiosity developed and he found a need to sort out and understand his past. At this point, the grandparents became a valuable source of information and provided him with an unusual perspective that he appeared to find fascinating. This initial improvement gives support to the views of others who have found the positive benefits of involving grandparents in family therapy (Ingersoll-Dayton, Arndt, and Stevens 1988).

In everyday life, grandparents are used by their children and grandchildren in a wide variety of ways, and vice versa. What Anthony and Benedek (1970) have referred to as "the last phase of parenthood" could be experienced as a nonambivalent and gratifying experience but is more often a "mixed blessing" and sometimes an emotional catastrophe. On the manifest level, grandparents can be regarded as experienced advisers and readily available baby-sitters or, more negatively, as meddlers, manipulators, and spoilers. Grandparenting may be regarded as a "new lease on life" or "parenthood once removed" without the daily hassles of parenting, but, in darker ways, it may become an emotional nightmare with a reactivation and reenactment of the deeper parental conflicts of the past. This is especially likely to occur when there is intergenerational pathology running through the family. Psychodynamically, this is best understood in terms of the "depressive constellation" in which the core of ambivalence is transmitted, relatively unchanged, from grandmother to mother to child. In certain situations, where there has been a total failure of parenting, the grandparents may be called on to undertake active parenting. They may welcome this, from unresolved feelings of guilt, and as a means of repairing their own bad efforts at previous parenting that resulted in the parental failure of their children. The move from grandparenthood back to parenthood is not without its load of trepidation, often requiring extensive reshuffling of stabilized lives. The transformation is by no means easy and evokes agonizing reappraisals. The generational gap may seem alarming in its extent. However, the process of reparation may render retreat impossible: they are making up for themselves, their children, and now their grandchildren. The children may feel that they are not "the parents we knew" because the grandparenthood is now infused with nuclear conflicts belonging to a different time and, therefore, somewhat anachronistic. Deeply buried memories from their childhood and from their parental experience may resurface and act as disturbing interpretations to current anxieties.

In the case of Vincent, a number of important insights emerged in one dramatic session when the boy complained to his grandparents about how he was feeling abused by a peer on the unit. This led to a discussion about his abuse at the hands of his father, the son of the grandparents. At one point, Vincent described a very sadistic game that his father used to play with him in which the father would pin him down and then dangle a strand of saliva over his face until he pleaded for mercy. On one occasion, father actually let go of the saliva, and it landed on his face. The grandfather was shocked and very upset to hear this story. He related his own experience with his son, Vincent's father, and recalled how he used to play the very same game with him, which actually originated in his own childhood. He had lived in a tough, rural area and remembered his peers pinning him down and doing the same horrible thing to him. The disclosure led to an intensification of interchanges between Vincent and his grandparents. The boy was anxious to learn about the past in a effort to make more meaningful sense of his own experience and history. The grandparents offered a good deal of information and insight into their son's development and subsequent problems in adulthood, and Vincent came to understand something more about the relationship between his parents and their divorce. A similar process ensued around his sense of guilt and badness for the sexual abuse with the father. Once again, the grandparents were supportive and helped him recognize that father, as an adult, was solely responsible for what happened.

The patient continued to work through feelings regarding both his parents in subsequent family sessions with the grandparents. He came to one session following a very upsetting phone call from his father and proceeded to give vent to his feelings of rage and hatred. This opened up a very productive dialogue between Vincent and his grandmother, who talked about her own experience with a disappointing and abusive father and her own efforts to cope with and resolve not only her painful feelings but also a chronically problematic relationship that continued into her adult life.

Although infrequent and somewhat tenuous contact was maintained with both parents throughout the course of treatment, the primary focus of the family therapy was on the development and strengthening of the relationship between Vincent and his grandparents. They had become the most constant and reliable objects in his life in terms of both present and future. While some reparative work was accomplished with the mother, a great deal of working through was achieved in the transference that developed with the grandparents. There were limits, however, on the extent to which the grandparents were available as transference objects. Grandmother, in particular, had a difficult time tolerating Vincent's expressions of rage that would surface frequently in family sessions. Her own experience of growing up with an out-of-control alcoholic father caused her to become extremely anxious in the face of Vincent's anger. Eventually, she was able to address this directly with the patient, who accepted that his feelings of rage, while understandable, would have to be worked out in his individual treatment.

The family work in this case predominantly involved the grandparents, although at different times efforts were made to include all the "significant others." For instance, while father never came for a session, there were several conference calls that attempted to address more directly some of Vincent's experiences with him. At one point, Vincent was motivated to set up a meeting with his father but became so anxious that it was postponed. In the past, he had been very jealous of the sibling who had stayed with mother. With the grandparents' support and encouragement, he was eventually able to establish a much closer and less conflicted attachment to her.

This case is presented as an illustration of the unusual family configurations that present themselves to family therapists at the Lodge and the flexibility with which these variations are handled. As in all therapeutic endeavors, it is often the difficult cases from which one learns the most.

Case Illustration 3[3]

As a newcomer to a long-term milieu, this particular therapist was able to bring a fresh viewpoint to the Chestnut Lodge experience. In her previous experience with short-term units, she had been struck by the constant crises, violent interactions, and upheavals. In her initial stage at Chestnut Lodge, she was most impressed by its relative serenity. As compared with former experiences, there was surprisingly little acting out, although, of course, suicidal gestures, fights, and running away did occur from time to time. Occasionally, it reminded her of a boarding school rather than a psychiatric hospital. From this first year's experience, it seemed to her that the strength of Chestnut Lodge lay in its capacity to contain the turbulences of disturbed adolescents without allowing them to go out of control. The competent, well-trained, and experienced staff seemed able to provide a nurturing and stable environment that gave the patients an opportunity to understand and master their anxieties. As she saw it, the crucial element was one of containment, a concept built on from Bion's (1967) work. Containment is the mother's capacity to take in the child's projections through the process of reverie and to accept the projections, thus conveying to the child that they are tolerable. This led the therapist to examine this process from the point of view of the therapist working with the family (a point of view elucidated by Box, Copley, Magagna, and Moustaki [1981] and Scharff and Scharff [1987]).

The Lodge provided the professional skills needed for containment of these adolescents who had been admitted because their families had failed to contain them. The contained thoughts and feelings were too powerful for the capacities of the container (Bion 1967), and a new container was needed. This was provided by institutional life with its greater resources, of which family therapy was one part. The family therapist was there to provide a particular experience of the process of containment. Scharff and Scharff (1987) have suggested that the therapist must create a space in which the family anxieties can be held while the family members tolerate looking at these fears and anxieties and learning about them. In this space, these anxieties have a place to reside while being examined and understood by the family members. These anxieties stem from suppressed rages that can now be uncovered and traced to their origins since the therapist is not afraid of them as the family members are and can help them understand and eventually modulate the rage.

It would appear that these families at Chestnut Lodge were lacking in their containment function and that the breakdown of this was what led to the hospitalization of their children. The goal of treatment could then be defined as an effort to strengthen this important familial function and to allow the families to hold their members at home. In short, the family therapist would, first, create a therapeutic space that would permit the families to experience their anxieties, understand them, and master them and, second, model the containing process and thus help the families strengthen their own containment functioning.

In the case of an eighteen-year-old girl admitted because of severe alcohol abuse and self-destructive acting out, not only was the family's containment capacity markedly deficient, but, in their first attempt at family therapy at Chestnut Lodge, engagement had failed around the issue of tolerating deviant behavior in an effort first to understand it and then to curb it. The parents had felt that Chestnut Lodge was not setting strong enough limits on their daughter's acting out and considered the therapist's handling of the situation as reflecting this. Before adequate containment could be developed, the parents, after a highly volatile session, walked out and refused to continue contact with the Lodge, although leaving their child to its care.

The treatment team accepted this setback as one of the inevitable hazards with such "noncontaining" families and appointed a different family therapist to undertake the delicate process of engaging this

153

disengaged and disenchanted family. The rest of the therapeutic milieu had continued its work so that Carol's alcohol problem had improved and she was no longer acting out as recklessly as before. Because of this, the parents relented and once again became available for family work.

The parents felt that their daughter could be helped only by extremely coercive and punitive action, although such measures had failed in their own management of her. They were skeptical of the leniency and kindness meted out to Carol and the consistent search to understand her better. Although their methods had failed, they wanted them applied. They remained convinced that Carol performed as expected when things were made difficult for her. They were aware of her passivity, her fearfulness, her self-hatred, and her inordinate self-doubts, but they could not connect these with their approach to her. When overwhelmed with these negative self-feelings, Carol would turn to alcohol to block out the pain. It was clear that in this behavior lay the road to eventual alcoholism.

The mother had grown up with a kind, weak, and somewhat masochistic mother, who was dominated and abused by a tyrannical, "always right" husband. Carol's mother identified strongly with her father's domineering rightfulness while rejecting her mother's weakness and vulnerability, presenting to the world an apparently tough, invincible exterior overlying her vulnerabilities.

The issue at stake was whether this mother could allow this eighteen-year-old daughter to separate from her, to have her own ideas and thoughts, and to make mistakes without being attacked severely for them. It was becoming increasingly apparent that mother, fearful of her own underlying weakness and vulnerability, was projecting these aspects of herself onto her daughter in order to control them and keep them out of her own self-awareness. Mother remained strong, self-controlled, and controlling while her daughter acted out her weakness and vulnerability. Having a scapegoat, mother was quite blind to her own acting out, such as more than social drinking.

The crucial question for the therapist was whether mother and her ally, the father, could be refocused to take a look at their own weaknesses and inadequacies and become more empathic with their daughter. Could the parents allow all these disturbing feelings to enter the therapeutic space and still allow the generation of a climate of containment? Would they be able to refrain from escalating every minor breech of rules through scathing criticism? Could they learn to talk out issues before exploding with rage? These were the containment problems that the therapist began to work with.

During the first few sessions, the parents expressed their concern about Carol's previous acting out and lectured her on the behaviors that they expected when she returned home. The patient said very little in response, trying hard to conform. In the third session, mother began an attack on Carol about her clothing, and the patient began to cry and ran out of the room. Rather than allowing the session to end at this point, as had occurred during the previous period of treatment, the therapist went out and brought Carol back into the office. She then told the family that this type of interaction had not worked for them in the past and had only led inevitably to Carol drowning her sorrows in alcohol. If they wanted to live together successfully, they needed to find new ways of dealing with their anger. In a recognizably maternal transference reaction, mother counterattacked with criticisms of the therapist's kindness and sensitivity to her daughter and predicted that this was doomed to failure. "She will only trick you or pay no attention at all!" The therapist said that she dealt with Carol the way she felt about Carol, not angry and critical, but wishful to help and to understand. It apparently became clear to mother that this statement held no pretense, no maneuvering, and no reaction to inner hostility. Her realization of this brought about some internal change that allowed her to respond more empathically to her daughter and, more important, to continue in treatment and share her own feelings of helplessness as to how to deal with the problematic relationship with her husband. For the first time, after a fight with her husband, her vulnerability was laid bare in the therapeutic space, unrepressed and available for work, with the growing confidence that the feelings involved could be contained. From this point on, the sessions became rewardingly productive, and mother's projections onto Carol were much reduced.

Conclusions

What has been described in careful detail is one important element in the long-term treatment of families with a hospitalized adolescent and the complexity of the processes involved. Unlike the usual therapist, the family therapist wears different "hats" associated with managing, mediating, and treating psychotherapeutically, integrating all these roles into a consistently helpful approach and coordinating it with the other therapies at work in the milieu. Notions of holding and containment, of transference and countertransference, of facilitating and reflecting, of family defenses, assumptions, fantasies, and needs—conscious and unconscious—and of therapeutic flexibility govern the practice of family therapy and weave it into the general philosophy of treatment prevalent in institutions, in itself no mean task. It is by no means easy to interpret deeply into the dynamic life of a family and also engage with them in a managerial discussion of allowances, jobs, and educational courses. "Ships and stars and sealing wax, and cabbages and kings!" Nothing lies outside the range of these skillful ombudsmen and therapists to the family.

NOTES

1. The therapist was Sandra Boots.
2. The therapist was David Goodman.
3. The therapist was Susan Loughman.

REFERENCES

Abelin, L. 1975. Some further observations and comments on the earliest role of the father. *International Journal of Psycho-Analysis* 56:293–301.
Anderson, C. M.; Reiss, D.; and Hogarty, G. 1986. *Schizophrenia and the Family*. New York: Guilford.
Anthony, E. J., and Benedek, T. 1970. *Parenthood*. Boston: Little, Brown.
Balint, M. 1968. *The Basic Fault (Therapeutic Aspects of Repression)*. London: Tavistock.
Bion, W. R. 1967. *Second Thoughts*. London: Heinemann.
Boszormenyi-Nagy, I. 1965. A theory of relationships, experience and transactions. In I. Boszormenyi-Nagy and J. L. Framo, eds. *Intensive Family Therapy*. New York: Hoeber.
Box, S.; Copley, B.; Magagna, J.; and Moustaki, E. 1981. *Psychotherapy with Families: An Analytic Approach*. London: Routledge & Kegan Paul.
Fairbairn, W. R. D. 1952. *An Object Relations Theory of the Personality*. New York: Basic.

Framo, J. L. 1970. Symptoms from a family transactional viewpoint. *International Psychiatry Clinics* 7(4): 125–171.

Goodrich, W. 1987. Long-term psychoanalytic treatment of adolescents. *Psychiatric Clinics of North America* 10(2): 273–287.

Ingersoll-Dayton, B.; Arndt, B.; and Stevens, D. 1988. Involving grandparents in family therapy. *Social Casework* 69:280–289.

Klein, M. 1964. *Contributions to Psychoanalysis*. New York: McGraw-Hill.

Klein, M. 1975. *Envy and Gratitude and Other Works*. New York: DelaCorte.

Masterson, J. F. 1972. *Treatment of the Borderline Adolescent: A Developmental Approach*. New York: Wiley.

Rinsley, D. B. 1980. *Treatment of the Severely Disturbed Adolescent*. New York: Aronson.

Scharff, D., and Scharff, J. 1987. *Object Relations Family Therapy*. New Jersey: Aronson.

Shapiro, R. L. 1979. Family dynamics and object-relations theory: an analytic, group-interpretive approach to family therapy. *Adolescent Psychiatry* 7:118–135.

Winnicott, D. W. 1965. *The Maturational Processes and the Facilitating Environment: Studies in the Theory of Emotional Development*. New York: International Universities Press.

10 LONG-TERM GROUP PSYCHOTHERAPY WITH ADOLESCENT INPATIENTS

DENISE FORT, LAURICE MC AFEE, ROBERT KING, WILLIAM HOPPE,
WAYNE FENTON, JUDITH ABRAMOWITZ, CAMILLE WOODBURY,
AND E. JAMES ANTHONY

The approach to groups in the adolescent and child division is psychoanalytically oriented, not only because this is in keeping with the other therapies at work on the campus, but also because the group supervisor derives his understanding from the work of British psychoanalysts who have specialized in group treatment (Bion 1977; Foulkes and Anthony 1984) as well as psychoanalysts from Britain whose work has a significance for group psychotherapy but who themselves have not been group psychotherapists (Bowlby 1977; Milner 1971; Winnicott 1958). To overcome this transatlantic prejudice, it should be noted that some of the members of the group seminar are more aligned with Yalom's (1983) model of inpatient group psychotherapy, which is more in accord with the interpersonal emphasis of Sullivan's influence on Chestnut Lodge. However, the so-called here-and-now interactions have a place, but not an exclusive one, in other group analytic models (Foulkes and Anthony 1984). Furthermore, feedback has been used by other group therapists who would, however, want to do more for the inpatients than enabling them to identify their problems and become susceptible to the "talking" therapy while reducing the anxieties inherent in hospitalization. The group analytic approach keeps a therapeutic eye both on the individual patient and on the group while deploying the group dynamic and the group relationships in the service of treatment.

The picture of the group in action has been drawn from different sources, all of which help clarify our understanding of the group. We will deal with different aspects in succession. The adolescent therapy groups conducted at the Lodge school as part of the adolescent and child division treatment program are small (six to nine members), with a gradual shift in numbers of members over the years due to intermittent admissions and discharges. The groups are heterogeneous in composition, with a mixture of genders, diagnoses, and ages. There is a sprinkling of day patients who have moved from inpatient to outpatient status on the way to rejoining the outside world. Each group has two therapists, who are drawn from a pool of four psychiatrists, one psychologist, one social worker, and one teacher. As presently constituted, each group has a psychiatrist as a therapist. The groups meet once a week for fifty minutes in one of the school's classrooms so that the therapeutic space is strewn with the instruments of education that can be used resistantly. Cotherapists, together with the director of adolescent psychotherapy and the school principal, also meet weekly to discuss the ongoing therapeutic process in each of the groups. The treatment is referred to by the patients as "group," and it is difficult to tease out what they understand by it. Some have attended group sessions in short-term facilities prior to their admission to the Lodge and contrast, often very critically, those structured, programmatic, and well-disciplined proceedings with the seemingly chaotic process to which they are introduced here—which one patient referred to as "a Mad Hatter's party!" For another patient with group experience, it was "like stepping into a different world where anything goes!" What the patients bring to the group is "a bereft incohesive quality" (Shapiro, Zinner, Berkowitz, and Shapiro 1975, p. 87) that finds the fluidity disturbing, understanding it as an invitation to regression.

The Group Therapeutic Space

To treat severely disturbed adolescent inpatients who have a marked propensity for acting out in a group, a special sort of psychological space is needed to accommodate them. To do this effectively requires the use of a theoretical model that delimits an area with well-defined boundaries and within which a variety of therapeutic processes can be activated. Given a space designated for therapy, the urge is to enclose it. For this purpose, one can make use of the image of frames with the understanding that what is inside the frame has to be interpreted differently from what is outside (Milner 1971). Thus, the frame marks off an area within which what is perceived has to be understood symbolically and outside which what is perceived is taken literally. An extension of this theory shows the space as a stage onto which the internal dramas of the different group members are projected. The stage is at first empty and devoid of psychic content, but, as treatment progresses, it is gradually filled with the outpourings of the patients. The image of filling the space evokes the association of containment— the container or group helps to contain the thoughts and feelings of the group members as they are generated in the way that the female contains the male, the mother the infant, and the therapist the patient. The container-contained model can also be used to represent projective identifications that are rampant in this type of group, in which the primitively structured patients are unable to detoxify greedy, envious, and hostile projections that become through introjection a nameless dread.

The Content of the Group Therapeutic Space

Occupying the therapeutic space is a matrix or network of all the individuals' mental processes and the psychological medium in which they meet, communicate, and interact, somewhat similar to the network of fibers and cells that make up the brain (Foulkes and Anthony 1984). The members of the group participate in the formation and creation of the interactional matrix, at the same time reestablishing the conditions of the individual's primary network as experienced in early childhood that is the group equivalent of the transference neurosis. The group, possibly universally, represents the image of the mother—hence the term "matrix." Even in groups with severely disturbed individuals, the maternal function may be apparent.

In this type of mother group, there is a predominance of preoedipal phenomena, requiring maternal types of management for regressed patients. This is the notion of the "good enough" group, one that holds, facilitates, promotes, mirrors, and shares experiences. If therapists forget this and become embroiled in the hostile interchanges, the group is likely to feel let down and misunderstood, with nothing to hold on to except one another. The nuisance value of the borderline patient is often exploited by the patient to the extreme for the purpose of stirring up a therapeutic space. Winnicott (1958) describes this well when he says that the patient's negative activities represent an effort to make the environment alert to danger and to organize it to tolerate nuisance: "If the situation holds, the environment must be tested and retested in its capacity to stand the aggression, to prevent or repair the destruction, to tolerate the nuisance, to recognize the positive elements in the antisocial tendency, to provide and preserve the object that is to be sought and found" (p. 314). These disturbed patients will often engage in dangerous and obscene activities in the spirit of playfulness in order to create space. In these situations, the therapist must be able to identify with the adolescent's inner struggles and respond empathically with the underlying needs that are being expressed in distorted fashion, even while exercising control and setting limits. The therapist, as well as the environment, is being tested and retested constantly, and he or she must accept the defiance, the silence, the ganging up, and the sarcasm, not as a personal attack, but as important expressions of the patients' negative feelings. The role of the therapist is to receive the projection, hold on to it, and find a way of handing it back in an acceptable form while remaining neutral and tolerant. The therapist, like the adolescent's mother, must go on being him- or herself. When the therapists are pushed beyond the limit, which can occur from time to time, and led to retaliation, this must all be contained within the therapeutic space and fully ventilated. The master of countertransference had this to say about therapists' reactions: "It seems to me doubtful whether a human child, as he develops, is capable of tolerating the full extent of his own hate in a sentimental environment, he needs hate to hate" (Winnicott 1958, p. 202).

The groups at Chestnut Lodge vary in their sentimentality. In some groups, hate makes an appearance in the countertransference and is dealt with without sentimentality. In such instances, the interchanges between therapist and group have been memorable and somewhat reassuring.

Within the space, some important therapeutic developments take place. At first, tentative, mistrustful, and insecure attachments begin to take place between members and between therapists and patients. The attachments fluctuate at times to the point of nonexistence and may cause the therapist to experience disappointment. As a therapeutic relationship is established over time and transference manifestations appear, there is the possibility for a secure base to be established from which even the most frightened patients can begin to explore and learn new patterns of relating. The therapists' attachments, understandably, vary with different members of the group. With some members, the therapists' attachments mirror not the patients' concerns but rather their own distressful reactions to the patients' concerns. The group, as a hall of distorting mirrors, at times aggravates self-doubt, and it is part of the therapists' therapeutic function to offer reliable mirroring.

The type of content that fills the space of a therapeutic group varies with the level at which the group is predominantly functioning, which in turn relates to the level of the individual's psychopathology. In the Chestnut Lodge groups, in which the psychopathology is mainly preoedipal, the levels are constantly shifting, although the major experience is less mature. A good deal of time in group is spent on the current level, at which everyday experiences with the milieu and the outerworld are in the forefront and may successfully exclude the therapists from the conversation. At the transference level, which corresponds to total object relations (in which the group represents the original family and the therapists the parents), the activity is fairly minimal. The material is not interpreted in this context, even though half the therapists are in psychoanalytic training. The group, for the most part, tends to function at the "projective" level (Foulkes and Anthony 1984) or the level of basic assumptions (Bion 1977), at which the primitive defenses of massive denial, splitting, and projective identification are paramount and there are narcissistic relations with part objects. At this level, the group represents the inner world of the individual self as well as the mother's body. In a group, some specific basic assumption function may take over and dominate the group activity, and the group may be divided by the extent to which each member goes along with the assumption. The individuals who take part seem to do so in an automatic and inevitable way, and some assumptions may so captivate the group that it appears as if a contagion has spread through it. When the group is operating at this basic level, the assumptions alternate. At their most dependent, the members look to the therapists for magical treatment that can rescue them from the predicament of hospitalization. At other times, the group may look for and find "enemies" within the group or out in the milieu, and their hostility may take many different forms. When conditions are right, pairing is established between two members, with the rest of the group not only tolerant of but also stimulating the relationship, as if they expect something very special to result from it. When the pair disbands or leaves the group, the members may come to ridicule the pairing and condemn it. The language at these levels is largely stripped of normal communicative value, for which the capacity for symbolization seems largely to be at fault. The language is used not as a vehicle of thought but as a form of action. The therapists may develop countertransferences in response to basic assumption activity, mostly in the area of frustration and anger. Their efforts to introduce reality into the proceedings are frequently sabotaged by the group acting with greater "craziness." The therapists may also struggle to create a work group to deal with the therapeutic task, but this effort may be frustrated by the patients' strong resistances to treatment. The resistances are often blatant and may become dominant features of the group. The patients resist any progressive movement, any attempt to clarify or interpret, any move toward coherence, any signs of therapeutic relatedness (particularly with the therapists), and any type of meaningful communication. New members coming into the group are relatively open to insight but are soon caught up in the resistances and embrace the group identity.

The primitive defenses, coupled with the resistances and the determination to disrupt all attempts at meaning, render treatment of the group a tough assignment. Curiously enough, the therapists have remained relatively unchanged over the past three years, have no wish to relinquish their jobs, and maintain a lively interest in the group seminars. They respond to the challenge constructively and, week after week, attend the seminar with process accounts of their groups and their efforts to understand them. To derive meaning from incoherence contributes to the general therapeutic climate that prevails.

The large groups are interminable groups and therefore do not have to work at termination and final evaluations of the group. As individual members leave the group, they can be separately assessed to determine whether the group experience has been beneficial, but this has shortcomings. The individual's group behavior might be much improved in terms of communicating and contributing to the life of the group, but his or her general adjustment might remain relatively unchanged. However, peer relationships on the outside may be observably better. The containing process, as judged by a diminution in the patient's impulsive acting out, may also show improvement, but individual, family, and milieu therapies can also claim some responsibility for this change.

Two Cardinal Elements Sensitive to the Group Process

The long-term inpatient group assembles a collection of incohesive selves that generate a high level of incoherence in the group as a whole that interferes with its therapeutic functional capacities. Freud (1923) described the ego as "a coherent organization of mental processes" (p. 17) that included some unconscious processes. In the patients described in this chapter, it would seem as if the chaotic, repressed unconscious had invaded all areas of the mental apparatus and the personality connected to it. Loewald (1980) sees the process of internalization as the factor involved in creating and increasing the coherent integration and organization of the psyche as a whole, and he sees repression as the factor working against coherence by maintaining parts of the psychic processes in a less organized and more primitive state. In these patients, a substantial portion of the psyche is kept in a disorganized and primitive state. When the group achieves, even episodically, a sense of "we-ness" and belongingness stemming from basic group processes, the evolving selves of the members may briefly experience a unity, a togetherness, not only of the group, but of the fractured elements of the personality.

Basic to the operation of the group, involving as it does an exposure of the self to others, is the appearance and reappearance of shame as a built-in production of the interpersonal situation. Among these inpatients, there is a painful recognition of being mental cases and of being stigmatized by being hospitalized. Thus, as Alonso and Rutan (1988) have stated, "The shame continues to flourish in a protected bubble" (p. 3). At any point in the proceedings, the suppressed feelings surface, and self-esteem, together with the anguish involved, plummets. The defense of denial is overused in such circumstances, exposing the patient to the narcissistic dilemma in which he or she swings between grandiosity and self-denigration and that isolates him from the group. In the group, shame is provoked by the presence of others, but it is also resolved by the presence of others as the elements of tolerance and empathy are generated by the group. Some of the patients never quite recover from the corrosive stigma and are locked into isolation and despair (Alonso and Rutan 1988). For others, the group provides a corrective experience that allows them to recognize their feelings as an everyday part of the human condition. As the shame diminishes, the sense of identity grows, and the constant mirroring in the group helps repair the primitive feelings and bring the patient out from silence and concealment. The "black humor" of the group has a special reparative power.

The four group experiences that follow underscore these various theoretical considerations and vividly bring to life the difficulties entailed in the therapeutic management of such long-term adolescent groups.

Group 1: The Issue of Containment[1]

The group has a history, and, many members would boast, a tradition, of tolerating and having to deal with primitive expressions of aggression along with explicit, aggressively charged sexual material. The issue of containment has been of foremost concern to the therapists in their weekly work with the group.

Almost all members of the group share three characteristics that have a significant effect on the group: their psychopathology is severe and of long-standing duration, they have a history of severe and often repeated childhood trauma, and they have failed to respond or have been resistant to previous treatment efforts. All have long treatment histories that include multiple hospitalizations. The members of the group entered adolescence with a seriously compromised capacity to trust and depend on caretakers and poorly equipped to negotiate crucial developmental tasks, particularly the modulation and integration of aggressive and sexual drives.

Inevitably, the interpersonal consequences of these deficits become evident in the group. The group affords a powerful opportunity for the reparation and modification of these deficits. Fostering a climate in which the reparative potential of the group can be realized is the major therapeutic task and challenge not only for the group therapists but for all group members.

The unfolding process through which the therapists endeavor to contain the group and, moreover, to promote the containing potential of the group itself is illustrated in the following review of an approximately three-month period of life and work in the group that included twelve weekly meetings. The group has been meeting weekly for three years. It is a mixed, open-ended group. The group currently includes four boys, four girls, Dr. F, and Dr. M. We meet in one of the school classrooms.

GROUP MEMBERS[2]

Derek, age eighteen, having entered the group two years ago, has more time in the group than any of the other adolescents. He considers himself the standard bearer of group traditions, the most important being, "The group doesn't mean anything. The group is useless." Derek has intense dependency needs that he defends against by maintaining a joking indifference to any effort to engage him. During the period of work reported here, Derek, about to be discharged, was in the process of terminating with the group.

Maggie, age sixteen, a member of the group for one and a half years, is our most volatile and explosive female but also probably the most powerful member of the group. She lends force to or initiates many of the potentially mutative interactions and confrontations. While her verbal threats and hostile gestures are intimidating and sometimes startling, she has never physically assaulted anyone in the group as she has in other settings, both in the hospital and before her admission. Maggie's power in the group derives from unbridled aggression that makes her a formidable opponent and from the ease with which she can align herself with various subgroups. She has a complex array of defenses, oscillating between sadistic attacks and masochistic reenactments, identifying with the aggressor or inviting abuse. These dynamics, although somewhat unpredictable, have a pronounced effect on the group.

Ben, age seventeen, has been in the group for one and a half years. He is by far the most difficult member of the group to contain, and a considerable amount of the group's time and energy has been expended in various efforts to contain him. In retrospect, his entry into the group seems prophetic. Soon after joining the group, he crawled into a closet in the room, and members of the group briefly blocked the door. Interestingly, he himself did not struggle to get out. He uses his good intellect to maintain a grandiose, contemptuous position vis-à-vis peers and authority figures. He often maintains center stage—literally— standing on furniture, pacing, twirling his chair in the center of the group, or instigating contemptuous verbal attacks on the therapists. He often subjects the therapists to an unrelenting barrage of graphic sexual remarks. Markedly fearful of any expression of aggression in others, he often takes on the role of group buffoon to divert the group's attention from emerging confrontations and hostilities.

Joe, nineteen, a member of the group for one year, is unique among group members because he is completely passive and withdrawn, only rarely speaking. When Joe first entered the group, he immediately laid down on the floor, dramatically signaling what was to become his customary mode of participation. He gradually moved to a position lying on top of a nearby sink counter, where he remained for many months, drawing attention to himself only when his foot would inadvertently bump the faucet, occasionally turning on the water. Joe is regarded as something of a sleeping dragon, an unknown quantity that the group is disinclined to engage. His occasional utterances of "Fuck you" suggest a dormant anger and reinforce the group's reluctance to confront him. His passivity places a burden on the other members of the group, who cannot rely on his support or participation.

Sally, age sixteen, has been in the group for one year. She craves physical contact and easily engaged the boys in typical preadolescent roughhousing. She eventually established herself as a kind of earth-mother, physically soothing and calming the more disruptive group members. She would, for example, brush Maggie's hair or let Ben sit on her lap. In controlling Ben, she made an important contribution to group functioning.

Tracy, age sixteen, a member of the group for one year, has maintained a distant, occasionally hostile position in the group. Tracy's active involvement in the group is limited to her participation in verbal attacks on the therapists. Otherwise, she is a self-contained, self-soothing unit and most often sits, sucking her thumb, rocking, reading, and listening through earphones to her radio—all at the same time. She obviously hears what is going on, as she will occasionally direct her attention to the group's interactions.

Gina, nineteen, in the group for seven months and a day student, is the only group member who lives at home, currently with her mother. Having previously had a purportedly positive group-therapy experience, Gina seemed initially a source of hope to our often disgruntled and struggling group. She quickly attempted to set the group straight, identifying the all too numerous shortcomings of the group, contrasting the group unfavorably with her earlier experiences, and pointing out how the group ought to be functioning. The group briefly rallied, trying to meet her expectations, but soon failed and proved a disappointment to her, after which she withdrew and was treated by the group as an outsider. She invited this role, ignoring the group by spending her time reading and generally responding with disdain when approached. Gina represents a harsh, critical group superego.

Jake, age fifteen, with four months in the group, is its newest member. Jake was surprisingly compliant on entering the group, in spite of a history of previous treatment failures, and it seemed that he might be a positive influence on the male subgroup. This hope was not realized as he readily joined in with and even exceeded the boys' disparaging commentary about the group and the therapists. Jake is invested in securing the group's approval and, in that regard, is a malleable, although not always constructive, group member.

Drs. F and M are experienced psychotherapists with a special interest in treating seriously disordered patients, particularly border-line adults and adolescents. When asked to run the group, both were interested in doing so.

The sessions are numbered to indicate the successive weekly meetings during this phase of the group.

SESSION 1

The boys find the wrench that opens the windows and proceed to open the windows and take off the screens. They stand partly outside the windows and yell at individuals passing by. The whole group is oriented toward what is going on outside the group. When Dr. F tries to retrieve the wrench, the boys are uncooperative and teasing, saying, "Let's play keep away." Ben finally relents. Dr. F gets the wrench and begins to close the windows. Jake stands on the window sill, interfering with Dr. F's attempt. Dr. M comes over to the window and tells Jake to get down, which he does. The boys become more agitated after the windows are closed. Ben threatens to drop his pants but instead turns his back to the group, unzips his fly, and puts a pencil in his fly opening, as if it were his penis. When the therapists comment that the group is having a great deal of difficulty dealing with what is going on in the group, the boys respond with, "Shut up, bitch. Shut up, dike." As the group ends, Ben walks over to Dr. F and taps her on the head, lightly, with a newspaper.

*Analysis.*This meeting came at a point when many confrontations, particularly between the boys and the girls, were beginning to emerge. Rather than confront one another, the group had been defensively criticizing and verbally attacking the therapists. This defense had been interpreted to the group and was weakening. At this juncture, members were quite anxious that the group would not be able to contain the expression of charged sexual and aggressive material. Ben produces a guaranteed distraction by threatening to expose himself. The association of the pencil with a small penis further heightens his anxiety, resulting in the unchecked aggressive impulse directed at the therapist. The group was tense, at times chaotic, and difficult for the therapists to manage.

SESSION 2

As the group enters the room, the windows are once again open. Gina will not come into the room, saying, "It's too cold." The therapists get one of the teachers to close the windows. With the windows closed, Gina comes in. Ben has something important to say to the group. He announces, "Now this is serious. Cut the crap, Derek. Listen to this. Dr. F, you're a coward. Last week when I hit you with the newspaper, you cowered. You're okay." Dr. F answers, "Oh, I'm the good therapist. Dr. M is the bad therapist." Ben responds, "No. It's not that. Now we've got you settled. We've got to work on Dr. M, get to her." Maggie agrees, but Sally is disinterested. Ben says, "Listen to this Sally. We've got to get Dr. M worked up." She tells him to be quiet. Gina feels that both therapists are cowards. At the end of the group, Jake says, "This has been a good group," to which Tracy responds, "Too good." Maggie says, "The anger's got to go."

*Analysis.*This is an interesting group in which Ben clearly articulates what is a condensation of two fears about the expression of aggression. First, he needs to know the therapists' psychological ignition point as well as the magnitude of their response. He wishes to agitate until they explode, and then he can confront the fantasied retaliation, allaying his anxiety, he hopes, by demonstrating that reality is less dangerous than fantasy. As he said to Dr. F, "You cowered. You're okay." The other condensed element, expressed by Gina, is the group's continuing anxiety about whether the therapists can safely contain the group's destructive potential. Gina signals this concern when she refuses to come into the room until the windows are closed, not wanting a repeat of the previous week's tensions. Jake is more involved, but Tracy is threatened by the group's work. Maggie succinctly reiterates the problem with which the group is struggling, "The anger's got to go."

The group is tense. Ben is hyperactive, playing with and touching various objects. He pokes at a map and some paintings hanging on the wall overhead. Both fall down, just missing him. Maggie, agitated, paces and then throws a book. Jake says to her, "Don't throw the book." She sits down, and Joe moves to sit next to her.

*Analysis.*Several significant events transpire. Ben's "accidents" lend immediacy to the group's concern about behavior run amok. The small miracle is Jake and Joe's response to Maggie. Jake, usually reluctant to take any constructive stance in the group, confronts Maggie, while Joe, who usually sits atop the sink, gets down from his perch and moves next to her. His action is dramatic in its singularity, and his presence provides an effective constraint. Thus, the group makes a fledgling and successful effort to contain one of its more explosive members.

The group begins on an extremely agitated, disruptive note. Derek, Ben, and Jake mount a sadistic verbal and, in a sense, physical attack on the therapists. The boys, with the exception of Joe, who is back on top of the sink, "jokingly" engage in a lengthy graphic commentary about the therapists' sexual proclivities. The girls, except Maggie, who intermittently joins the boys in their attack, say nothing. Derek and Ben, escalating, take paper clips and rubber bands from the desk and sail them in the direction of Dr. M's chair. Efforts by Drs. M and F to get them to stop are unsuccessful.

*Analysis.*This was a difficult group for the therapists. Ben realized his wish to "get Dr. M worked up." Both therapists felt immobilized and uncertain about how to handle the group and were unclear as to how to support one another. Nor were they communicating effectively with one another during the group. Dr. F did not know how Dr. M wanted to handle the situation and tried repeatedly to interrupt the boys. Dr. M was hampered by her feeling that Dr. F would not want to put the boys out of the group. The therapists met briefly after the group, and some dissension between them was apparent. A further miscommunication occured that was to have later consequences. Dr. F was annoyed at Dr. M when she indicated that, because of an unavoidable scheduling conflict, she would be unable to attend the group supervision that day. Unfortunately, Dr. F was going to be late coming to the supervision but did not mention this to Dr. M. When Dr. F subsequently arrived at the supervision, Dr. M *was* there and had already described the group, a situation that further annoyed Dr. F. These tensions between the therapists notwithstanding, a clear consensus emerged from the group supervision. The therapists needed to establish limits for the group, specifying behaviors that were unacceptable. It was agreed that at the next meeting the therapists would inform the group that anyone engaging in behavior that physically endangered others would be asked to leave (for that day).

SESSION 5

The therapists begin the group stating that any behavior that physically endangers others will not be tolerated and anyone engaging in such behavior will be asked to leave the group for the day. Maggie is absent, so she does not hear this announcement. Jake begins to play with a classroom projector. Someone turns out the lights so the group can watch the movie that Jake is trying to start. The projector stops working. A lengthy discussion follows about who will pay for the broken projector. Dr. F maintains that it is the group's responsibility since the group did nothing to stop Jake from playing with it and that therefore the group should share the expense of having the projector repaired. Other members of the group adamantly disagree with this position, including Dr. M. Ben says, "I'm not worried. I know what I'll say. Jake did it." Ben begins to talk about his close friendship with Derek. Derek says Ben is not a close friend.

*Analysis.*With the projector breaking and the tacit disagreement between the therapists as to what should be done about it, group tension was still running high, even though the group seemed to accept, with surprising equanimity, the rule prohibiting physically threatening behavior. The group readily became interested in watching the movie, hoping to avoid further hostilities. However, for the first time, Derek challenges Ben. Perhaps of even greater significance was a confrontation between the two therapists, not in the group, but after the group, when they met briefly. During this short but heated exchange, several important areas of conflict surfaced. Unable to resolve their differences quickly, they agreed to meet at a later but unspecified time.

171

SESSION 6

The therapists inform Maggie, who was absent the previous week, about the rule prohibiting physically threatening behavior, after which they fall silent, reflecting, in part, the fact that they have not yet resolved their own differences. Jake repeatedly comments on how quiet the therapists are and speculates that they are harboring a conspiracy. Jake asks Ben to explain how electricity works and, although Ben provides a good explanation, continues to ask increasingly detailed questions until Ben is stumped. Jake is pleased that he has prevailed. Ben turns away from Jake and joins Sally and Tracy, who are playing a marriage game. When Ben plays, they derogate him, making the game turn out so that it predicts, "Ben will live in a hole, have sex in a toilet, and have an ugly baby." Ben then shifts his attention to Derek, who ignores him. When Ben persists, Derek calls him a faggot. Turning back to the girls, Ben flicks a lighter near Sally's face. She pushes him into the wall and calls him a faggot. He cowers in the corner, then says, "Let's attack Dr. M and Dr. F." The group provides no support for this idea, and, in fact, when Ben approaches Dr. F, several members gather around her, protectively. Dr. F says, "I feel safer with the whole group around me than with just Ben alone."

*Analysis.*The group makes a concerted effort, in a variety of ways, to challenge Ben, who has been one of the main instigators of aggressive eruptions. Additionally, the therapists met after the group to discuss their conflict. While acknowledging respective personal issues activated by the group, the therapists focused mainly on the dynamics of the group and the difficulties in working with such primitive material. Clearly, the group had projected onto the therapists a number of salient conflicts around good and bad, weak and strong, and dominance and submission, and it seemed that some significant gains might be made if the therapists could deal with and try to understand these projections better. They agreed to reinstitute their weekly lunch meetings.

SESSION 7

The group did not meet the previous week because of the spring vacation. Members assemble slowly, and inertia settles over the group. Ben and Tracy set up a small radio with two miniature speakers, reassuring Dr. F, "We won't play it too loud." The group criticizes the radio station Ben picks. Almost everyone is sitting, reading quietly, listening to the music. Joe has joined the group, sitting in a chair in the circle. The therapists comment about the depressed feeling in the group. Derek says, "What do you expect? Look at the weather." No one went home over the break. Tracy and Sally discuss their reading for health class, a chapter on marriage, teenage pregnancy, family violence, and child abuse. Tracy says, "I want to read that." Ben asks, "Can you have sex when you're pregnant?" Sally answers, "Yes, but you shouldn't." Ben says, "It's better then because the woman's breasts are bigger." Sally tells him he's stupid. He retorts, "Scratch my crotch." She responds, "Is that all you ever think about?" Ben says the group is boring and stands on top of the sink, tapping his feet. Sally tells him to stop it. "You're making too much noise." He gets down. Derek hopes the music shop will be hiring by summer. He just quit a job and cannot find another. Dr. F remarks that there is not much time left until school ends. The group ends, and everyone leaves quietly.

*Analysis.*The group is depressed. No one went home because most of their home situations are untenable, a fact alluded to in the assigned readings for health class. Nor are they adequately equipped to find employment and support themselves, an issue that Derek has to struggle with when school ends.

SESSION 8

As the group begins, Jake and Derek are absent. This group composition in which Ben is outnumbered by the girls makes him anxious, and he defensively launches into a barrage of obscene comments about dicks, cunts, and getting a hard-on. Maggie reprimands him, "I'm getting tired of the way you treat me like one of the guys, saying all these things in front of me. I'm getting sick of it." Jake arrives and quickly joins Ben. When Dr. M encourages Maggie to continue, Jake tells Dr. M to shut up and adds, "What a stupid haircut you got. It really looks awful." Maggie admonishes Jake, "Did it ever occur to you that they get tired of hearing that stuff from you? They listen to it all the time. Don't you think it ever hurts their feelings?" Jake and Ben continue their sexual banter, inviting further criticism from Maggie, Tracy, and Sally. Jake begins to play with a pile of leaf

173

pods he has brought with him, squirting the juice from the pods at Maggie. She repeatedly tells him to stop, he continues, sometimes squirting Ben as well, and she finally threatens to hit him. He leaves the room to get a drink of water, and Maggie persists in expressing her anger about the boys making obscene, degrading comments about women. Jake comes back but finds the door locked. No one will get up to let him in. Finally, someone in the hall unlocks the door. Dr. M remarks, "The group didn't seem to want to let you back in, Jake." She encourages Maggie to continue. Maggie does, acknowledging that she brings some of this on herself. As her confrontation with Jake intensifies, Ben's anxiety escalates, and he begins twirling his chair in the center of the circle. Dr. F comments that Ben is feeling anxious about the group's confrontation of Jake and is "trying to distract us by acting like a clown." Maggie says Ben is not so bad. "Sometimes he listens." Sally lets Ben rub her back. This calms him, and Maggie continues her work with Jake, which becomes quite moving. She points out his good and bad aspects. She is hurt by the way he has changed because he used to be very supportive and she needs his support. Jake responds, "That's just Maggie's complaint." Dr. F comments, "No, it's not. Maggie is speaking for the other girls in the group, too." Maggie adds, "Gina doesn't count. She's not really part of the group." Maggie states that Gina is disappointed in the therapists because they take so much verbal abuse. Both Jake and Ben are quiet as the group ends, and everyone leaves in silence.

*Analysis.*The girls are able to capitalize on the group's previous efforts to contain disruptive members. They function more cohesively, are more active, and are not as fragmented. Real gains in the girls' capacity to challenge the boys' sexualized aggression are evident. Maggie's leadership in this effort is crucial. Important too is Sally's ability to calm Ben. Maggie's integration of good and bad and her move away from a masochistic position are important changes.

SESSION 9

The group is tense, and the windows are open once again. This time, however, no one yells out or stands near the windows. Maggie is angry about the possibility that she will be enrolled in regular classes at the local public high school (mainstreamed) for summer school. Maggie is both upset about the prospect of mainstreaming and hostile toward Dr.

M when she wonders if Maggie is really ready for such a move. Ben says he too might be mainstreamed for the summer. Gina comments that she might fail gym, which could jeopardize her graduation plans. Ben insists that the therapists guess what grade he is in.

*Analysis.*The open windows, leitmotiv of the group's ongoing concern with containment, herald a possible or approaching denouement of the containment issue. So too does the movement in the material from concerns about containment in the group to concerns about whether members will be able to contain themselves outside the group—Ben and Maggie in the public school and Gina after graduating. Ben's insistence that the therapists guess what grade he is in expresses a concern about how he will appear to others outside the group.

SESSION 10

From the onset the group is settled. Sally is absent. Derek is sick and complains about having to come to school and the group just to be able to go out in the evening, by which time he knows he'll be feeling better. Jake, lying across two desks, says he is daydreaming. When someone asks, "Oh, about sex?" he says, "No. Just a daydream." Dr. F asks, "What about?" Maggie tells her, "Stop acting like a shrink." Derek hates his housemother. Dr. M wonders if his mood is connected with graduation. He responds with a vigorous criticism of the group, announcing, "With all my heart, I won't miss this group." Dr. F mentions former group members who continue to ask about the group. Maggie adds that Jack, a former member, has said that he misses the group. Derek describes an unsuccessful attempt to get together with two friends, who eventually left without him because he was late. Having no other place to go, he returned to the hospital. Maggie wonders why he did not just go somewhere else. She worries about not fitting in with the cliques in the school where she is to be mainstreamed. She tells the therapists that they have taken too much abuse from the group and says that if she were a doctor she would not take it. Dr. F asks her, "What would you do?" She answers, "I'd beat the shit out of them, one by one." Gina tells the therapists that, because they are cowardly and poor disciplinarians who do not follow through, their children will become drug addicts. Drs. M and F reiterate their interest in keeping members in the group, working on their problems. Gina disagrees, "People should be thrown out for using abusive language.'' Maggie says, "No, not for saying 'fuck.' " The therapists point out that with such a rule no one would be left in the group. Gina says, "I'd still be here." Throughout, all the group members, except Ben, have been attentive. He leaves the room, and, when he returns, Maggie says, "Don't open the door for him." Tracy does let him in but leaves herself. Maggie briefly refers to a fight she had with Ben the previous evening and, in the group, accepts an apology from him, which she had been unable to do the night before.

*Analysis.*The group evinces a readiness to work on issues confronting departing members, signaled both by the climate established at the beginning of the group and by Maggie's rejection of Dr. F's focus on Jake, who is not leaving the group. A unifying dynamic underlies the seemingly disparate topics under discussion. Although each of the departing members is struggling with his or her individual problems, they are all problems that have been expressed and elaborated in the group. Derek defensively avoids attachment both in and out of the group and consequently has no support system and "no place to go." Maggie's beat-the-shit-out-of-them response to conflict could easily result in exclusion from the cliques she anticipates encountering. Gina's intolerance isolates her from the group and leaves her at risk for continuing alienation from peers. Ben will be shut out, as he is in the group, if his disruptive behavior persists. Maggie actively fosters and promotes the reparative potential of the group. In affirming the importance of the group to former members, she challenges Derek. She counters Gina's rigid position with a more tolerant one. With the support of the group, she and Ben are able to resolve their differences.

SESSION 11

The group starts on a tense note. Jake sits at the desk, playing with items he has removed from the desk drawer. The therapists remind him that the teachers do not want group members to go into their desks. He says, "Shut up," and continues to root through the drawer. Finding a paper a student has written, he reads it to himself. Dr. F tells him to put it back and close the drawer. Ignoring this directive, he takes out the teacher's grade book and starts to read the grades out loud. Dr. F tries, without success, to take the grade book away from him. The therapists maintain that the grades are confidential. Jake polls the group, asking if anyone wants him to stop. Most members are either unresponsive or say that they do not care. Joe, however, dissents, "Don't read my grades." Jake, persisting, announces Joe's grade. Joe asserts, "I told you not to read my grades." Dr. F wonders if Jake should be asked to leave. Jake then takes some rubber bands and with them slings paper clips toward Dr. M. Drs. F and M quickly agree that Jake cannot stay in the group, and he is sent out. The remainder of the group is quiet and uneventful, with members reading or resting on the desks.

*Analysis.*The paper clip incident is a repetition of the attack on the therapists in session 4 and graphically reintroduces one of the major group issues—the containment of aggression. This group provides a good example of the effect of the group and group dynamics on the therapists. Having dealt with the previous paper clip episode and its repercussions, the therapists are better prepared to respond, less uncertain, more able to communicate with one another in the group and to act in concert. Their lead in removing Jake benefits the group, which, at this point, is unable to confront him directly. The therapists may also be experienced by some members of the group as responding constructively to the criticism that they take too much abuse. At yet another level, the therapists' collaboration contrasts markedly with the chronic parental discord, particularly around child management issues, present in most of their families.

SESSION 12

This is a productive group. Maggie, not Joe, is on the sink top. Joe sits in the group circle. Ben stands near the sink closet, sorting through a large stack of old newspapers. He said, "It's so much fun to look back over this old stuff." Derek describes how he plans to use his weekends after he is discharged. He will hunt and fish, preferably with a friend, but alone if he cannot find a friend to go with him. He would like to blow up squirrels with an M-16. The nursing supervisor said that he cannot hang around the unit after he is discharged. He plans to obtain vocational training but will not use the county job placement service. He will feel better if he can find a job on his own. At first he will have to live at home. This entails abiding by his parents' rules, one of which is, "Respect the family name." Dr. F asks, "What's that mean?" He does not know. He does not want to continue in treatment. Dr. M wonders who he will talk to when he is having problems. "Friends," he answers. Jake is lying on the floor, and Dr. M jokes with him, "All this talk about being out really has you floored." Gina laughs and tells the group about her plans to move to California and attend school there. She acknowledges that change is anxiety provoking but claims that leaving the Lodge school is not. Derek imagines the food he will keep in his refrigerator—butter, soft drinks, and steak sandwiches—but demurs, "You can't live just on steak sandwiches." He wonders what will be served for lunch at the hospital that day. A detailed discussion ensues about what is needed to set up an apartment and live alone. Maggie moves her seat near Derek's and offers him advice. Maggie tells the group about her summer school plans. Ben adds that he will also be taking summer courses at the local public school. Sally, Tracy, Joe, and Jake, none of whom will be leaving the group, listen quietly. Group members are still talking as the group ends.

Analysis. The productivity of this group is attributable to the interaction of two significant dynamics, operating in tandem. First, the historically disruptive members of the group are well contained. Ben is reviewing old newspapers and putting them in the closet. Reviewing is itself a meaningful metaphor for this group, with four of its members moving on. Noteworthy too, perhaps more incidentally, is Ben's use of the closet—at this point to store the papers, not himself, as he once had on entering the group. The act of reading the papers contains him. Jake has settled down, literally, on the floor, and Maggie actively interacts with Derek. Second, departing members are considerably less defensive about sharing their concerns, and the group, being free of disruption, is able to hear and respond to these concerns. These concerns revolve around caring for and containing themselves when the support, nurture, and containment provided by the hospital is no longer available.

What transpired during this three-month period of work? A number of group trends are observable. Defensive, hostile attacks on the therapists diminish in intensity and frequency. Group members become increasingly adept at confronting one another. Strategies for dealing with disruptive members are gradually developed and deployed. The sadistic-masochistic polarization between boys and girls shifts. The therapists develop more effective means of dealing with aggression. Members become more able to expose their vulnerabilities and share their concerns. The power of the group, acting in concert, is effectively mobilized in the service of containing a highly disruptive member.

From another perspective, changes in each member of the group can be identified. Maggie's gains are evident in her increased capacity to integrate good and bad and to modulate intense affect and in the modification of her masochistic-sadistic defenses. Ben is clearly more contained and his tolerance for confrontation enhanced. Joe has joined the group. Sally has relinquished her giddy defense and more readily acknowledges feelings of depression. Tracy has taken off her earphones, reversing her massive retreat from the group. Gina too has become a more active participant, abandoning her role of disinterested outsider. Jake is less defiant and oppositional and shows a greater degree of comfort with his dependency needs. Derek gradually reveals more of his anxieties and works more actively with the group. His poignant comment is strangely telling. "With all my heart, I won't miss the group." We like to believe and, in a way, need to believe that this resolutely ungrieving heart was at least briefly touched by our group.

The therapists are well served by having a clearly articulated, overriding treatment philosophy or theoretical orientation. In our group, the principle of attempting, if at all possible, to keep members in the group, rather than resorting to extrusion, serves this purpose. A corollary to this is our belief that the group itself, acting in concert, is more powerful than any one or two members, and our main therapeutic strategy is to try first to mobilize the group, particularly the containing potential of the group as a whole. When functioning cohesively, the group is the best possible container.

Group 2: Issues of Isolation and Control[3]

The group has been in operation for several years. For the past three years it has had two male cotherapists: a teacher at the Lodge school (Mr. H) and a member of the psychiatric staff (Dr. K). Although the membership of the group has almost completely changed during this time, the group culture has remained relatively stable. The "official" group philosophy and the most salient group defense is one of stubborn alienation—from the cotherapists, from one another, and from the milieu. The tradition of estrangement is historically transmitted without apparent intention or purpose. Although members will sometimes admit to being close to a particular patient, a staff member, or their individual therapist, this is presented as a private matter, in no way mitigating the fact that they have nothing to say to us or to each other in group. Hence, the frequent complaint, "Group sucks!" or the sarcasm with which one of the members ritually heralds the beginning of each group: "Another exciting day of group!"

Maintaining physical safety and order has never been an issue in this group. Periods of silence and somnolent dejection alternate with giddily crude and deliberately tangential cross talk on a few members' parts. Reflective, inquisitive, or interpretive comments from the therapists are met with the ultimate opprobrium, "There you go analyzing again." At such moments of resistance, the cotherapists' attempts to move the group toward more positive interaction may engage one or two allies, but these are easily discouraged in the face of other members' seeming apathy or opposition.

The members are also often deeply mistrustful of each other. They frequently complain, "You can't trust anyone in this place," "All people do is gossip around here," or, "There's no one worth talking to," as though they were speaking of someone other than themselves. The group has a high tolerance for impulsive, addictive, or oppositional behavior in its members and peers, but even a whiff of schizotypy arouses ostracism or mockery. For a period of time, the group's tendency to scapegoating, splitting, and defensive clique formation was apparent in the institution of the self-styled "power group," a faction of higher-status, narcissistic members who sat at one end of the room with their feet up on a common chair. Similarly, over a period of time, the group revolved around a succession of "queen bees"—modish, self-absorbed young women who dominated the group, rewarding admirers with attention and seductive strokes and zapping challengers with bolts of sarcastic contempt. The group was thus often divided into the "ins" and the "outs." The group's kaleidoscopic style and shifting pairings and rejections are illustrated in the details of the following session.

The group assembled when Kathy, one of the last to enter the room, arrived. Characteristically regarding herself in charge, Kathy turned the lights off as she entered but relented at Mr. H's request and turned them back on. We commented that it was Tina's first meeting and welcomed her to the group. Kathy launched into an animated, scathing description of a housemate, Lily, who had disgusted everyone by sitting in the parlor with her legs agape. The boys joined in with a chorus of revulsion about Lily's genitals and those of women in general. Tina was about to sit down, but, in the course of her dramatic account, Kathy peremptorily seized the chair from Tina's hand, saying, "I'll give it back in a minute." Kathy proceeded to demonstrate Lily's position with her legs draped apart on the chair. Tina stared in wide-eyed amazement. After Kathy returned the chair, Tina was able to sit down. Kevin solicitously invited her to sit closer to him, and for most of the remainder of the session they talked quietly together, looking occasionally at Dr. K, who sat next to them.

Sam and Sheldon, who sat next to each other, immediately plunged into the flamboyantly lewd repartee that was their characteristic presentation but that had yielded to a more serious, reflective style over most of the preceding several sessions. This provided a bass (and base) continuo for the entire session. In this session, there was less talk of their girlfriends, more joking about homosexuality, and more mock fondling of each other, often with raucous imitations of masturbation and ejaculation. For a while, they dominated the group with tales of shopping at a local erotic emporium specializing in sexual apparatus. Flamboyant in his punk attire, Sam announced that he was looking forward to his new bondage suspenders. No longer the center of attention, Kathy read, sometimes silently, sometimes aloud, from her *People* magazine, alternately ignoring the boys, expressing her disgust at them, or egging them on. Somewhat deferentially, Sam asked Kathy whether she could help him get a job as a stock boy at the shop where she worked, but she demurred that they wanted a stock boy who looked like a stock boy. Sam complained about his present movie theater job, protesting about the clothes he was required to wear. There was also much joking about the sort of "job" he wanted (homosexual blow job).

Kathy turned to Dr. K to inform him cuttingly that he had been discussed in other groups and was regarded as "boring." She then launched into a diatribe about how other groups got to do what they wanted. Why did this group "always have to act the way you want, to do what you say?" (Needless to say, this was news to us!) Mr. H observed that it seemed to him that it was often Kathy who called the shots. Kathy interrupted him contemptuously and dismissively, complaining that she did not like the way he acted in group because he always sided with Dr. K. Looking about and seeing that others were not joining in, she complained that no one was listening. Somewhat taken aback by her diatribe and perhaps disappointed at the group relapsing into a more chaotically regressive mode, we commented that there had been several sessions of people talking seriously and listening to each other but that the group seemed in a different place today. This drew no response other than some more desultory grousing from Kathy; she then broke off with an expletive and an air of futility and lapsed back into silently reading her magazine. Meanwhile, Kevin and Tina continued to murmur together in an increasingly intimate fashion. At one point, looking up and seeing Dr. K looking at them with amiable interest, Kevin said half apologetically, "It's not about group." Dr. K retorted that, if it was during group, it must be about the group in some way. Feeling that there was little image in censoriousness, Dr. K observed that one reason why Kevin and Tina were chatting together was that Kevin was trying to make Tina feel at ease and welcome, which the others had not done. With great mock chivalry, Sam and Sheldon rose, bowed, and intoned sardonically, "Welcome to the group!" In fact, however, this did draw Tina into the group, and she and the boys started chatting animatedly about the previous day's volleyball game, where they had teased her. Kathy, who remained aloof from this, suddenly turned to Sam, interrupting him in mid-sentence, and peremptorily began to talk at him about a totally unrelated matter, abruptly cutting Tina out again. We commented that it seemed as though Kathy did not want the group to take notice of Tina having joined us. Sam started to say something to Tina, but Kathy leaned forward disdainfully, sticking her chest out and blocking Sam's view of Tina. Sam said, "There you go, putting your tits in the way." He then walked around her, sat down next to Tina, and said to Kathy with mock defiance, "So screw you. I'll talk to her if I want to." He then asked Tina with mock solicitude what she had been saying. Rather bewildered, Tina said that she did not remember, whereupon Sam said, "Well, screw you too," and returned to his seat next to Sheldon. In passing Kathy, he pretended to front himself against her outstretched foot and make crude sexual noises.

Sam turned to Kathy and asked, "Did you dream you were in bed with me last night?" Kathy: "No. Why? Should I have?" Sam: "Well, I dreamt I was getting it on with someone and I'm damned if I know who." Sheldon added that indeed she should have; she did not know what she was missing. Sam asked her, "When are we going to have that *ménage à trois*?" Much suggestive repartee between them followed. We asked who was the third side of the triangle and was told "Lily."

Sam continued to chat with Sheldon, Kathy read, Tina returned to conversations with Kevin, Dolly remained with her head down (as she did all session), and Ken sat quietly in a corner. After many more minutes passed in this mode, we futilely commented that, after several weeks of really being able to talk together, something now seemed to be in the way, breaking us up into isolated groups. Characteristically, this drew no apparent response. Sometime later, Sheldon twice imitated the flamboyantly eccentric behavior of Robert (a former group member who had been transferred for assaultive behavior). Sam whined in Robert's tone, "Mr. H, make him stop it." We commented that it was hard to forget that we had not only a new member but a missing member.

Despite its studied "attacks on linking" and meaning, the group nonetheless managed many moments of significant interchange and communication. Some of these moments of increased intimacy and cohesion were in response to external events. Thus, on one occasion, when Robert had become wildly assaultive at a unit meeting, he was transferred to the adult hospital and hence out of group. Group members sat close together and were extremely solicitous of each other; they talked about the need for people in the division to stick together and look after each other; they were indignant toward their assaultive peer and denounced him as "psycho," while protesting how different his problems were from their own. On another occasion, group members pulled together when a member, whose compulsive bodybuilding masked deep insecurities, came to group black and blue, having been beaten up in a fight in town the night before the "Mr. Rockville" physique contest. Beyond expressing sympathy, several usually contemptuously aloof patients spoke near tearfully of their own repudiated feelings of vulnerability. Although such moments strengthened a sense of commonality, it was often technically difficult to move from external events to the "here and now" of the group.

On other occasions, moves toward greater intimacy and self-revelation stemmed from developments intrinsic to the group. For example, June, one of the "queen bees," usually spoke as though the Lodge were simply the latest in a long line of fashionable boarding schools to which her parents had sent her. However, in response to one member's concern over a sibling who remained at home, June spoke of her worries about her sister and finally told the story of her own losses, depression, and serious suicide attempt that led up to her hospitalization. The group listened with rapt and sympathetic attention.

Following such sessions, however, the group would often defensively retreat to "trashing" the next meeting, acting affectively as though the previous meeting had not occurred. Much of the therapists' efforts were directed toward maintaining a sense of continuity (i.e., there had been moments of warmth and closeness) and toward exploring the nature of the anxieties that led to members isolating themselves and trivializing their interactions. Indeed, following one serious discussion, a defensively sardonic member unwittingly echoed the lines of a Samuel Beckett character, saying, "You don't suppose we're starting to mean something, do you?"

Two sessions, one and a half years apart, illustrate the group's movement around issues of isolation and control. One recurrent grievance was the complaint of not being understood or listened to by others. Indeed, members made only intermittent attempts to be attentive to or supportive of each other. Some lacked social skills and experience in communicating or responding appropriately; for most, issues of envy and competitiveness, intolerance of painful affects, and a propensity for projection were major impediments. However, members tended to see the problem as external; that is, it was the other person, the cotherapists, or people outside the group who were insufficiently empathic. Over time, however, members came to grapple more directly with this issue, with some decrease in their sense of isolation.

A second persistent issue was the resentment of adult authority and limit setting. Characteristically, the group presented itself as though unambivalently on the side of id impulses, with any (self-) blame or realistic needs for restraint put onto the staff and attacked. Over time, members became able to own their concern over each other's self-destructive behavior and to see the struggle for the containment of impulses as an internal, rather than an external, struggle.

The first session followed a weekend when the parents of John, who came from an impoverished background, had brought a picnic for the entire house. As the weekend was being discussed, John commented, "I don't know why my parents did it; I wouldn't have; we don't deserve it." A member protested that they had been appreciative. One of the more disturbed members made a tangential comment, and the conversation became fragmented. John, looking upset, complained, as he had in the past, "That's the trouble with this group; no one ever listens." Someone retorted, "Why should we? Who cares?" One of the cotherapists remarked that being heard was something everyone wanted and needed, like food, but that we were talking about it as though such things had to be deserved. John responded, "That's right, but look, no one except you guys [the therapists] is listening: Dolly's reading, Kevin looks like he's sleeping." We suggested that here was an opportunity to find out right now what got in the way of our hearing one another. John confronted Dolly, who put down her book and protested that she was listening. After John confronted Kevin, Kevin retorted, half sarcastically, "I sleep to keep from going crazy. . . . People are so difficult to deal with. There are only a few people like John, out of millions, that you can relate to." John retorted that sleeping was a lousy way to do so. At this point, Ken pulled out his wallet and wanted to show some photos: his old house, two dogs from old times, and a former "girlfriend." (Ken, one of the youngest and most immature members of the group, had been shuffled through a variety of foster homes.) John and Kevin woofed derisively; Ken looked hurt but responded characteristically with obscenity. We remarked that people talked about not being heard but that Ken was trying to tell people about old times and people important to him and not having much success. Members listened more attentively to Ken and responded with recollections about moves and displacements in their own lives. At this point, John picked up a globe from the nearby science equipment and began tossing it in the air (much like Chaplin in *The Great Dictator*). We commented that he had got the whole world in his hands. "I'm God," he replied, first twisting the two hemispheres apart and then trying to realign them. Asked what he would do as God to set the world right, he answered virtuously, "If I were the president, I'd bust all the dealers, use the army to stop drugs; I wouldn't spend money on space, I'd spend it on people here at home first." We remarked that the solution to a lot of our problems probably did lie right at home here in the group. For example, we had seen today that the problem of not hearing each other was not just something out there but was inside each of us. Conversation continued. Usually the school bell was eagerly anticipated, but this time it took everyone by surprise. Some remarked, "Gee, time goes fast when we're talking."

The second session took place shortly before graduation and the impending discharge of several students. One outpatient, Sally, was absent, having run away from home. The group opened with Sheldon announcing that he was preparing a petition to the director for redress of grievances. He read from his verbose and grandiose document, calling for an end to restrictions on patients' sexual conduct and weekend activities and denouncing administrative actions taken without ironclad "proof" of wrongdoing. Kathy deplored Sally's parents, whom she accused of being arbitrary and overly restrictive. (In reality, Sally was given to periods of psychotic dissociation when, belying her usual school-girl appearance and deportment, she would become involved in dangerous, potentially life-threatening activities in unsavory parts of town.) A debate followed about how much worry was appropriate about Sally.

After much fragmented side conversation, the group began teasing Kevin about his "hicky" and how he had gotten it. Implicit in this was concern about Kevin's intermittently drinking himself into a stupor, after which he could remember little of what he had done. As usual, Kevin dismissed others' concerns, claiming that his drinking was not a problem. We commented that we seemed to be talking about what sort of help and limits people needed when they acted in self-destructive ways and seemingly could not control themselves. Sheldon began working on his petition again, urging members to sign. Kathy pointed out that his demands were unlikely to be met and that his "freedoms" were curtailed because he had messed himself up amply enough outside to show that he could not handle them yet. "You ought to get to work to straighten things out with your dad, or get your act together enough to make it on your own, like George did, without messing yourself up; then you can have the freedom to do what you want." She launched into a further spirited defense of the hospital's rules. We observed that Kathy had not always felt that way (to put it mildly). Kathy reflected that she guessed her impending discharge had something to do with it; she was going to have to make it on her own at home and at her new school; maybe if she were staying she would still feel as Sheldon did.

Despite their defensive stance of alienation, cynicism, and mistrust of adults' helpfulness and authority, these adolescents remained hungry for meaningful contact and assistance in bringing order to their chaotic inner and outer lives. Material from two sessions illustrates the usefulness of the group in progressively fostering the corroding sense of isolation and internalizing the locus of control.

Group 3: Issues of Basic Assumptions: Fight/Flight and Pairing, Group Security, and Termination[4]

The group is now in its fourth year. To understand its present functioning, one need go back to its beginnings since early events left a particular stamp on the group's "culture." When we arrived, out-of-control behavior seemed to be the group norm. A particularly menacing male, with grandiose pretensions, often led the group in virulent, verbal attacks on the therapists or in activities designed to provoke constraining reactions from them. His grandiosity was amplified by the fact that his individual therapist was a very senior member of the hospital staff and the patient seemed inclined to trade on this.

At this early stage, insecurity was at its height, and the group could hardly guarantee the physical safety of its members. As incoming therapists, we announced that, while living in a mental hospital afforded many opportunities for "acting crazy," there was little to be gained in providing yet another opportunity for doing so. We wanted the group to be a place to talk about and share this pressing problem. To do this effectively, we would stay in the room, keep to our seats, and listen to one another. We should not, as a group, tolerate physical violence or destruction of property since this would work against the treatment. Departure from these ground rules was understood by the therapists as a sign that the member concerned wished to address the group and verbalize his wishes and urges. From that juncture forward, each manifestation of disruptiveness was taken up and examined with the invitation, often the demand, to *put it in words*.

Early on, paradox was sometimes useful in mobilizing group change. The onset of each session, for example, had been regularly disturbed and delayed by members stomping out to the bathroom and staying there for various periods of time. The therapists, parents of toddlers, made a ritual of beginning each group by asking if anyone who had to "go pee pee" would now do so. This preamble lasted for several weeks until, disgusted with the therapists, the members began using the bathroom before the sessions. The nursery school technique was then put to rest and was never again required.

Changing the "cult of violence" that had possessed the group prior to the arrival of the new therapists was more dramatic. The grandiose and assaultive patient had managed to lure a school aide into the group

187

room with provocative obscenities and the threat of murderous retaliation if restrained. The male therapist interposed himself bodily between the patient and staff member and defused the escalating struggle, insisting that the aide leave the room because "we want to handle this patient in the group." Later, the therapist found himself caught in a cross fire between staff and patients, with the former feeling that the therapists were meddling in what was essentially a disciplinary problem and the latter expressing the view that the member was out of control and should have been restrained as he deserved. Nevertheless, it was a vivid demonstration at a critical time in the group's development that therapists and patients stood together and worked together as a whole in taming the violence and bringing it under the group's control. It was the last time that an aide was needed to quell any behavior in the group. This mutative experience seemed to change the group culture. Patients stayed in the room, kept to their seats, and began to talk. An atmosphere of safety and expectability developed, and the group became a comfortable rather than an intimidating place for both therapists and patients. Over the years, the tradition consolidated, and the group began to be known as the "good" group because of the absence of behavior problems. Patients were referred who were higher functioning and who were judged likely to fit into a group that was largely operating on a verbal level.

As talking became the main mode of expression in the group, loneliness and sexuality became the main topics of discussion. Mostly male, the group often felt like a boys' locker room session. This phase began with reading from a lurid novel some detailed descriptions of the consummation of adolescent longings. At that time, all the group members were quite shy and withdrawn, and many were despairing of ever having a date. One member of the group obtained employment outside the hospital and actually began meeting girls. He would return to the group with tales of his experiences. The contrast between the idealism of the novel and the awkwardness of reality became a theme for the group. Nonetheless, it became clear that many of the boys, too shy to have relationships themselves, were living vicariously through the group member who was able to function on the outside. The group's euphoria grew as our protagonist learned by experience that girls were as interested in him as he was in them. This became less abstract when an attractive female patient was admitted to the group. They immediately paired, taking a place on a shelf in the corner of the room. Having felt that it had created the perfect romantic couple, the group entered a period of therapeutic euphoria that ended with the couple eloping from the hospital and getting married. Once this drastic action was taken, it was acknowledged by nearly all the group members as a poor move, demonstrating bad judgment. This assessment was borne out by subsequent events.

Pairing took on a more menacing quality in the following year. One sixteen-year-old male patient, the son of a schizophrenic mother, was quite preoccupied with fantasies of murder, rape, and mutilation. He occasionally composed poems on these themes that he read to the group. As the lone deviant in the group (in relation to his open expressions of murderousness), this patient was remarkably able to rise to the level of his peers. However, when another patient who shared similar interests became a group member, they immediately formed a subgroup of two. Within several weeks they had stimulated each other to the point of actually getting out of their seats and enacting a "playful" form of rape and murder. That evening they went AWOL and were actually involved in an assault. To a larger extent, the shocked group felt that their actions could have been prevented had we been more attentive to their communications in the group. In a general sense, group members came to feel that future events in the community might be predicted, as it were, by their representation in some form or other in the group.

By the third year, the composition of the group had changed from nearly all boys to nearly all girls. Questions of who is friends with whom, who is whose enemy, and who is talking behind whose back were never far off. The question of confidentiality was tested by various members confessing sordid misdemeanors to the therapists to determine whether the confessions would be passed on to the treatment team. Our position has been that what is said in group remains entirely in the group. An interaction typifying the girls' group phase concerned a patient who was having very severe conflicts with her roommate, leading to several physical attacks. Two boys who were housemates with Della insisted that she talk about her roommate situation in the group, perhaps with the hope of solving it and avoiding further violence. It became clear as the discussion unfolded that Linda and Bess, themselves close friends, felt quite differently about Della's relationship with her roommate. Bess tended to feel that Della was being scapegoated and mistreated on no other grounds than the fact

189

that she was relatively new to the hospital. Linda, on the other hand, felt that Della was playing the role of victim up to the hilt to gain people's sympathy. She had nothing but contempt for such an attitude. Before too long, Linda and Bess were arguing themselves over which view of Della was more accurate. This quickly drifted to complaints about each other, Linda feeling that Bess passively acted the victim in her relationship and Bess accusing Linda of being domineering and aggressive. Meanwhile, Della had moved entirely from the center of attention to a peripheral position while the fighting took place around her. The two friends had turned to enemies before our eyes while discussing a third party with whom neither was particularly involved. Our only intervention was to point out this pattern and comment on how remarkable it was. The group experienced therapeutic euphoria, feeling that perhaps it could actually solve the problems underlying the girls' tendencies toward shifting relationships and allegiances. More often, this euphoria had its counterpart in despair, as many problems were unsolvable, and at times it appeared that the most one could do would be to look at a situation and bemoan it.

At times, being the "good group" itself came to be experienced as a burden. On one such occasion, the group "decorated" the entire room with rolls of toilet paper. Nonetheless, by the end of the hour, it was all picked up and thrown away in the trash cans. On another occasion, a more playful scenario evolved, in which the girls paired off with the female therapist to compile a detailed rating of the physical attributes of all the boys in the division. Disgruntled and left out, the male therapist and three boys in the group tried to ignore them. When this became impossible, one of the boys pushed his way into the middle of the girls' group, grabbed the list, and a playful wrestling match ensued. Escaping from the girls, the thief ran out through another room in which a class was taking place. The teacher placed him on detention for that afternoon. Returning to the group sober and sullen, it was negotiated that he would return the list to the girls if they, as a group, would plead his case with the teacher who had given him detention. At the end of the group, the girls made an earnest plea, claiming the disrupter was not responsible for his actions since they were a product of the group at large. They were successful in winning him a reprieve.

At the end of each school year, a large percentage of group members leave because of graduation from high school or discharge from the hospital. These endings mark significant transitions to new and often uncertain living situations and have been particularly challenging for our groups. Staying involved with peers whom one may never see again is a difficult task. A tension develops as the group wavers between withdrawal and fragmentation or using the last hours together to experience parting fully. Several recent sessions illustrate this tension.

As year's end approached, two-thirds of the group were slated to be discharged or otherwise move from the area. The group began to slip into what seemed like a depressive and hopeless state of dejection. Walkmans and earphones began to appear, isolating the wearers into states of seemingly autistic self-stimulation. Comments of the members were generally confined to denigrating the group ("This group sucks"), with occasional remarks of, "It used to be good, but that was a long time ago." The therapists, too, began to withdraw, abandoning hope that anything could be accomplished as the end approached. In earlier times, optimism had prevailed, but those times seemed long gone. It was hard to remain interested in a group doomed to disbandment.

In the supervisory group session, the therapists' depletion became noticeable. Was the therapists' withdrawal fueling the group deterioration? Had the individual group members sensed the therapists' loss of interest and responded themselves with withdrawal? Or, alternatively, were the therapists themselves swept into the group process, influenced by the general tone of despondency and despair? One could not tell. Nonetheless, the therapists were admonished not to abandon ship, to try to remain the group's therapists to the very end.

With new therapeutic enthusiasm from the supervision, we returned, interpreting the group's withdrawal as related to impending good-byes faced by the members. The group's task appeared to be to remain involved with each other, knowing that relationships among members would end in several weeks. We questioned whether there was unfinished business for the group, suggesting that the good-bye might be a fuller and richer one if this could come out. Indeed, the impending end of the group might even represent a unique opportunity to speak more candidly than before. This idea was picked up by a powerful group member. "I think Fenton is absolutely right. We could really benefit from a serious talk before the end. There are a lot of tensions, still, among us." Other members agreed, and slowly the Walkmans came off. The dangers of such a plan were raised by group members. Things might get out of hand; emotions might run too high. Someone might be ganged up on. Feelings might be hurt. A member suggested that rules were needed. One person was to talk at a time. Two people would not be allowed to gang up on one. No one was to be allowed to get up and leave the room in the heat of the discussion. There must be order. By the end of the session, the organizers of the plan solicited each member's agreement to attend the next week, form a close circle, and adhere to all the stated rules.

The following week, the group convened promptly. Linda and Bess, whose formerly close friendship had dissolved over the course of the year, began. Linda said that her feelings had been quite hurt by what she saw as Bess's withdrawal from her several months earlier. Bess felt that it was Linda who had begun to withdraw, and she herself had felt hurt. A tangled story emerged. Bess had become pregnant months earlier. Linda, who considered herself to be Bess's best friend, had found out about the pregnancy from a third person on Bess's unit. Linda had felt insulted that Bess, whom she hoped would confide in her, had not herself told Linda. Bess was evidently under the direction of her unit chief not to discuss the pregnancy with anyone, although the teenagers in her house, including the one who had told Linda, knew about this. Bess's boyfriend, who had impregnated her, was jealous of Bess and Linda's relationship and threw tantrums whenever Bess expressed her intention to spend time with Linda. At that time, Bess had chosen the boyfriend. It seemed that a simple misunderstanding had gotten out of hand, but other aspects of the situation began to emerge. During the pregnancy, Bess had become withdrawn and suicidal. After she finally did tell Linda, she admonished Linda to tell no one else. During one of Bess's absences from the group, however, Linda revealed the secret to the group. This, of course, later got back to Bess, who felt that Linda had betrayed her confidence. Linda, in turn, argued that she had done so not out of a wish to perpetuate gossip but rather out of the belief that to bring it up in the group over Bess's objections would be best for Bess. Other group members began to relate experiences analogous to this with Linda. Several months earlier, Casey, an outpatient, had begun drinking and abusing drugs. Linda had taken a hard line with her, refusing to go out drinking. Further, she had spoken to Casey's administrator and told her that Casey was drinking and using drugs and was out of control. The administrator gave Linda two days to confront Casey face to face, which Linda was unable to do. The administrator finally confronted

Casey herself, informing her that one of her peers had "told on her." Casey went to each of her friends, including Linda, asking them if they had done it. Linda denied that it had been she. Casey later found out otherwise. She, too, felt that her trust had been betrayed by Linda. A discussion ensued regarding "telling." There was nearly complete agreement that there were circumstances under which "telling" was justified but that Linda's inability to confront the people whom she "told" on was unacceptable. Linda admitted her cowardice, agreeing that this was a problem for her, and the session ended on what seemed to be a conciliatory note.

To the therapists' surprise, the next group began even more fragmented and chaotic than those before the therapists' intervention. Ginny, a group member, placed herself in the back room. Linda was absorbed with the computer. The boys admonished the therapists for "really fucking up this time." An atmosphere of tension prevailed. One by one, the girls drifted into the back room with Ginny, finally asking the female cotherapist to join them. The council of women, including the female therapist, emerged five or ten minutes later. They reported that they could not bear the tension of the group and that the group's last meeting had been very upsetting to each of them. The therapists were astounded. We had thought that the discussion had been productive and the tone conciliatory. Each of the girls expressed their fearfulness of Linda, evidently fearing some sort of retaliation as a result of what seemed, to the therapists, to be last week's relatively mild confrontation. We had underestimated the group's fear of its own anger, now projected onto Linda, who had become in fantasy a fearsome and menacing figure.

The last group session of the year arrived and the question raised, "What shall we do with it?" "Let's be destructive; remember when we toilet-papered the room?" "Let's go outside and smoke." The group, absent the therapists, moved toward the windows, removed screens, and opened the windows, and several members hopped out onto the lawn, lighting cigarettes. "Are we going to get into trouble? What are you going to do?" "We're trying to be therapists, not disciplinarians," we replied. Having smoked, the group came in, closing the windows and replacing the screens. "Well, we have to say good-bye," Linda said. "Everyone should make a speech." She went around the group saying good-bye to every member. Jack, who was leaving to return to an unstable home situation, said that he could not make a speech but could only scream. Standing on his desk, he did so, loudly. Casey, who was graduating the next day, had been a quiet and withdrawn group member during her four years at the Lodge. Remarkably, she too stood on her desk and gave a short good-bye speech: "I know I haven't talked very much in the group, but I hope everyone recognized that it's not because I don't care or haven't paid attention. It's just that I'm self-conscious and think what I have to say is stupid." In turn, each group member gave what seemed to be the best good-bye speech they could. Bess's speech, delivered from desk top, seemed to sum up the year well: "I want to thank everyone for being in this group with me. Sometimes it's been very distressing and sometimes it's been enlightening. Sometimes it's been just plain boring, but I think we've learned that that's what you have to expect from a group. I will miss you." As therapists, we left feeling satisfied that we had traveled with the group, albeit, with many detours, to a good end. At least for this year.

What conclusions have we arrived at from our experiences with the group? First, like the individual teenager, the group is moody: one day euphoric with romanticism, the next sullen and withdrawn in a manner that defies prediction or adequate understanding. In the face of this, once a safe environment is assured, the best therapeutic attitude is a phenomenological one. That is, approach each group freshly, with as few preconceived notions as possible, with the aim of understanding what is going on at the moment. Therapists' comments are best confined to things that are quite obvious and have been observed by all. The group is poised to blame its difficulties on the leaders and similarly place enormous pressure on the leaders to become disciplinarians and oppressive authorities. Direct efforts at maintaining discipline seem only to gratify the group's wish to experience itself as mistreated victims of an oppressive adult regime. The therapists' responsibility is to guarantee a safe environment where issues can be discussed in confidence; beyond this, the group determines its direction. If a feeling of security can be created, we have been impressed with the extent to which, underneath various sorts of behaviors, the adolescent longs to open him- or herself to the group or to a group of peers.

Group 4: Issues of Being Different and Victims of Fate[5]

This adolescent group has been conducted by two female therapists—a psychiatrist and a social worker—for about one and a half years. Currently, there are seven members: four inpatients (Carl, Sairy, Louise, and Leslie) and three day students (Doris, Tom, and Martin). Sairy is very much the dominant member of the group, with up and down affects and a capacity for rage that makes her much feared both in the group and in the milieu. When she is "good," she is charming and contributing, but, when she is "bad," she can totally disrupt the group. She is also one of three adoptees in the group and the one with the most disturbed preadoption and adoption history. Her sense of being different (in the group, in the milieu, at home, and in the world in general) is also episodic, and, when she feels different, she becomes inimical and destructive. She has her favorites in the group and holds court among them. In the cottage, her room is designated the "Empress Suite."

In the past years, the group was exposed to an administrative change that had reverberations for some time. Carl had been discharged from the hospital to his home after only eight months and then attended the Lodge school as a day student. This was quite unusual since most of the inpatients stay a minimum of two years. The group, led by Sairy, interpreted this as meaning that, unlike the rest of them, he was well adjusted and had a home and family to go to. Well adjusted Carl was not. The fantasy life that he acted out from time to time made him dangerous because he played with explosives. His personal myth ran a different course: he empathized deeply with the victims of terrorist attacks and pondered ways of exterminating the perpetrators. He came from a military family that had set up rigid rules for him to follow, and he conformed to their expectations. When his violent inner life was externalized occasionally, as when he blew up the mailboxes of people he disliked, it brought him into trouble with the police and eventually got him hospitalized. When Carl was admitted to Chestnut Lodge, he conformed to the rules and regulations, was civil but never close to his peers, studied well, and did well at school, took special care of his health, and cooperated well with his individual therapist.

He accepted the need for his hospitalization and made no complaints about it since this was what the authorities had decreed. He accepted the need for group psychotherapy and participated actively in the group, talking about his problems of depression and anger. He told the group that in the past he would often lose his temper and punch holes in walls. This was surprising to the other members since he habitually appeared calm and controlled. He was outraged by the overt hostility and nonconformity of his fellow patients and questioned the need for Sairy and Louise to be so persistently mean and hypercritical. As a result, both girls toned down their negative comments for a while. Carl always listened attentively to others in the group and offered them feedback. He seemed to be a very good group patient except that his inhibitions had an inhibitive effect on the members. In one instance, Doris began sharing with the group her infatuation for an older, unavailable man, a very sensitive topic for her. Several of the male members not only paid no attention to her but drowned out her remarks with raucous interchanges. After a while, Doris left the group, and, in her absence, Carl admonished the rowdy members. When Doris returned, he pressed her to continue her story, but she refused to discuss the matter any further. Toward the end of the session, both Doris and Carl were angry but tight lipped, and one of the therapists asked them to tell how they felt. Carl blurted out, "Talking doesn't help; it's better to punch holes with your fists!" It was clear that his rescue fantasies had not worked out in practice and that this had infuriated him.

Carl became more reluctant to discuss his feelings but managed to control his anger during the group sessions. In the milieu, however, his aggression was liberated from its straitjacket, and he took a punch at Sairy. The therapists wondered what he had to say about this and suggested that it might do both parties good to settle their differences in the group, but verbally. The therapists explained that it was preferable to express anger verbally and personally rather than blow up installations impersonally. Both patients then presented their case to the group. It became clear in the discussion that both had a share in the blame. The group became not only a forum for resolving conflict but a temporary repository for conscience. When Carl acted out in the milieu in other ways, he would report back to the group. When he went AWOL, for instance, he brought the behavior in for scrutiny. He had gone because he had felt a nostalgic yearning to visit his old haunts and friends and had returned because it was the right thing to do. His protagonist, Sairy, recalled going AWOL in the past but now judged it to be unproductive. It was better to work with the staff toward a proper discharge from the hospital. That sounded a little too good to be true coming from the tempestuous Sairy, but it had the advantage of putting Carl in his place. He was no longer the paragon of mental health, slumming with the "screwed up kids," but someone who could do with a longer period of inpatient treatment. If he was going to leave, which the group now found was imminent, they had no further interest in him and excluded him pointedly from their interactions. They punished him not only for leaving but for feeling, in contrast to them, that he was well enough to leave. With this anger and resentment directed toward him, Carl struggled not to overreact to the segregation and ridicule. Under pressure, he broke the group rule of confidentiality, was soundly taken to task, but accepted responsibility for the breech of conduct and apologized. But nothing he could do at this point could compensate for his terminating. When he spoke about his experiences in the outside world (he was now a day student living at home but continuing to attend the group), the other group members would not listen to him. He no longer belonged to the group as far as they were concerned. He was too different or thought he was. In their opinion, he was being discharged only because the hospital staff had been taken in by him and was too soft with him. What was unfair was that others, like themselves, were being kept in hospitals forever. The attack was fueled by the envy, jealousy, and sadness of the "interminables."

The theme of victimization was sparked off by this discussion. Life was so unfair. Louise talked about her predicament. She was adopted, and her adopting parents divorced when she was four years old. She felt that she was first thrown out of her adoptive mother's home and later from her adoptive father's home when she was sent away to Chestnut Lodge. She realized that she had problems and had to work them out, but she felt that it was hard to do so so far away from home. The group resonated to the thought that parents often give up their children to hospitals and relinquished the responsibility of caring for them. Sairy mentioned that her adoptive father and stepmother were very rejecting of her and that she could not get on with her adoptive mother. The theme of victimization continued to occupy the group since each member's parents had either given them up or given up on them. At this point, Louise and Sairy began an angry tirade against the group therapists, whom they perceived to be as uncaring as their parents and as easily forgetting the group after work hours and on the weekends, when the therapists could enjoy themselves and be with their families while the patients remained stuck in the hospital, feeling isolated, abandoned, and bored. Louise began to cry and said, "It is so unfair." She added, "People put you in a hospital when they don't care about you. . . . A lot of people on the outside do things wrong, and yet they are not hospitalized." The group was fervently in agreement.

When Carl was discharged from the group, everyone denied that they would miss him even though he had been with the group for a year. At the time of discharge, Carl was better able to verbalize his feelings of anger instead of acting out. The members dealt with his departure by elaborating a shared group fantasy pertaining to why they were where they were. According to this, they were victims of fate, innocent and helpless in the face of oppressive forces, beginning with rejecting parents, traumatic environments, and endless physical and psychological stresses, with everything culminating inevitably in hospitalization. Thus, they had every right to protest against their plight and every right to compensation in the way of attention and sympathy to counteract their misery. The fantasy (not without underpinnings in fact) was especially appealing to the adoptees with their histories of abandonment. This piece of personalized mythology arose with the impending departure of Carl and was reinforced by the entry of Ted, an adoptee with a severely conflicted relationship with his adoptive mother. The climate of the group at this stage was therefore highly congenial to Ted, and he made the most of it. He was unwanted at home, different from his parents, who had a natural and favored daughter, dumped in a hospital, and placed in a group for reasons beyond his comprehension. It was all grossly unjust. The group could not agree more, and they joined in blaming parents who were unable to care for their children and were not meant to have children in the first place. They had been born different, had lived differently, and had been treated differently by their families, and the differences were being further accentuated by hospitalization.

The shared group fantasy (with its emphases on difference and abandonment) served several purposes for the members: they were not responsible for getting better since they were not responsible for getting ill in the first place; they could experience some degree of togetherness in sharing the fantasy; they could externalize through the fantasy their feelings of resentment, envy, and an aching sadness onto scapegoats, like Carl, who had the effrontery to have things going for him rather than against him; and the fantasy served, for a while, as a token of admission for new members into the group. Some months later, it seemed as if the transitional fantasy had been worked through and disappeared from the scene. Sairy was able to tell a newcomer who came in with a chip on her shoulder that this was the place to get well and become similar to other adolescents on the outside and that one should make good use of the treatment opportunities offered. Sairy had now rejoined her family and continued to attend the Lodge school and the group. She had vacated the "Empress Suite" and her cottage and seemed altogether less infused with the admixture of grandiosity, self-abasement, and self-absorption than at the beginning of the group. She no longer controlled the group to the same extent with her vitriolic attacks and vilifications, and the group consequently opened up considerably.

Conclusions

The therapists themselves are the single most important therapeutic instrument brought to bear on the life and work of the group. They need to be open to experiencing the wide range of often intense feelings evoked in the course of working with the adolescent group. There is little doubt, as well, that the cotherapists' ability to talk calmly with one another, in the midst of the powerful primitive affects generated in a group of disturbed adolescents, facilitates a processing and working through that must take place within the group therapists in order for them adequately to contain the group.

The therapists cannot hope to be certain about the meanings of all the events unfolding in the group but, rather, must be able to tolerate a moderate degree of ambiguity. Nor can they anticipate what will develop in the group or be prepared adequately to deal with every conceivable contingency that may arise. They must have a certain amount of flexibility and sometimes may even seem to be inconsistent.

The adolescent group is rich in metaphorical expressions, and therapists are well advised to attend to these expressions closely. Actions and exchanges that seem incidental on one level often reveal significant group dynamics. The therapists should seek to understand the meaning that details and seemingly offhand remarks have for the group.

It is useful to interpret group defenses and to identify the roles that group members assume in order to avoid conflict. These defensive maneuvers are highly varied across members but, at the same time, highly consistent for specific individuals. That is, each member has his or her own repertoire of avoidance behaviors. Interventions that predict group or individual responses are quite effective. Once the therapists are able to discern that, when A happens, B invariably follows, they are in a position to make interpretations that have a high probability of being accurate and accepted.

Projection and splitting are common in groups of seriously disordered adolescents. The therapists need to recognize and accept these projections. By accepting and examining what they come to feel in the course of working with the group, the therapists have an opportunity to process, modify, detoxify, and articulate these affective experiences for the group.

One of the most potentially demoralizing problems confronting adolescent group therapists is the strong resistance and therapeutic nihilism that often permeate the group. Disturbed adolescents in particular will repeatedly and vigorously assert that the group is useless. Therapists would be mistaken and misled in concluding that the group is unimportant and ineffective. More than anything else such statements reflect the troubled adolescent's own sense of futility.

Analytically oriented groups have become an integral part of the Chestnut Lodge experience for adolescent inpatients, and, in keeping with the long-term perspective, the same therapists have been in action for some years. Between them, they have accumulated a good deal of technical experience that they share weekly with one another. The different vignettes presented indicate very clearly the different therapeutic styles that have emerged over time despite the theoretical and technical biases of the group supervisor. The therapists are experienced in their own right and in the world of individual therapy, and a large part of the management of their group stems from acquired therapeutic skills. In this sense, the group seminars are very much a peer experience in a learning group in which everyone seeks to learn and to teach. The group therapies and the group seminars thus proceed hand in hand for the benefit of both patients and therapists. For the patients, not only does the group offer space for holding, supporting, facilitating, sharing, containing, mirroring, experiencing, and deframing, but it is also in the nature of a transitional phenomenon, and, in time, as Winnicott would have predicted, it is destined to be discarded unmourned, having played its essential part in integrating the patients into their social milieu.

NOTES

1. The cotherapists and reporters are Denise Fort and Laurice McAfee.

2. Group members are listed in their order of seniority in the group.

3. The cotherapists and reporters are Robert King and William Hoppe.

4. The cotherapists and reporters are Wayne Fenton and Judith Abramowitz.

5. The cotherapists and reporters are Camille Woodbury and Judith Abramowitz.

REFERENCES

Alonso, A., and Rutan, J. S. 1988. The experience of shame and the restoration of self-respect in group therapy. *International Journal of Group Psychotherapy* 38(1): 3–27.

Bion, W. 1977. *Seven Servants*. New York: Aronson.

Bowlby, J. 1971. *Attachment and Loss*, vol. 2. New York: Basic.

Foulkes, S. H., and Anthony, E. J. 1984. *Group Psychotherapy*. London: Maresfield.

Freud, S. 1923. The ego and the id. *Standard Edition* 19:19–27. London: Hogarth, 1961.

Loewald, H. 1980. *Papers on Psychoanalysis*. London: Allen & Unwin.

Milner, M. 1971. *On Not Being Able to Paint*. London: Heinemann.

Shapiro, R.; Zinner, J.; Berkowitz, D.; and Shapiro, E. 1975. The impact of group experiences on adolescent development. In M. Sugar, ed. *The Adolescent in Group and Family Therapy*. New York: Brunner/Mazel.

Winnicott, D. W. 1958. *Collected Papers*. New York: Basic.

Yalom, I. 1983. *Inpatient Group Psychotherapy*. New York: Basic.

11 PERSONALITY AND DEMOGRAPHIC DIFFERENCES AMONG DIFFERENT TYPES OF ADJUSTMENT TO AN ADOLESCENT MILIEU

RICHARD C. FRITSCH, ROBERT W. HOLMSTROM, WELLS GOODRICH, AND REBECCA E. RIEGER

This exploratory study examined the relation between different styles of adjustment and selected patient characteristics as a way to generate hypotheses about the interaction of different subgroups of patients with the therapeutic milieu. The first task of this study, therefore, was to derive clusters or types of adolescents with similar behavioral responses to the structure and program of the milieu. The characteristics of patients who populated each adjustment subtype were then examined, with an eye toward common personality variables or demographic characteristics within each cluster. A second, more theoretically based goal was to determine whether a measure of maturity of object representations would shed some light on clusters that appeared to contain dissimilar patients, especially where the adjustment was not of resistance but rather of cooperation and compliance.

When an adolescent is admitted to a long-term, psychodynamically oriented residential facility, the initial task of the treatment staff is to make an assessment of the milieu's capacity to contain the patient's behavior. This involves an assessment of the severity and dynamics of the adolescent's disturbance along with a prescription for how the therapeutic milieu can make a contribution toward ameliorating the problems. The primary diagnostic question is an assessment of the state of the ego. Misdiagnosis and misapplication of treatment modalities can have serious negative consequences. Underestimating the severity of the dysfunction and the inappropriate use of expressive treatment can convert a severely disturbed adolescent into one who is intractably ill (Miller 1980). Overestimating the level of the dysfunction can mean that an adolescent will miss the opportunity to use expressive treatment to make substantial character changes and stabilize at a lower level of adjustment than otherwise might have been the case.

The nursing staff has an important role in the assessment of the psychological capabilities since they have contact with the adolescents twenty-four hours a day. The milieu is the site of the therapeutic action in the initial stage of treatment for severely disturbed children and adolescents (Masterson 1972; Redl 1972; Rinsley 1980) and has been seen as the most salient therapeutic agent for the initial treatment of the disruptive adolescent (Crabtree 1982; Davis and Raffee 1985; Rossman and Knesper 1976). Characteristically, the nursing staff tends to form its own assessment of the treatability of the newly admitted adolescents based on the level of management problems the patient creates. Acting-out adolescents are typically viewed as more seriously disturbed than cooperative, compliant adolescents. Concerns about violence and runaway behavior take priority over other less disruptive adjustments. Disorganized, psychotic adolescents form a subgroup of their own. Based on these categories the prescription for the milieu worker is relatively clear: support the disorganized adolescent's adaptive functioning, contain and confront the acting-out adolescent's behavior, and reward those adolescents who comply with the ward regimen.

Apart from the overtly psychotic patient, we need to ask whether the most difficult patients on the unit are the most disturbed and whether they carry the poorest prognoses. Very little has been written about the interaction between diagnosis and behavioral presentation in the milieu. In adult populations, the organizing and calming effects of the structure and support of the hospital for borderline (Brown 1981) and psychotic (Gunderson, Will, and Mosher 1983) patients have been documented. For adolescents, resistance is viewed as axiomatic for patients with borderline-level personality organization (Goodrich 1987; Masterson 1972; Rinsley 1980). Other types of adjustment, such as the disorganized, compliant, or model adolescent patient, have not been similarly described. It is our view that the relation between the patient's behavior and the state of his or her ego is complex and multiply determined and that there is a paradoxical relation between severity of illness and behavioral difficulties on admission. Active resistance in the initial stage may augur for increased capacity to benefit from treatment rather than for a negative outcome.

Outcome studies have identified the positive prognostic value of an assessment of an adolescent's capacity for interpersonal relationships (Garber 1972; Logan, Barnhart, and Gossett 1982; Masterson and Costello 1980). In each of these studies, there was a direct relation between improvement and a higher capacity for interpersonal relatedness at follow-up. The patient's capacity for interpersonal relationships, however, was not always apparent to the treatment staff on admission or throughout the course of hospitalization. Logan et al. (1982) examined the components of interpersonal relationships as prognostic indicators. Using measures of interpersonal closeness in several domains, they found that the adolescent's peer popularity and his or her capacity to form a relationship with a member of the nursing staff were predictive of good outcome. They failed to find a relation between the *staff's* assessment of the nature or quality of their relationship with the adolescent and the patient's outcome. The authors speculated that the staff ratings might have been influenced "by the youngster's apparent conformity to institutional goals and procedures" (p. 491). This finding raises an interesting question about the relation between presence or absence of resistant behavior as a barometer of psychopathology. Compliance may mask more severe pathology, while resistance to the staff in general, when accompanied by good peer relations, may be indicative of healthy object relations and therefore greater potential for positive outcome. What may appear to be trust and relatedness may be passive dependency and fear of autonomy in disguise.

Diagnosis from an Object Relations Perspective

In resolving the apparent paradox, an assessment of the adolescents' levels of object relations, determined independently from their peer and staff interactions, should prove useful. One potentially fruitful paradigm for categorizing adolescents on the basis of their level of object relations ego rather than on symptoms or behavior has been proposed by Rinsley (1980). He divided adolescents into two groups on the basis of their level of object relations rather than on diagnosis or symptoms. The first group, the "presymbiotic group," failed to advance beyond a symbiotic relationship with the maternal object. This group is characterized by a weak, easily disorganized ego, lack of autonomy, and an inability to form reliable reality constructs.

Individuals in Rinsley's second group are called "symbiotic." They have failed to achieve ego autonomy or to differentiate from the symbiotic attachment to the maternal object. Here, representations of self and other are split along the affective dimensions of "good" or rewarding self- and object representations and "bad" or frustrating self- and object representations. These patients act out to maintain the split between the rewarding and the frustrating aspects of the self and the object as a defense against the experience of the negative affects associated with attempts at the integration of the frustrating and the rewarding introjects.

Logically, a third group would be called "postsymbiotic." Rinsley does not describe this group since he feels that most adolescents who require residential treatment generally have not reached this level of personality development. For this group, self- and object representations are stable. Repression replaces splitting since the primary defense and conflict involves more evolved psychic agencies (superego, ego, and id) rather than preoedipally structured object relational units.

The general usefulness of this type of subgrouping over the more traditional categorization of psychotic, borderline, and neurotic, which it closely resembles, is questionable. Nevertheless, characterizing adolescents in object relational terms does allow for some differential predictions about their response to the milieu.

An object-relations perspective suggests that, on critical indices, the response to hospitalization will not be a linear function of increasingly more adaptive or prosocial responses that correlates with decreasing severity of illness. Instead, this object-relations perspective suggests a more complex relation for those indices that relate to the adolescent's employment of oppositional, acting-out, or hostile behaviors as means of resistance.

The symbiotic adolescent directly or covertly resists the influence of the hospital program and personnel. The predominance of negative introjects and the use of splitting, denial, and projection (Kernberg 1975) that characterize this pathology from an object-relations perspective is expected to be manifested by acting out against the perceived oppressor (e.g., the staff) in an attempt to maintain reunion or refusion fantasies with the object. Although the acting-out behavior is the most difficult to control, it is not developmentally the most disturbed. Therefore, we would expect those groups in which acting out or resistance are the distinguishing characteristics to be populated by adolescents with relatively more maturely developed object representations.

It is hypothesized that, for adolescents whose pathology is more severe and for whom the basic problems are at the level of differentiating inner world versus outer reality, the hospital environment will act as an external, auxiliary ego that can help the patient organize and respond with more appropriate behavior. The central struggle for this group, according to object-relations theory, is in maintaining adequate reality testing. In these adolescents, there may be little capacity for empathy or an inability to engage in meaningful interpersonal relationships with both peers and adults. They will, however, manifest less disruptive, antisocial, and rebellious behaviors than adolescents operating at the part-object level. Therefore, we would expect adolescents with very low levels of object relations to be overrepresented in groups in which disorganization and withdrawal are the distinguishing characteristics.

Additionally, adolescents with less mature object representations who have other ego strengths and who can use the structure of the milieu to reorganize will be found in groups in which the presentation is one of compliance, trust, and engagement. This prediction is paradoxical to the usual direct relation between level of maturity of object relations and more adaptive or socially acceptable behaviors.

For adolescents who have achieved a degree of object constancy and operate at the level of whole objects, it is hypothesized that they will have the capacity to make immediate use of the supportive and therapeutic functions of the milieu and of the treatment staff. These adolescents will be able to view the staff in more differentiated, less distorted ways, and cooperation and engagement will be evident. It is hypothesized that these adolescents will respond to the residential milieu with cooperative and organized behavior.

These hypotheses suggest that a significant portion of the variance associated with adjustment to the milieu can be explained by the maturity of the patient's object representations but that the relation will not be a straightforward, linear one between increased capacity for relationships and prosocial adaptation on the unit. Instead, it is hypothesized that patients with the most primitive object representations would be found both in the most disorganized group and in the most compliant and cooperative group.

206

While we believe that a measure of object representations will make a contribution toward understanding adjustment types, an adolescent's entry into a residential milieu is a function of many variables in addition to personality variables, of which level of object relations is only one. Social psychological factors such as conscious motivation for treatment, experience in other institutional settings, the culture and climate of the unit when the adolescent arrives, and the treatment philosophy of the staff all contribute to the variance associated with adjustment. Other patient variables that we believe influence adjustment are age, gender, level of intelligence, intactness of sensorium, and adoptive status (Fullerton, Goodrich, and Berman 1986). Though we could not measure social psychological variables in this study, we did attend to a number of demographic and personality variables as a way to understand, in addition to object relations, what can account for variance associated with different adjustment patterns.

An understanding of the patient characteristics of adolescents who populate different subgroups of adjustment to the milieu would clarify the accuracy of the milieu-developed assessments, which presuppose a direct relation between disruption and severity of illness. Through the examination of different subtypes, we hope to provide information that would generate new hypotheses about treatment interventions for different groups.

Procedures

SETTING

The study was conducted in conjunction with the treatment research program at the Chestnut Lodge Research Institute, Rockville, Maryland. Chestnut Lodge is a long-term residential facility with a capacity of thirty adolescent and/or child beds. The adolescent/child service is a self-contained unit of the hospital and has been described in detail elsewhere (Goodrich 1987).

SUBJECTS

Subjects for this study were chosen from consecutive admissions to the Chestnut Lodge Adolescent and Child Division from 1978 through

207

1984. Of the 119 adolescents who were admitted during this time, eighty-one met the following criteria for inclusion in the study: age between thirteen and nineteen; no evidence of mental retardation; and valid Rorschach and Chestnut Lodge Adolescent Interaction Report (CLAIR) protocols. In achieving interpretable clusters, the sample was reduced by ten subjects. The remaining seventy-one subjects were almost exclusively from white upper- and upper-middle-class families, with nearly equal numbers of males (thirty-seven) and females (thirty-four). Age at admission, by design, ranged from 12.5 to 18.5 years, with a mean age of 15.6 years. The IQ level of the sample was slightly higher than that of the normal population ($M = 104$, S.D. $= 12$). These demographic characteristics are quite representative of the overall sample of adolescents receiving treatment at Chestnut Lodge.

In addition to the high socioeconomic level, there are several distinguishing features of the adolescents at Chestnut Lodge. In a majority of cases, the adolescents have had a previous psychiatric hospitalization (75 percent). It is not uncommon for these patients to have had multiple short- or moderate-term stays prior to admission. Second, while there is a range of diagnoses present among the adolescent patients, including severe neurotic disorders, impulse disorders, affective disorders, conduct disorders, and various schizophrenic disorders, the largest diagnostic group can be described as chronic, moderately severe borderline, narcissistic, or mixed personality disorders.

INSTRUMENTS

The data in the study included (1) verbatim Rorschach protocols, (2) an experimental version of the (CLAIR), (3) the Global Assessment Scale (GAS) and (4) demographic information.

MEASUREMENT OF MATURITY OF OBJECT
REPRESENTATIONS

The Concept of the Object on the Rorschach Scale was developed by Blatt, Brooks, Brenneis, and Schimek (1976). It provides a score on a continuum from primitive to mature object representations (ROR-SCORE) derived from an analysis of the structural components of the subjects' human responses to the Rorschach. This scale was applied to human content responses from verbatim Rorschach data. Details of the scoring procedures are presented in Appendix A.

This score was used in two ways. As a continuous measure, it was included in discriminant analyses. Second, the patients were subdivided into four equal-number groups on the basis of this object representation score. These groups represented low, low-middle, high-middle, and high levels of maturity of object representations.

SEVERITY OF ILLNESS

The GAS, a widely used 100-point global rating scale for evaluating the overall functioning of a subject over a given time period, was used as a measure of severity of illness. The GAS has been incorporated into DSM-III-R as Axis 5. Adequate reliability, especially with trained raters, has been established, with interjudge correlations reported between .61 and .91 (Endicott, Spitzer, Fleiss, and Cohen 1976).

The GAS ratings were completed retrospectively from admission notes by two trained raters as part of the research program at Chestnut Lodge. Reliability of these raters was determined to be similar to the reliability reported in the literature (Pearson $r = .82$).

MEASUREMENT OF REALITY TESTING

A measure of reality testing was obtained by using the $X + \%$ (X plus percentage) from the Rorschach protocols. The $X + \%$ was determined by summing the total number of good form responses within the domain of all responses using form as a determinant and dividing by the total number of responses in which form was used. (The determination of what constituted good form was based on the criteria established by Beck [1949].) It is important to note that this percentage, therefore, was based on a different set of responses than were those that were used to calculate the Object Representation score (RORSCORE).

MEASUREMENT OF BEHAVIOR

The CLAIR (Yates, Fritsch, Fullerton, and Goodrich 1988) is a behavioral checklist on which two dimensions of patient behavior, socialization and symptomatology, are recorded by the nursing staff.

The CLAIR is based on a combination of the Inpatient Multidimensional Psychiatric Scale (IMPS) (Lorr, Klett, and McNair 1963) and socialization behaviors and psychiatric symptoms constructed by the Chestnut Lodge Research Institute on the basis of behavior identified by the nursing staff as clinically relevant for hospitalized adolescents. After the patient has been in residence for one month, it is completed by the member of the nursing staff who best knows the patient. As it was used in this study, it had nine scales (see table 1). A reliability study of the instrument conducted in 1979 found adequate reliability.

CLUSTER FORMATION

In order to identify subtypes of adolescents in terms of admission behavior, a cluster analysis was employed. Cluster analysis divides a sample of cases into relatively homogeneous subgroups or clusters on one or more dimensions. Cluster analysis attempts to minimize differences within each subgroup while simultaneously maximizing differences among subgroups or clusters. After a sample is divided into discrete clusters on certain specifically designated characteristics, the clusters can be examined more closely on a variety of other dimensions. The analysis, essentially a statistical means of creating a classification or a taxonomy, has been used to identify patient types in psychiatric outcome studies (Coyne, Whitmarsh, Clarkin, and Canfield 1986).

A cluster analysis (BMDP P2M) was performed to sort patients into types using five of the CLAIR scales as dependent variables. Since we were interested in looking at different behavioral adjustments to the

TABLE 1
CHESTNUT LODGE ADOLESCENT INTERACTION REPORT SCALES

1. HOS	Hostile actions and verbal expression
2. EXC	Excited, restless, and pressured behavior on the unit
3. OBEYS	Compliance with unit rules and routines
4. TRUST	Trust and engagement with staff and peers
5. PEER	Engagement with the peer group
6. RTD	Psychological withdrawal (includes motor retardation and interpersonal isolation)
7. DEPRES	Symptoms of depression
8. PCP...........	Symptoms of perceptual distortion
9. GRN	Grandiosity, grandiose ideals, delusions of grandeur

milieu, only those scales that focused on the response to the milieu were used. These were HOS (hostility), EXC (excited, pressured behavior on the unit), OBEYS (compliance with unit rules and routines), TRUST (trust and engagement with adults), and PEER (engagement with the peer group). The scales that measured symptoms of severe psychopathology were excluded from the cluster formation on the basis of the assumption that inclusion of these variables would tend to sort patients primarily by level of psychopathology rather than by response to the milieu.

A number of procedures were employed in the attempt to achieve discrete clusters for this small sample. Outliers were eliminated by running analyses with large numbers of clusters and eliminating those cases that formed clusters of only one case. Analyses of smaller numbers of clusters (four to eight) also were performed, and a decision to use a solution using six clusters was made on the basis of ease of interpretation of the clusters, percentage of variance accounted for, and division of cases into clusters that had reasonable membership frequency. Outliers from these clusters were also eliminated, deleting those cases from each cluster that deviated considerably from the cluster seed (distance > .30). These procedures reduced the number of cases from eighty-one to seventy-one, as mentioned previously.

Results

Given the nature of the statistical techniques employed, the relative arbitrariness of the decisions used in constructing the clusters, and the small sample size, the results of this pilot study should be viewed as speculative and hypothesis generating.

The description of the salient characteristics of each of the six clusters generated by this cluster solution and the differentiation of the personality and demographic dimensions across clusters involves multiple comparisons. Figure 1 provides a profile of the behavioral, demographic, and personality variables for each cluster. An inspection of these profiles shows the similarity between clusters 1 and 2, 3 and 4, and 5 and 6. Values for demographic, behavioral, and personality variables for each cluster are shown in Appendices B–D.

To determine which of these variables maximally discriminate among the six clusters, the cluster solution was subjected to a stepwise discriminant function analysis. A stepwise discriminant analysis first

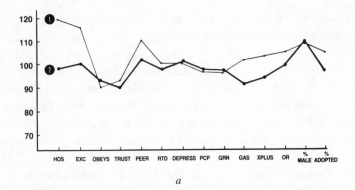

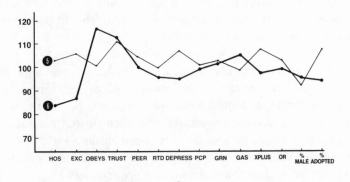

Fig. 1.—*a*, Clusters 1 and 2, borderline. *b*, Clusters 3 and 4, presymbiotic. *c*, Clusters 5 and 6, mixed complaint.

enters the variable that explains the most variance of the dependent variable into the discriminant function equation and adds other variables to the equation in the order of the magnitude of their explanatory power so long as they meet criteria for entry ($p = .05$ in this case). The following variables were used as possible discriminants: maturity of object representations (RORSCORE), intelligence, GAS score (GAS), gender, reality testing ($X + \%$), history of previous hospitalization(s), adoption, and age. The variables that significantly discriminated (Wilks Lambda = .4033, $p = .0002$) among the clusters were (in order of their entry into the discriminant function) GAS ($p < .002$), gender ($p < .001$), reality testing ($p < .001$) adoptive status ($p < .001$), and maturity of object representations ($p < .001$).

It is interesting to note that several measures of severity of illness (GAS, reality testing, and object representations) proved to be the most powerful discriminating variables, suggesting the cluster solution was based, in part, on the intensity of disturbance even though the variables directly associated with more disturbed behavior were not included. The solution also suggests that male and female adolescents and adoptees versus nonadoptees have significantly different adjustment styles.

Figure 2 graphs the relation between cluster type and number of adolescents in each of four levels of maturity of object representations. Inspection of this figure shows that clusters 1 and 2 were, for the most part, populated with adolescents from the higher levels of object representations. Adolescents in clusters 3 and 4 had scores almost exclusively from the lower end of the spectrum of maturity of object representations. Clusters 5 and 6, however, had adolescents with quite primitive object representations.

The typology generated by the cluster analysis provides interesting qualitative data about the possible types of adolescent responses to admission to the hospital. Each of the six clusters will be described in two ways to highlight the different types of patients represented in each. First, the commonalities among the cluster membership derived from the cluster analysis will be described (summarized in table 2). Second, the senior research psychiatrist and third author of this chapter, Wells Goodrich, was asked to review each cluster. Since he was familiar with most of the patients, he was asked to describe the various dynamic and diagnostic commonalities from a clinical perspective. Goodrich was blind to the behavioral characterizations. In this

213

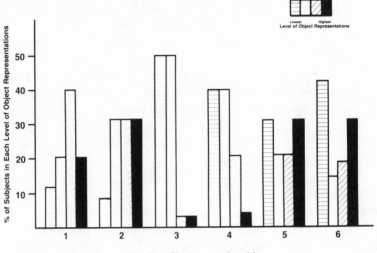

Fɪɢ. 2.—Cluster membership

way, the richness of the adolescents who populate each cluster can be preserved.

Cluster 1 is a cluster composed mostly of males (76 percent) who fall in the middle to upper level of object relations for this sample. This cluster has the highest mean global functioning score (GAS), a high level of reality testing, and a moderately high object-relations score. A high percentage (29 percent of the cluster, 38 percent of all adoptees in the sample) of these adolescents were adopted. In terms of behavior, the cluster is characterized by hostile, acting-out behavior with a strong propensity for peer interactions. There are few instances of symptoms of severe psychopathology. In general, it appears to represent a high-level, action-oriented, male adolescent. Goodrich had the following to say regarding a cluster 1 patient: "This is a fairly well-integrated mild borderline or fully functioning psychotic character who has narcissistic defenses against attachment and whose passive-aggressive, acting-out, and manipulative behaviors often work well, except episodically under stress."

Cluster 2 is composed mostly of girls (69 percent) with moderate to high levels of maturity of object representations, good reality testing, and high levels of general functioning (GAS). A large percentage of these adolescents were also adopted (38 percent of the adolescents in this cluster were adopted; 38 percent of all adoptees in the sample were

TABLE 2
Subjects by Maturity of Object Representations and Cluster

	Maturity of Object Representations				
Cluster	Low	Low Middle	High Middle	High	Total
1. Boys adopted, high HOS, high EXC, high PEER, low OBEYS	2	4	7	4	17
2. Girls adopted, high PEER, low TRUST, low OBEYS ...	1	4	4	4	13
3. High PCP low HOS high RTD low OBEYS low EXC low PEER	2	2	0	0	4
4. High HOS, high RTD, low OBEYS, low TRUST, low PEER	2	2	1	0	5
5. Boys high DEPRES, high TRUST, high IQ	3	2	2	3	10
6. High TRUST, low EXC, low HOS, high OBEYS	8	3	4	7	22
Total	18	17	18	18	71

Note.—HOS = hostility; EXC = excitement; OBEYS = obeys rules and routines; TRUST = trust and engagement; PEER = peer relatedness; RTD = psychological withdrawal; DEPRES = symptoms of depression; PCP = perceptual distortion; and GRN = grandiosity.

in this cluster). Behavior is characterized by moderate oppositionality, low trust, and moderate attention to the peer group. The clinical picture of the group is as follows: "Pretty, sexually appealing females who are manipulative but more psychotic characters or severe borderlines—more severe than milder narcissistic or borderline patients. They are dependent but with severe identity confusion. Only one or two formed good working alliances. Most have a rigid need to control the object."

Cluster 3 has a small membership and is heterogeneous by gender. The group has very low level of object representations and very low GAS scores; reality testing is moderately low. The behavior in this group is characterized by a high level of perceptual disturbances, absence of interpersonal relatedness, and a relatively low level of hostility. It appears to represent a group of very confused individuals who are able to use the milieu to organize, at least to the point of not actively resisting the staff. The clinical clustering suggested by Goodrich was that of "a

215

compliant, dependent, chronically psychotic, and, at times, fragmented group of patients. There were very marked cognitive disorders, but they were not paranoid in the sense that this blocked attachment."

Cluster 4, by contrast, contains individuals who have scores on measures of interpersonal interest comparable to cluster 3 patients but demonstrate high level of hostility. Reality testing and object relations are low, but average GAS scores are slightly higher than in cluster 3. This cluster appears to represent a group of significantly disturbed adolescents who resist the effect of the milieu by verbally hostile behavior and turning away from both staff and other patients. Acting out, however, is not a principle characteristic, as evidenced by the low excitement score. Goodrich states, "This group has a poor outcome. They are very damaged, helpless, personality disordered patients. All *eventually* attached well, but continued with damaged schizoid or grandiose selves."

Cluster 5 is populated mostly with males (80 percent). This group had the highest intelligence level among the clusters and the highest level of depressive symptoms. Behavior is characterized additionally by a good capacity for trust and above-average peer relationships. There was a higher than average level of hostility in the group. The patients had poor reality testing scores, moderately low GAS scores, and moderately poor reality testing. There was a range of maturity of object representations. Goodrich says, "These are very disorganized, very anxious, schizophrenic or developmentally disabled patients as well as borderline patients. Most formed strong alliances in treatment (more trusting than cluster 1). Some improved greatly. Those who did not did not improve because of biological deficits or very early developmental trauma." (Note that this group is difficult to categorize from a clinical perspective.)

Cluster 6 represents the largest cluster of the sample. It is composed mostly of girls (63 percent), especially at the two higher levels of object relations (73 percent). On the basis of behavioral data, it can be seen that this group makes the most prosocial adaptation to the hospital. A high level of trust and obedience, low levels of hostility and excitement, and few symptoms of severe psychopathology characterize the behavior of all members of this group. The cluster also has a bimodal distribution of object-relations scores, which include a group of very low level and a group of moderately high levels. This cluster represents a mixed group of adolescents who appear to approximate the hypothesized relation between level of object relations and "good" adjustment. That is, adolescents with less mature levels of object representations will organize around the structure of the milieu, while adolescents with more differentiated, articulated, integrated, and accurate intrapsychic schemata will form an attachment to staff and, to a lesser extent, the peer group. It is important to note that only girls with more mature object representations fit this pattern, while both boys and girls with lower levels of object representations appeared to be able to make a prosocial adjustment.

The clinical description of cluster 6 is also bimodal: "Most of these are interpersonally warm, appealing, not distrustful adolescents who make good attachments. But they vary greatly in structural damage and chronicity. Several are very high-functioning adolescents who were considered by some staff to be at a neurotic level. Others are chronically psychotic or chronically severe depressive patients, some of whom looked good on admission."

Discussion

The results of this exploratory study point to novel patterns of inpatient adaptive responses. While the demarcation of these clusters in terms of demographic, psychological, and psychopathological variables is far from certain, the results do challenge any simplified concept about the relation between prosocial adaptation in the hospital and increased psychological health. These patterns integrate the nursing staff's observations of behavior with projective test responses and combine a focus on overt adaptive functioning together with a focus on dimensions of personality variables. Even though these clusters involve less parsimonious explanations, we believe that they increase our understanding of the resistances and treatment processes that emerge across time in a very different fashion for contrasting groups of severely disturbed adolescents.

The cluster analysis suggests that Rinsley's (1980) distinctions between presymbiotic and borderline groups may be valid and useful conceptualizations. Using only milieu-related variables (OBEYS, HOSTILITY, TRUST, PEER, AND EXC), the cluster analysis separated two of the groups (3 and 4) where, with one exception, all members were from the lowest two levels of object relations. These groups showed similarly high levels of autistic withdrawal from both adults and peers, had problems following rules, and had low levels of excitement. They differed on level of hostility and degree of perceptual

217

distortion. These two groups appear to correspond to the descriptions of the presymbiotic group, where the capacity to differentiate self and object is grossly impaired. While these adjustments appear to have been poor, it is important to note that, for both groups, the behavior is not associated with action against the milieu. Instead, the behavior is associated with the decathexis of the external world, something that Rinsley has associated with the presymbiotic level.

The other four groups, two of which (5 and 6) included adolescents with low levels of object relations, all demonstrated behavior that indicated a potential for relatedness. These four groups (1, 2, 5, and 6) may constitute what Rinsley calls the symbiotic group or, more commonly, "borderline" adolescents. Resistance, however, was not the modal presentation in groups 5 or 6. For groups of adolescents who are not actively psychotic or severely schizoid, the milieu can meet dependency needs and offer support, encouragement, and new benign objects for identification from the outset. For some adolescents with higher levels of object relations—mostly girls in this sample—the hospital provides an opportunity to use their developed capacity for positive interaction. As noted, there are fewer members of this "healthier" cohort than those who populate either the healthy and resistant group or the compliant and more disturbed group.

These findings are in agreement with the object-relations-derived hypothesis that "good" adjustment, that is, cooperative, prosocial behavior, was not always associated with the highest maturity of the internalized object representations. In both boys and girls, the more oppositional adolescents were from the higher object-relations levels. This suggests, as predicted, that the most "positive" adaptation to the unit is not necessarily an index of the most developmentally advanced level of object representations.

In this sample, hostile, acting-out adjustment was associated with a group of boys with higher-level object-representation scores. Girls with approximately the same distribution of object-relations scores showed what could be characterized as a passive-aggressive adjustment. While both serve the same defensive purpose of negating the effect of the milieu, the presentation is quite different.

In this sample, after severity of illness, gender had the most discriminating power. The results indicate that boys are most likely to turn to hostile acting-out behavior even if (as in cluster 5) they demonstrate the capacity to follow rules and trust the staff. Girls, on the other hand, showed either a compliant, trusting adjustment or a passive-aggressive, manipulative adjustment. Boys who resist the milieu and the initial attachment through hostile action, however, are not the most primitive in terms of personality organization. They may be defensively resisting attachment to maintain their fragile sense of masculinity. Therapeutically, this may mean allowing and/or understanding the need for these adolescents to find more active solutions to their current conflicts and that verbal psychotherapy and transference-based interpretations may be initially impossible and, perhaps, counterproductive.

Girls, though not following the rules, were not hostile or acting out in general. Instead, they turned to the peer group and away from the staff to resist the effect of the milieu. Again, the adolescents who defensively use the peer group appear to be "healthier" than many compliant, trusting girls.

One way of understanding the gender differences found in the sample of adolescents with higher-level object relations would be to consider the generalized institutional transference to the hospital with its dual tasks of nurturing and protecting while, at the same time, controlling and punishing, as a kind of representation of the preoedipal, maternal object. The results then would be consistent with the understanding of the differential conflicts that confront males and females as they enter adolescence.

Blos's ideas (1962, 1967, 1970) on the second individuation at adolescence are applicable here. He states that the onset of puberty rekindles conflicts originally associated with the oedipal situation. For girls, the foremost anxiety on reaching adolescence is loss of love of the object, while, for adolescent boys, it is castration anxiety. It is Blos's contention that girls turn to pseudomaturity and heterosexuality as a defense against the regressive pull of the preoedipal mother as a means of maintaining a feminine identity. Boys, on the other hand, turn to activity and acting out as a defense against the castration fear that is associated with the regressive phantasies of the preoedipal mother. This leads to different behavioral presentations. The girl can adopt either a tomboy approach or a vampishness as a means of dealing with the conflict. Preadolescent boys turn away from the opposite sex and are generally in a state of restlessness and motility. Blos (1970) states, "From the beginning of adolescence, the girl is far more preoccupied with the vicissitudes of object relations than the boy. His energies are directed outward, toward the control of and dominance of the physical environment'' (p. 28).

Conclusions

The approach taken in this exploratory study was to adopt a complex, multiply-determined model to understand the adaptation of adolescents to a residential unit. While simpler explanations of functioning based on relating health-sickness dimensions to a prosocial adaptation may be easier to handle methodologically, these data suggest that the interaction between ego functioning, dynamics, and unit behavior is better understood through more complex approaches. Clinically, it is important to note that these data suggest that resistance, despite its toll on the staff, may be a better prognostic sign than compliance. Furthermore, the data suggest that containment and support of the milieu may have different meanings for different subgroups of patients. The eventual story of these clusters will be told when we have outcome data for these adolescents and can make a determination of which types of patients and which courses of hospitalizations resulted in better long-term adjustments to the world.

Appendix A

Scoring Procedures for the Measure of Maturity of Object Representations

An adaptation of the Concept of the Object on the Rorschach scale devised by Blatt et al. (1976) was used to provide a score of maturity of object representations. This scale, based on the developmental principles of Werner (1948), provides a rating of verbatim Rorschach responses in three categories: (1) differentiation (the ''nature of the response,'' e.g., full human figure, human detail, quasi-human detail); (2) articulation (to what extent the response was elaborated, e.g., articulation via perceptual characteristics such as posture, size, clothing, etc. or articulation via functional characteristics such as sex, role assignment, or identity); and (3) integration (the manner in which the response is integrated, either with other percepts or into a context of action). Integration is scored in three subcategories: (*a*) type or presence of motivation for the action in which the object is involved (unmotivated, reactive, intentional); (b) extent to which the action and the object itself are integrated (fused, incongruent, nonspecific, congruent); and (c) quality of the integration of the interaction of the object with another object (malevolent-benevolent, active-passive, active-reactive, active-active).

For each of these categories, a continuum based on progressively higher levels of development has been established. For example, in the area of articulation, the hierarchy proceeds from quasi-human detail response to human detail to whole quasi-human response to whole human figure. The whole human figure is proposed as the highest level of articulation. Similar continua have been established in the other two areas as well.

ADAPTATION OF THE CONCEPT OF THE OBJECT SCALE

In order to create a single, overall score of maturity of object representations, plus and minus weights were assigned to each response on the basis of good versus poor form level. Poor form levels were given a weight of -1 and good form level responses were given a weight of 1. The subject's object-relations score was, then, a sum of the total number of weighted responses, some of which were positive and some of which were negative. The formula for computing the score for each subject is:

RORSCORE $= [(gX) + 1)] + [(pX - 1)]$,

where g equals the developmental score for each good form response, and p equals the developmental score for each minus form response.

Following previous research of this type (Shaffer, Graves, Mead, Thomas, and Pearson 1986), a protocol needed to yield two responses that could be scored in such a way that they could be included in the sample. Of the eighty-nine potential protocols, five had one or zero responses that could be scored and were therefore excluded.

RELIABILITY OF THE CONCEPT OF THE OBJECT
ON THE RORSCHACH SCALE

Previous work with the Blatt scale has shown that raters are able reliably to rate responses on the scale. Agreement has ranged from 75 to 95 percent, with most percentages in the 80s and 90s. The interrater

221

agreement between the two raters in the present study ranged from 76 to 96 percent, with a mean percentage of agreement of 88.

CONTROL OF RESPONSE PRODUCTIVITY

Researchers (Blatt, Berman, Bloom-Feshbach, Sugarman, Wilber, and Kleber 1984; Shaffer, Graves, Mead, Thomas, and Pearson 1986) using the Rorschach have advocated controlling for response productivity by computing residualized scores. This method was used in this study. The Residualized Object Representation Score (RORSCORE) was the object-representation score residualized for overall response productivity (i.e., the number of responses in the entire Rorschach record).

Appendix B

TABLE B1

MEAN SCORES FOR DIAGNOSTIC AND DEMOGRAPHIC VARIABLES FOR SIX CLUSTERS

Variable	Cluster					
	1	2	3	4	5	6
RORSCORE	10.02[a]	7.92[a]	−20.49[b,c]	−24.36[c]	1.30[a,b,c]	1.28[a,b]
X + %	83.17[a,b]	85.57[a,b]	84.50[a,b,c]	70.60[c]	74.10[c]	75.45[a,b,c]
GAS	41.31[a]	39.15[a,b]	29.25[c]	41.20[a,b]	36.60[b]	42.33[a]
IQ	104.64[a,b]	104.61[a,b]	104.25[a,b]	96.20[b]	109.50[a]	103.31[a,b]
Age	15.46[a]	16.03[a]	16.23[a]	15.94[a]	15.85[a]	16.01[a]

NOTE.—Means with the same superscripts are not significantly different at the level of trends ($p < .10$, least significant difference test).

Appendix C

TABLE C1

PERCENTAGES FOR GENDER AND ADOPTIVE STATUS FOR SIX CLUSTERS

Variable	Cluster						χ^2	p
	1	2	3	4	5	6		
N	17	13	4	5	10	22		
Gender (%):								
Boys	76	31	50	40	80	36	12.01	<.05
Girls	24	69	50	60	20	64		
Adoptive status (%):								
Adopted	29	38	0	20	10	4	9.08	N.S.
Not adopted	71	62	100	80	90	96		

Appendix D

TABLE D1

MEAN SCORES FOR CLAIR VARIABLES FOR SIX CLUSTERS

Variable	Cluster					
	1	2	3	4	5	6
HOS	119.75[a]	98.00[c,d]	94.57[d]	111.37[b]	103.25[c]	84.34[e]
EXC	117.98[a]	100.22[b,c]	91.40[d,e]	97.32[b,c]	106.52[b]	86.41[d]
OBEYS	89.91[c]	93.72[b,c]	86.00[c]	82.63[c]	101.54[b]	116.12[a]
TRUST	93.09[b]	90.79[b]	85.75[b,c]	77.12[c]	111.91[a]	112.44[a]
PEER	110.70[a]	102.19[a]	66.68[b]	70.99[b]	105.64[a]	100.39[a]
RTD	100.83[a]	97.68[a]	110.35[a]	110.17[a]	100.05[a]	96.89[a]
DEPRES	100.18[a]	100.93[a]	95.30[a]	103.18[a]	108.82[a]	95.76[a]
PCP	96.96[b]	96.99[b]	122.56[a]	101.95[b]	101.53[b]	99.10[b]
GRN	96.21[a]	96.65[a]	107.11[a]	97.46[a]	103.69[a]	102.44[a]

NOTE.—Means with the same superscript are not significantly different ($p < .05$, Ryan-Einot-Gabriel-Welsh Multiple F-test). Scores are standardized to distribution with mean = 100, standard deviation = 15. HOS = hostility; EXC = excitement; OBEYS = obeys rules and routines; TRUST = trust and engagement; PEER = peer relatedness; RTD = psychological withdrawal; DEPRES = symptoms of depression; PCP = perceptual distortion; and GRN = grandiosity.

NOTE

An earlier version of this chapter was presented at the thirty-first annual meeting of the Association for Children's Residential Centers, New Orleans, Louisiana, October 15, 1987. The authors wish to acknowledge the help and support of many people associated with the research project within the Adolescent and Child Division of Chestnut Lodge: Dexter M. Bullard Jr., medical director; Jaime Buenaventura, clinical director; Mary-Louise Schmidt, director of nursing; Phyllis Stang, nursing coordinator; Maureen Cavanaugh, assistant nursing coordinator; and Ginny Embry, Nancy Mornini, Michael Gleason, Mildred Hamacher-Bennett, and Vivian McCrimon, houseparents. In addition, we would like to thank our colleagues at the Chestnut Lodge Research Institute for their review and support of this project: Thomas McGlashan, director of research; Robert K. Heinssen, research coordinator; David Feinsilver, symposium chairperson; Linda Beth Berman, editorial and research assistant; and Carol Thompson and Patricia Inana, secretaries.

223

REFERENCES

Beck, S. J. 1949. *Rorschach Test*. Vol. 1. *Basic Processes*. New York: Grune & Stratton.

Blatt, S. J.; Berman, W. ; Bloom-Feshbach, S.; Sugarman, A.; Wilber, C.; and Kleber, H. D. 1984. Psychological assessment of psychopathology in opiate addicts. *Journal of Nervous and Mental Disease* 172:156–165.

Blatt, S. J.; Brooks, C. B.; Brenneis, J. G.; and Schimek, J. 1976. A developmental analysis of the concept of the object on the Rorschach. New Haven, Conn: Yale University. Typescript.

Blos, P. 1962. *On Adolescence*. New York: Free Press.

Blos, P. 1967. The second individuation process in adolescence. *Psychoanalytic Study of the Child* 22:162–186.

Blos, P. 1970. *The Young Adolescent*. New York: Free Press.

Brown, L. 1981. The therapeutic milieu in the treatment of patients with borderline personality disorders. *Bulletin of the Menninger Clinic* 45:377–394.

Coyne, L.; Whitmarsh, G.; Clarkin, J.; and Canfield, M. 1986. Patient and hospital treatment clusters. *Psychiatric Hospital* 17:181–189.

Crabtree, L. 1982. Hospitalized adolescents who act out: a treatment approach. *Psychiatry* 45:147–58.

Davis, M., and Raffe, I. H. 1985. The holding environment in the inpatient treatment of adolescents. *Adolescent Psychiatry* 12:434–443.

Endicott, J.; Spitzer, R.; Fleiss, J.; and Cohen, J. 1976. The global assessment scale: a procedure for measuring overall severity of psychiatric disturbance. *Archives of General Psychiatry* 33:766–771.

Fullerton, C. S.; Goodrich, W.; and Berman, L. B. 1986. Adoption predicts psychiatric treatment resistances in hospitalized adolescents. *Journal of the American Academy of Child Psychiatry* 25(4): 542–551.

Garber, B. 1972. *Follow-up Study of Hospitalized Adolescents*. New York: Brunner/Mazel.

Goodrich, W. G. 1987. Long-term psychoanalytic hospital treatment of adolescents. *Psychiatric Clinics of North America* 10:273–287.

Gunderson, J. G.; Will, O. A., Jr.; and Mosher, L. R. 1983. *Principles and Practice of Milieu Therapy*. New York: Aronson.

Kernberg, O. 1975. *Borderline Conditions and Pathological Narcissism.* New York: Aronson.

Logan, W. S.; Barnhart, F. D.; and Gossett, J. T. 1982. The prognostic significance of adolescent interpersonal relationships during psychiatric hospitalization. *Adolescent Psychiatry* 10:484–493.

Lorr, M.; Klett, C.; and McNair, D. 1963. *Inpatient Multidimensional Psychiatric Rating Scale: Manual.* Palo Alto, Calif.: Consulting Psychologists Press.

Masterson, J. T. 1972. *Treatment of the Borderline Adolescent.* New York: Wiley.

Masterson, J. T., and Costello, J. L. 1980. *From Borderline Adolescent to Functioning Adult.* New York: Brunner/Mazel.

Miller, D. 1980. Treatment of the seriously disturbed adolescent. *Adolescent Psychiatry* 5:468–481.

Redl, F. 1972. The concept of a "therapeutic milieu" in residential treatment of emotionally disturbed children. In G. Weber and B. J. Haberlein, eds. *Residential Treatment of Emotionally Disturbed Children.* New York: Behavioral Publications.

Rinsley, D. B. 1980. *Treatment of the Severely Disturbed Adolescent.* New York: Aronson.

Rossman, P., and Knesper, D. 1976. The early phase of hospital treatment for disruptive adolescents. *Journal of the American Academy of Child Psychiatry* 15:693–708.

Shaffer, J. W.; Graves, P. L.; Mead, L.; Thomas, C. B.; and Pearson, T. A. 1986. Development of alternate methods for scoring the Rorschach Interaction Scale. *Educational and Psychological Measurement* 46:837–844.

Werner, H. 1948. *Comparative Psychology of Mental Development.* New York: Wiley.

Yates, B.; Fritsch, R.; Fullerton, C.; and Goodrich, W. 1988. The Chestnut Lodge adolescent interaction report. Rockville, Md.: Chestnut Lodge Research Institute. Typescript.

12 THE SEVERELY DISTURBED ADOLESCENT: HOSPITAL TREATMENT PROCESSES AND PATTERNS OF RESPONSE

WELLS GOODRICH

This chapter addresses four questions. What services constitute a basic minimum within a long-term adolescent hospital program? What concepts are useful to guide therapeutic interventions and evaluate whether positive personality changes are taking place during the hospital stay? Which severely disturbed adolescent patients do well with such a program, and which patients do we find often improve considerably less than we had hoped? Finally, what might be done in the future to improve our results with those patients who currently present difficult resistances to the change process?

Before discussing these questions, however, let me clarify what patients we are really talking about here. Who are the severely and chronically disturbed adolescents? Recent studies (Almqvist 1986; Milazzo-Sayre 1986) suggest that approximately 3 percent of the population will enter a psychiatric hospital for treatment at some time during their adolescent years. Of these adolescents, approximately 10–20 percent are sufficiently ill to require repeated or long-term hospital treatment of from one to four years' duration.

Psychopathology in severely disturbed adolescents follows symptom patterns and disturbed behavior that is remarkably stable from one hospital to the next. A recent study of 800 adolescents (Miller and PACTE 1988) who were admitted to over a dozen private psychiatric hospital units revealed a uniformity in the types of presenting problems. The most common difficulties bringing patients into hospitals for a minimum six months' stay were inability to learn in school (85 percent), self-destructive and assaultive behavior (50 percent), drug or alcohol abuse (50 percent), and difficulties with the law (40 percent). Over one-third of the patients had presenting symptoms of sexual acting out or running away from home. Only one-fifth presented with grossly psychotic behavior.

Most of these private hospital psychiatric units also reported a uniform pattern as regards admission characteristics. Approximately 55 percent of the adolescents were male and 45 percent female. While the median age was fifteen years old and 50 percent of the disturbed youngsters were fifteen to eighteen years old, the younger 50 percent of this population ranged in age from five to fourteen years old. That is to say, most adolescent units included a significant number of eleven- to fourteen-year-olds, with occasionally an even younger child.

Most patients reported serious symptomatic behavior for a duration of four years, with an average outpatient-plus-inpatient treatment experience totaling two years. Adolescents living with both natural parents constituted approximately one-third of the sample; close to 50 percent of the patients had been living with a single parent, and 10–20 percent had been living with neither biological parent. The frequency of adoption was high among these hospitalized adolescents—ranging from 20 to 30 percent among private hospital inpatient populations. Patients in the Adolescent Unit at Chestnut Lodge display similar characteristics.

Developmentally, studies of many of these adolescents reveal that significant stress, anxiety, and behavioral symptoms occurred during the first five years of life (Kernberg 1977; Rinsley 1980). Among the patients who tend to have a better result from long-term hospital treatment, one often discovers that this early developmental psychopathology has been followed by reasonably adaptive behavior from ages six to twelve. Among the more difficult patients to treat, however, it is usual that the history will describe ongoing, interpersonal, and developmental difficulties during the latency phase. Severe symptomatology emerges as most of these patients enter preadolescence.

Nearly all come from families in which one or both parents have suffered from either severe personality disorder or some variant of a psychotic process. In relation to the peer group, either these adolescents have been schizoid and avoidant, with very few experiences of

227

close attachment to peers, or the peers whom they have chosen also were severely troubled. Finally, most of these patients have received outpatient or brief inpatient treatment prior to being admitted for long-term hospitalization, but without significant improvement. This raises a question as to how skillful we are in perceiving the potential for outpatient and brief inpatient treatment failure. Could adolescent clinicians identify those adolescents who have the observable characteristics that require long-term hospital treatment earlier in their illnesses?

Diagnostically, these adolescents are heterogeneous: conduct disorders; oppositional disorders; chronic, severe depressions; borderline, schizoid, and schizotypal personality disorders; narcissistic personality disorders; and schizophreniform and chronic schizophrenic illnesses. Such severely disturbed adolescents suffer from multiple intrapsychic disturbances as well as interpersonal dysfunctions on genetic, early maturational, and familial bases. These adolescents demonstrate a variety of disturbances in self-concept, in their perceptions of adults or peers, in their value systems or ego ideals, in their ability to observe correctly and to evaluate interpersonal relationships, and in their abilities to modulate impulses and to regulate their own social behavior. Regardless of the specific diagnosis, nearly all these patients have been attached to a chronically and severely disturbed parent. These adolescents often have become rigidly patterned in experiences of high anxiety or guilt, of despair, and of delusional grandiosity or persecution. Maladaptive aggression or social withdrawal tends to have become extreme and habitual.

The normally expected healthy psychosocial developments have not been achieved. The secure attachment experience has not occurred in infancy (Mahler 1979). For years, many of these patients have internalized a depressive state accompanied by the pervasive sense of feeling abandoned, unsupported, or worthless. The self is often experienced as deprived and excessively needy for special gratifications; adults usually are perceived as insensitive, hostile, or rejecting. Not having a reality-based "good self" and healthy guilt, the patients may be caught in a conflict between excessive impulsiveness and an internalized punitive superego. Later in treatment, when gratifying and close attachments do emerge, these patients then tend to experience, in treatment, extreme possessiveness and separation anxiety in relation to these new significant persons, much as a younger child would have experienced normally.

Hospital Treatment Processes

These patients have structured internalized conflicts centering around infantile developmental issues. In order to free them up for further ego growth, Chestnut Lodge promotes a dependent attachment and a reworking of these early issues that, typically, a healthy child would have mastered between ages one and four years. In order to do this, it is useful to provide an environment that fosters a sense of containment, support, and protective timelessness. At Chestnut Lodge, a psychodynamically oriented team approach orchestrates six program elements (see fig. 1): a special school, a nursing milieu designed for adolescents, family therapy, intensive individual psychotherapy, some combination of group therapy and rehabilitation, and, when indicated, psychotropic medication.

Psychotropic medication is required less as part of a long-term treatment situation than it is as part of shorter-term inpatient treatment or outpatient work since the relationship bonds may become meaningful enough during the long-term inpatient experience to reach many adolescents without medication. In deciding about medication, consideration is given as to whether the patient's work in psychotherapy is being blocked by a cognitive deficit (as with hallucinating or delusional patients) or by suicidally depressed or manic states. When participation in psychotherapy is not severely blocked by such extreme cognitive or affective deficits, it is well to keep in mind that medication may dull the patient's perceptual sensitivity, thus detracting from the work of insight. When employed, the medication can be reduced over

FOCUS ON TREATMENT	TREATMENT PROGRAM
1. Improving cognitive skills	School
2. Improved role functioning; affect and impulse modulation	Milieu, school
3. Change in self-other percepts and conflict resolution	Individual psychotherapy
4. Improved self-esteem; self-expression in peer relations, work, and avocations	Group psychotherapy, recreation, and rehabilitation
5. Family pathology and adaptation	Family therapy
6. Psychophysiology	Medication

Fig. 1.—Model for hospital treatment

time, as the patient's symptoms improve, and sometimes it can be discontinued before discharge.

Family therapy is also an essential component. During the early weeks of the adolescent's stay, the family may best be engaged separately from the patient. Initially, the family may experience relief from this enforced separation from such a disruptive adolescent, although a symbiotically tied parent will find the adjustment to separation extremely painful. This way of introducing family work provides a useful opportunity for the family therapist to explore the origins of the patient's difficulties as they are perceived by each family member as well as to investigate those chronic patterns of family conflict that have actively served to promote and maintain the patient's individual pathology. After the patient has formed an attachment to the nursing unit, the patient will then join these weekly family therapy meetings.

A primary consideration in family work is whether the parent or others who are most pathologically attached to and involved with the patient can relinquish or modify these attachments. When long-term hospital treatment fails, many times it will fail during the middle phase of treatment as the patient is beginning to improve. Genuine improvement in the adolescent is usually threatening to the overly involved family members. Thus, when the patient improves, the family may provide unexpected resistances to further treatment. They may support and collude with the patient by clinging to denial of conflict, splitting, and projective identification. Transferentially, they may distort their perceptions of the staff's goals and interactions. The family therapist will then confront such family members with their need to resolve their side of these conflicts involving the adolescent. At such a time, a disturbed mother or father needs to experience a mourning reaction having to relinquish a disturbed introject that has been projected onto the patient over a period of many years and has promoted, unconsciously, the patient's anxiety and immaturity. The mother or father then needs help to form some new goals or attachments to replace this disturbed introject. If these family changes cannot occur, such a failure of treatment may lead to the adolescent leaving the hospital against advice, running away from the hospital, or rejoining the family in order to resume old patterns of defensive operations and maladaptive behavior. Much of the early work of family therapy is aimed at preparing the ground for this crucial therapeutic encounter, which can be expected during the middle phase of treatment.

The school program, the individual or group psychotherapy, and the unit milieu program each emphasizes different treatment aims. The school necessarily focuses on containing and reducing the patient's symptomatic behavior during class to a level at which behavioral disturbance does not block learning. Thus, the school finds itself with goals of both cognitive improvement and improvement in social behavior. All but a very few disturbed adolescents enter the hospital one to three grades behind the achievement level expected for their abilities. Within the protected hospital environment, most non-brain-damaged patients catch up academically, provided the teachers have the requisite educational and therapeutic skills and provided the nursing unit can support the learning processes collaboratively with the school. A rough index for judging the rigidity of the patient's internalized pathology is the rapidity, after hospital admission, with which the patient catches up academically. Patients whose admission pathology is derived largely from overwhelming but relatively recent environmental stress blossom early in the school program. Those whose pathology is more severe and whose core conflicts were internalized during early development respond more slowly. There is little opportunity in school to help the patient gain insight into unconscious or denied conflicts other than using the school setting to identify for the patient his recurrent patterns of symptomatic behavior that require further therapeutic work. The school also is a setting within which most patients begin to entertain new and healthier identifications. As treatment progresses, improving adolescents often model themselves after a teacher who is perceived as empathic and helpful.

On the nursing unit, there are special opportunities to work on improving social responsibility and on fostering a collaborative and mutually supportive pattern of behavior in relation to both peers and adults. The modulation of aggressive, sexual, or dependent needs becomes a major goal of the nursing staff. The use of the "life space interview" (Redl 1959) is a useful tool for nursing and child-care staff. When disturbed behavior has been interdicted, the patient becomes anxious. The nursing staff then provides a combination of confrontation, inquiry, and clarification, about "what are the real issues that led to this upset?" At the same time, the staff demonstrates emotional support and a wish to understand the patient's own perceptions of this episode. As an outcome of such repeated supportive confrontations with the patient around the containment of symptomatic behavior, an attachment can emerge. As this attachment grows, so also grows the patient's awareness of his or her own contribution to these entrenched relationship difficulties, which now have been transferred from the family environment into the patient's relationships within the hospital.

Finally, in the individual and group psychotherapy, there is the greatest opportunity for the patient to verbalize and reflect about past and present experience. At Chestnut Lodge, all patients are provided with four-times-per-week, fifty-minute individual therapy sessions. During the first phase of treatment, these adolescents often resist insight-oriented communication with the psychotherapist. The first phase of individual and group psychotherapy tends to be involved with testing the therapist's acceptance of the patient and testing the therapist's commitment to understanding. Usually, the patient makes transferential attempts to get the psychotherapist to reject him or her. These provocations may take dramatic forms such as stubborn silence, setting small fires in the office, falling asleep, threatening to damage the therapist's office furniture, or simply demanding that the therapist "prove you care!" When the attachment does finally begin, it usually takes the form of what Winnicott, Feinsilver, and others have termed "a transitional relatedness" (Feinsilver 1983). That is to say, the communication pattern in interviews expresses the patient's need for a prolonged period of playful activities or shared fantasies as a way of beginning to make interpersonal contact in a positive, but primitive, mode. It may not be until the middle phase of treatment, approximately the second year, that the patient can tolerate being evaluated directly or can contribute his or her own self-observations about how memories of past experiences are affecting present experience and behavior.

This process of insight is facilitated, as in all psychoanalytic therapy, by the interpretation of transference (Kernberg 1977; Price 1983). From the beginning, it is useful for the therapist to clarify the various ways the patient resists the relationship and avoids talking about himself or herself. During the second phase of the work, the patient may be able to tolerate, from time to time, comments about how his or her interaction in the session itself replicates family patterns and how the same patterns led to hospitalization. A fifteen-year-old girl, symbiotically attached to her depressed, possessive, borderline mother, may have repeated difficulty leaving the individual psychotherapy session at the scheduled time. After a preliminary period of bringing such transference separation feelings to the patient's attention, the therapist might speculate out loud, questioning whether the patient may be feeling something similar, here and now, to what she had experienced at home with her mother. This intervention embodies an analytic approach to the transference, which is couched cautiously and tactfully in terms tolerable to the adolescent. Overall, the individual psycho-therapist pushes for a collaborative review of self-perceptions, fanta-sies about others, perceptions of others, defensive behavior, and the basic conflicts defended against.

Over the two or more years average stay in the hospital, the patient's individual therapist, the unit administrator, a representative from the school, and the family therapist meet regularly to formulate the emerging information about conflicts and defenses as revealed in each of these four settings. This ongoing exchange of observations assists each member of the treatment team to be mindful of what issues are being addressed elsewhere and to refine current interventions appro-priate to the specific work of individual psychotherapy, milieu man-agement, and family therapy. Toward the end of the hospital stay, the family will participate in planning for discharge and in the patient's decision whether to live with a peer group in a halfway house or to return to the family.

It is useful to conceive of the treatment processes as occurring over time in three phases (Goodrich 1984, 1987; Masterson and Costello 1980; Rinsley 1980). During the first six to nine months in the hospital, the staff seeks to reduce the severity of symptomatic behavior and to form a trusting bond and working alliance with both patient and family. During the middle phase, which begins toward the end of the first year in the hospital, significant personality restructuring is sought. The goals for this middle phase include the attainment of significant insight by both patient and family into their disturbing conflicts and defenses. These insights will also promote new identifi-cations and life goals for the adolescent as well as for his most involved family members. If and when those changes have occurred, the patient can make plans appropriately and gradually to reenter the community. This reentry phase, or separation-individuation process, begins during the months preceding discharge from the hospital and continues over the first two or three years after discharge. Each of these loosely delineated phases places relative emphasis on different treatment goals in order to respond appropriately to the patient's changing developmental needs.

233

Four Patterns of Response

Clinical observation of 150 severely disturbed adolescents treated at Chestnut Lodge during the past decade has suggested grouping together patterns of adolescent and family pathology according to their responses to our ability to engage them in the work of treatment (see fig. 2). How does each patient respond, in the earliest period of treatment, to our goals to contain symptomatic behavior and anxiety, to foster a regressive attachment, and to promote an alliance? Further along in time, how does each patient tolerate and respond to transference clarifications and interpretations? Later still, do new positive identifications and ego strengths emerge? Finally, is the separation process from the hospital negotiated in a collaborative manner, with the patient demonstrating appropriate adaptive behavior in the community rather than becoming disorganized, self-destructive, or regressed under the stress of losing the supportive hospital structure?

While reviewing discharged patients' courses in the hospital, four patterns emerged that appear to apply to many patients. (1) Younger adolescents with good prognoses who are positively attached to a disorganized but not totally rejecting parent and who have experienced repeated environmental dislocations during late childhood and pread-olescence may show early improvement over a six- to twelve-month period. (2) Adolescents who experienced significant trauma during infancy and early childhood but who also have shown significant ego strengths during the latency stage may improve significantly in treat-ment, but this occurs slowly and often with an ambivalent alliance. (3) Adolescents achieving limited improvement who have suffered severe early psychosocial trauma and/or congenital deficit, often accompanied by malignant family psychopathology, tend toward a less satisfactory outcome. (4) Adolescents whose intrapsychic structure involves rigid needs for interpersonal control, for devaluing others, and for avoiding attachment may remain defensively disengaged from a meaningful treatment experience. Interestingly, these four patterns of response to psychoanalytically oriented, long-term, residential treatment do not correspond to DSM-III diagnostic groups or to Kernberg's (1976) descriptions of four levels of severity for borderline personality organization.

Disturbed
concepts

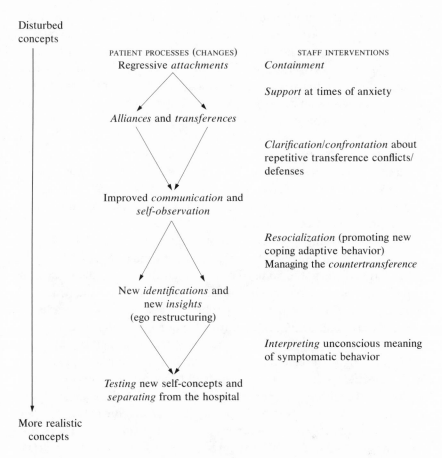

PATIENT PROCESSES (CHANGES)   STAFF INTERVENTIONS
Regressive *attachments*   *Containment*

                                        Support at times of anxiety

Alliances and *transferences*

                                        Clarification/confrontation about
                                        repetitive transference conflicts/
                                        defenses

Improved *communication* and
self-observation

                                        Resocialization (promoting new
                                        coping adaptive behavior)
                                        Managing the *countertransference*

New *identifications* and
new *insights*
(ego restructuring)

                                        Interpreting unconscious meaning
                                        of symptomatic behavior

Testing new self-concepts and
separating from the hospital

More realistic
concepts

Fig. 2.—Work of treatment: Psychoanalytic residential treatment for adolescents. For staff interventions, cf. Goodrich and Boomer (1958).

ONE TYPE OF "GOOD PROGNOSIS" ADOLESCENT

Patients who respond positively during the first six months often are younger adolescents whose symptoms were moderately severe prior to admission. Such adolescents have maintained a positive attachment with one parent who may still show considerable reality orientation and a sense of responsibility for the patient. In many of these cases with a good prognosis, the need for long-term hospitalization has arisen because of repeated changes in the environment around the parent-child dyad. Usually, these

235

changes have been brought about by divorce or marital separation of the parents and a tenuous economic situation. Often, this patient is a younger adolescent living with the mother: the mother has changed jobs and residences many times over the previous three to four years; she herself may suffer from a primitive personality disorder; and the preadolescent child's normal need for a stable peer group to attach to has not been provided for because of these repeated and disruptive changes in the social and physical environment. Often these have been latchkey children, wandering the streets without supervision. These children come home to an empty apartment at the end of a school day, have no sitter, and have to prepare their own meals. They may become so anxious, depressed, and full of rage as to set fires and engage in other antisocial behavior such as shoplifting, sexual promiscuity, or vandalism.

In other cases, there is more disruptive warfare between the parents. The single mother may have had a series of male lovers who have moved in and out of the home. These changes have been distressing to the child, who has repeatedly formed expectant, dependent attachments to this series of potential parent surrogates, only to be disappointed again and again. Gradually, all these stresses—the economic changes, the geographic moves, the mother's own conflicts with the father or with other male companions, the lack of parental supervision, and the patient's rage and anxiety—lead to more and more disorganization in the already vulnerable preadolescent. A fire, an arrest, a suicide gesture, or self-cutting may be the final cry for help.

These rageful, severely depressed, and impulsive youngsters are burdened by an internally structured "bad self" and a persecutory view of adult relationships. Yet they have internal strengths and often have a history of early good childhood functioning. When they arrive in the hospital, they often are diagnosed as conduct or dysthymic disorders (Goldstein 1988), and the therapeutic environment may have an early healing effect. Within six months, these children have caught up to their expected school achievement level. Not uncommonly, they form meaningful attachments to selected adult staff and to peers. While they are burdened with intense and primitive transference conflicts and affects of rage and depression, which may take from two to four years to resolve (on the basis of the memories and conflicted introjects from the past), they may not be burdened by severe narcissism or primitive defenses such as projective identification and splitting or by deficits in reality-testing capacities. Thus, they do not fulfill all the criteria described by Kernberg (1977) for the borderline syndrome.

Informal follow-up information on a small number of these children is that they complete high school, attend college, and may go on to graduate school and marriage. We believe that, while family and individual psychotherapy has been essential, perhaps the most healing attributes of the program have been the nurturant containment, the social order, and the emotional support that have been brought into the patient's life.

"SLOW IMPROVEMENT" ADOLESCENTS

The second group of patients responds less dramatically and may be left with certain psychological deficits after treatment. Their intrapsychic organization is borderline (Kernberg 1977) or primitive (Robbins 1983). Their adaptive-defensive patterns may present as schizoid, schizotypal, narcissistic, or oppositional behavior. These patients, in DSM-III-R (American Psychiatric Association 1987) terms, may also carry diagnoses of dysthymic disorder, conduct disorder, or oppositional disorder. They do appear, however, to have identified with healthier functioning in at least one parent. Many have histories of reasonably good adaptation during the elementary school years. They tend to have experienced severe environmental stress before the age of five as well as after the latency period. The symptoms may be extreme; often such histories include brief psychotic episodes or suicidal, self-cutting, drug abusive, or violent behavior. Usually, they have had more hospitalizations and more disappointing efforts at treatment prior to Chestnut Lodge admission than have the first group. Their parents may still be together but are bound to each other with sadomasochistic attachments or psychotic bonds. These patients appear less trusting and less available for immediate attachment than the first group. They are more hesitant to engage in a treatment alliance. Instead of forming a meaningful alliance within the first three to six months, this group of patients takes a year or more to engage in insight-oriented psychotherapeutic work.

Female patients in this group may have escaped from the family by attaching themselves, at the age of thirteen to fifteen years, to narcissistic, psychopathic, drug-addicted, or drug-dealing males. They have used their sexuality in the service of gaining a pathologically dependent attachment. Masochistic behavior, violent behavior, or both may have taken extreme forms. They have often cut themselves repeatedly or made suicidal attempts. Substance abuse and joining with an antisocial peer group has been common. Alternatively, withdrawal into brief psychotic episodes has been another pattern. Still another pattern has been schizoid withdrawal into fantasy or schizotypal and semidelusional preoccupations as a refuge from the unbearable confusion of family relationships.

Their capacity for relatedness has developed to the stage of search for symbiotic or intense, mutually dependent ties. This search may be accompanied by intense narcissistic wounding or persecutory rage should it meet with frustration. Their positive introjects tend to be few and their negative introjects rigidly internalized. This leads to persistent attitudes of pessimism, fear of new attachments, sadomasochistic fantasies, helplessness or hopelessness, and intense anxiety in the face of new challenges. Because of their potential for positive attachment and treatment alliance formation, these patients do begin to improve slowly during the second year of hospitalization. They continue to be somewhat suspicious of their assigned administrators and therapists, continue to be willing to "go along," as it were, with the school program and with certain efforts at insight, but always reserve a part of themselves in private rebellion or distrust. The result is that some leave the hospital somewhat prematurely, but still after having gained a good deal. Others, who stay on with the program for three and a half or four years before returning to the community, on follow-up appear to be adapting quite well. Some are able to continue their education or to find meaningful employment consistent with their abilities. Certain of these patients, eventually, are able to find stable, intimate relationships.

DEFICIT DISORDERS

The third group is the patients with more severely damaged personalities. The damage may be from various sources (Bemporad, Hanson, and Smith 1981). We have seen adolescents who as infants were abandoned and had numerous foster homes. We have seen others who suffered chronic sexual abuse by a parent. We have seen unusually rigid, psychoneurotic patients, as in the case of a very severe obsessive-compulsive adolescent who actually became more disabled than most schizophrenic patients. And we have seen patients with malignant forms of chronic schizophrenia or schizoaffective disorder who mobilize sufficient inner resources to gain partial recovery.

Strangely, adoptees seem to fall into this third "limited-improvement" category. The adoptees show good improvement in the first year to eighteen months in the hospital; then they seem not to be able to tolerate the middle phase, the insight process. Insight into separation anxiety and expressed dependent transferences is experienced by the adoptees as too humiliating and intolerable and as an experience too reminiscent of the intense real abandonment they have experienced. Just at the time when the adoptee's dependent transference has become a most intense attachment and anxiety over their fantasied rejection by the therapist is at its height, should any type of vacation or reality-determined absence on the part of a valued staff person occur, these patients may become enraged and need to put great distance between themselves and the therapist. Over half our adoptees terminate treatment by running away from the hospital, mostly in the middle phase (Fullerton, Goodrich, and Berman 1986).

To summarize, whether the ego damage is in the area of cognitive deficit (as with the chronic schizophrenic patient) or distrust and rage (as with the repeatedly abandoned child or adoptee), or whether it takes the form of severe helplessness (as it often does in the case of the abused child), one sees that certain adolescents do not have the inner resources to build a new, healthy self prior to discharge. Their structured deficits may not interfere with the eventual dependent attachment and treatment alliance processes, but those deficits do limit gravely these adolescents' capacities for self-observation, for communication about transference experiences, and for positive new identifications.

In these cases, discharge should be approached more gradually, usually after three to four years in the hospital. Discharge plans must be made that contain more support systems (such as a halfway house living plan) and more active, continued, therapeutic interventions following discharge. Our impression is that certain of these appear to maintain better adaptation following discharge; others seem rather rapidly to regress and to return to a condition not too dissimilar to their admission presentation.

DEFENSIVELY DISENGAGED ADOLESCENTS

Finally, there is a fourth group of patients who, even though admitted to the hospital, either quickly or after a prolonged period of time demonstrate that they have been unable to engage the program meaningfully. In very few of these situations, it can be seen retrospectively that either the family or the patient never intended that the patient remain with the program. Many have intended to be treated but are identified with an extremely narcissistic parent. Despite earnest therapeutic efforts by the psychotherapist, the family therapist, and the clinical psychiatric administrator, the narcissistic or other patterns of primitive defenses shared between patient and family may prove unmodifiable. Certain of these patients suffer from what Kernberg (1984) has described as "malignant narcissism," in which grandiosity is linked with sadism and/or masochism and the patient takes triumphant pleasure in cruel or self-destructive acts. Others evince antisocial personality traits.

These patients may leave the hospital early, after two to three months. The departure is often initiated by the adolescent trying to find a way to make the parents anxious and suspicious: anxious about their own separation from the patient and suspicious about the hospital's conduct of the treatment. Some patients gain a sense of reward through a determined and consistent battle against any type of self-observation or any type of therapeutic communication, thereby defeating the staff. Some of these patients do show, despite their own conscious efforts at opposition, some degree of improvement, but, in the end, they resist the opportunity for new, positive identifications or insight into their defensive avoidance of positive relatedness. In one such case, a sixteen-year-old girl, who was lied to by her parents (unbeknownst to us) in order to manipulate her into the hospital, set about, carefully, cautiously, and with considerable skill, arranging for herself to be rescued from the hospital by an older lesbian lover. The patient was careful enough not to have this escape occur in the first two months: she correctly surmised that it would be easier to carry off such an escape if she presented herself as a compliant, "well-attached" patient for three months before she would attempt such a successful deception. She used the lesbian lover as a way of escaping from her powerful father and mother who had controlled her and demoralized her in power struggles over many years. We have little information, even of an informal nature, about the condition of this last group of difficult patients after they have left treatment.

Discussion

Over the last twenty-five years, more communities have been providing specialized inpatient units for the psychiatric treatment of adolescents. Clinicians who have compared the results of treatment on these specially designed units with treatment on units where adolescents are mixed with adults have concluded that the results of such treatment are superior (Gossett, Lewis, and Barnhart 1983). Over 80 percent of adolescents who require hospitalization apparently can receive sufficient benefit to return to community-based treatment within sixty to ninety days with the support of a careful treatment plan that continues family, individual, and psychotropic treatment that were initiated in the hospital. Nevertheless, 10–20 percent of adolescents admitted for inpatient psychiatric treatment will require long-term inpatient treatment varying from one to four years in duration. Our experience at Chestnut Lodge suggests that we can move beyond treatment planning based on each patient as a unique entity to predicting, for certain diagnostic subgroups of adolescents, the course of treatment, the relative difficulty of treatment, and the probable outcome five years after hospital discharge.

This chapter has presented a parsimonious psychodynamic process model of treatment that potentially can serve as a clinical guide as well as a basis for research evaluation. Early in treatment, we attend to whether the patient maintains an attachment to others and whether he or she demonstrates a collaborative treatment alliance. In the second phase, we note whether the patient can communicate observations about his or her own psychological functioning, especially transference manifestations, and whether these self-observations have led to any useful insights into the determinants of symptomatic behavior or have led the patient to form new self-concepts. Has the patient been able to identify with the positive attributes of others in the hospital? In the third phase, the model suggests that the patient should gradually test out these new self-concepts as he or she is beginning to make plans to separate from the hospital, emphasizing that this separation should be gradual. In this final period, supportive and interpretive interventions aim to modify the regressive return to admission symptomatology, which often appears transiently as patients attempt to overcome anxiety over separation from the hospital.

As noted, there do seem to be certain adolescent disorders in which the family and the patient can readily grow and change within this framework without the appearance of destructive resistances. There is also a second group of adolescents with severe pathology or deficits whose progress continues, but with periodic delays. There are also a number of different syndromes in which pervasive damage to executive ego functions arising from physiological causes or deficits arising from severe psychosocial trauma during early personality development deprive the patients of a full response to this treatment program. Finally, there is a small group of adolescents and their families who are so rigidly locked into primitive or narcissistic defenses that their resistances to a therapeutic alliance seem impenetrable, even by skilled and patient clinicians.

These less responsive types of chronic adolescent patients require more investigation as well as experiments with new and focused interventions. Following the early assessment and treatment planning, the treatment team carries out regular reviews of patient progress. However, these periodic reviews may, in practice, serve only to reinforce the original treatment plan. Moreover, it is unusual to attempt to predict ultimate treatment outcome before the time for discharge planning. Since, for the reasons described, approximately one-third of our patients do not improve as greatly as one might have hoped, such an early formal reevaluation and outcome prediction should be added to our treatment routine.

POSTHOSPITAL DISCHARGE PLANNING

Approximately one year after admission, enough clinical experience will have accrued that such a judgment can be made about the patient's and the family's potential for ultimate improvement. This judgment will be based on how much change has been possible during the first twelve months. This initial baseline of change can be used to project future change and anticipate continuing unusual resistances to change. With certain groups of patients, such as adoptees or patients who have unusually strong passive-dependent needs or oppositional defenses or who have more serious cognitive deficits, it is relatively easy to foresee, by one year, who is going to progress slowly, if at all, during the second and third years. Therefore, to introduce a formal "outcome assessment" into the treatment program seems appropriate.

This reevaluation should engage the family and the patient openly in a frank and honest review of what has happened and what has not happened during the first year of treatment and what more can be anticipated between that point and the projected hospital discharge. After one year of hospitalization, it should be possible to anticipate those patients who may need to have a halfway house placement for two or more years between hospital discharge and autonomous living in the community. It also should be possible to alert adoptees and other chronically oppositional patients and their families to the losses in personality development that would accompany a premature disengagement from treatment by running away from the hospital or by giving up because the search for self-understanding does indeed mobilize, at times, high levels of anxiety. Collaborative inquiry with the patient and with the family needs also to be undertaken about their sense of what may be missing from the program in the way of support or interventions that have not been provided—what additional help, if it were provided by the hospital, would make the family and the patient more receptive to persisting in treatment? For example, adding a monthly evening multifamily group discussion of treatment problems has also been found to be a nonthreatening way of strengthening the treatment alliance. Our studies suggest the need to introduce more individualized approaches to treating specific forms of psychopathology. Individually tailored behavior modification or cognitive therapy interventions can be provided in a manner that is not necessarily incompatible with psychoanalytic process and may ameliorate specific ego deficits.

Following discharge, the routine application of a five-year follow-up study can provide meaningful outcome data if such data are evaluated using admission and treatment process observations as predictors. Published follow-up studies of hospital treatment have shown that the patient's condition at the time of discharge is not a useful basis for predicting the patient's level of functioning at the time of five-year follow-up. Therefore, discharge status does not provide an adequate basis for evaluating the effectiveness of hospital treatment (Gossett, Lewis, and Barnhart 1983).

Conclusions

In this chapter I suggest that the evaluation of psychoanalytic hospital treatment and its effectiveness for various psychopathological syndromes will be advanced through longitudinal investigations that link admission diagnosis to follow-up status and, at the same time, consider the patient's participation in the essential treatment processes as intervening variables between admission status and outcome. We need to increase the rigor, reliability, and standardization of our admission classification of patients. Eventually, this will improve our clinical consensus about adolescent disorders and our understanding of adolescent disorders beyond what is available from DSM-III-R. We need also to evaluate in an increasingly structured and standardized manner each patient's positive or negative response to the major treatment processes: attachment and alliance formation in phase 1; insight and new identifications in phase 2; and the transferential separation-individuation process during hospital discharge. The effectiveness of discharge planning and the adequacy of follow-up and rehabilitation services also need more rigorous study. If these principles can be implemented, these new observations should stimulate new therapeutic interventions.

NOTE

This chapter is a revision of a lecture presented to the Indiana State Psychiatric Society, April 21, 1988, Indianapolis.

REFERENCES

Almqvist, F. 1986. Psychiatric hospital treatment of young people. *Acta Psychiatrica Scandinavica* 73:289–294.

American Psychiatric Association. 1987. *Diagnostic and Statistical Manual of Mental Disorders.* 3d ed., rev. Washington, D.C.: American Psychiatric Association.

Bemporad, J. R.; Hanson, G.; and Smith, H. F. 1981. The diagnosis and treatment of borderline syndromes of childhood. In *American Handbook of Psychiatry,* 2d ed. New York: Basic.

Feinsilver, D. B. 1983. Reality, transitional relatedness and containment in the borderline. *Contemporary Psychoanalysis* 19:537–569.

Fullerton, C.; Goodrich, W.; and Berman, L. B. 1986. Adoption predicts treatment resistances. *Journal of the American Academy of Child and Adolescent Psychiatry* 25:542–551.

Goldstein, W. N. 1988. The depressive impulse-ridden character and the core borderline personality. *American Journal of Psychotherapy* 42:28–39.

Goodrich, W. 1984. Symbiosis and individuation: the integrative process for residential treatment of adolescents. *Current Issues in Psychoanalytic Practice* 1:23–45.

Goodrich, W. 1987. Long-term psychoanalytic hospital treatment of adolescents. *Psychiatric Clinics of North America* 10:273–287.

Goodrich, W., and Boomer, D. S. 1958. Some concepts about therapeutic interventions with hyperaggressive children. *Social Casework* 39:207–213, 286–291.

Gossett, J. T.; Lewis, J. M.; and Barnhart, F. D. 1983. *To Find a Way: The Outcome of Hospital Treatment of Adolescents.* New York: Brunner/Mazel.

Kernberg, O. 1976. *Object Relations Theory and Clinical Psychoanalysis.* New York: Aronson.

Kernberg, O. 1984. *Severe Personality Disorders: Psychotherapeutic Strategies.* New Haven, Conn.: Yale University Press.

Mahler, M. 1979. *Infantile Psychosis and Early Contributions.* New York: Aronson.

Masterson, J., and Costello, J. 1980. *From Borderline Adolescent to Functioning Adult.* New York: Brunner/Mazel.

Milazzo-Sayre, L. J. 1986. Use of inpatient psychiatric services by children and youth under age 18, United States, 1980. Mental Health Statistical Note, no. 175. Publication no. (ADM) 86-1451. Rockville, Md.: U.S. Department of Health and Human Services.

Miller, P., and PACTE (Hospital Coalition for Psychiatric Adolescent and Child Treatment and Education). 1988. Child and adolescent admission profile, 1985 and 1987. Paper presented at the annual meeting of the National Association of Private Psychiatric Hospitals, Phoenix, Arizona, January.

Price, R. 1983. Development of a relationship capacity in an atypical child. *Residential Group Care and Treatment* 1:3–21.

Redl, F. 1959. Strategy and techniques of the life space interview. *American Journal of Orthopsychiatry* 29:1–18.

Rinsley, D. B. 1980. *Treatment of the Severely Disturbed Adolescent.* New York: Aronson.

Robbins, M. 1983. Toward a new mind model for the primitive personality. *International Journal of Psycho-Analysis* 54:127–148.

245

13 ADOLESCENT INPATIENT ATTACHMENT AS TREATMENT PROCESS

RICHARD C. FRITSCH AND WELLS GOODRICH

Research on the effectiveness of inpatient residential treatment of adolescents has focused on admission or discharge patient characteristics as predictors of outcome (Gossett, Lewis, and Barnhart 1983; Grob and Singer 1974; Herrera, Lifson, and Solomon 1974). In the most comprehensive study, Gossett et al. (1983), defining outcome as the patient's adaptation in the community five years after discharge from the hospital, found that the most powerful prognostic sign was the severity and chronicity of the patient's symptoms at admission; other admission characteristics could also predict outcome. High IQ, a locus of control score indicating a sense of ego autonomy, and the posthospital continuation of psychotherapy predicted good outcome; severe family pathology was associated with poor outcome.

While these studies have made useful contributions by identifying some important prognostic indicators, they have generally ignored what transpires during the treatment to contribute to differential outcome within groups of patients with similar admission characteristics. With the possible exception of the family pathology variable, the other admission characteristics could be subsumed under the general category of severity of illness. The validity of these results, therefore, could be questioned on the grounds that better outcome only reflects the initial baseline differences documented at admission and that better functioning at outcome represents a maturational rather than a treatment effect.

On the basis of our clinical experience at Chestnut Lodge, we assume that many individual psychological and relational processes within the hospital have a great deal to do with whether the patient improves within the hospital and whether the patient maintains significant improvement after hospital discharge. Fineberg, Sowards, and Kettlewell's (1980) review of outcome research on residential treatment specifically states the need for process-oriented research and the absolute absence of any studies. It is our belief that a significant portion of the variance associated with differential outcome, above and beyond the variance explained by admission characteristics, can be explained by these process variables. This chapter will present some preliminary data that support these assumptions.

As described elsewhere (Goodrich 1987; Masterson 1972; Rinsley 1980), successful, long-term, inpatient treatment of adolescents involves negotiating three phases of hospitalization: (1) a resistance or testing phase, during which the adolescent resists separating psychologically from the family and resists forming attachments to the personnel in the treatment milieu; (2) a working through phase, during which interpersonal and intrapsychic conflicts are addressed in the various psychological therapies; and (3) a termination phase, during which new identifications and self-concepts are tested prior to discharge.

The residential treatment model suggests that initial improvement involves the partial replacement of outside emotional attachments with the establishment of affectional, ambivalent, or hostile attachments to peers, staff, teachers, and therapists within the hospital. The formation of new attachments in the hospital is seen as a prerequisite for more insight-oriented work. These new attachments are based on real people and relationships but also involve the transference of feelings and identifications from the early infantile and current family relationship patterns. The complexity of these relationships with the new caretaking figures in the hospital—the degree to which the early inhospital relationships are reality based—is a function of the maturity of the adolescent's object relations, his or her cognitive resources, and the qualitative history of his or her previous attachments as well as the patient's psychosexual development, intrapsychic defensive structure, and identity formation. While the patient's difficulties with close attachments have contributed to the clinical disturbance at admission, paradoxically, it is the patient's capacity, willingness, and demonstrated ability to form attachments and develop an alliance that we believe are salient predictors of the patient's psychological availability for intensive residential treatment.

From the clinical point of view, we are used to making prognostic judgments based on the attachment and alliance concepts. The adolescent's behavior during the initial interview as self-disclosing and comfortable in acknowledging inner conflict is seen as a sign of a "workable patient" and may become a clinical admission criterion. Similarly, the patient's ability to accept emotional support and limits from the staff, to tolerate separation from the family, and to form relationships with staff and peers all may be considered indicative of a favorable prognosis.

The concept of an attachment or an alliance has been advanced as a prerequisite for successful treatment to occur in almost all forms of psychosocial interventions (Bordin 1979). Outpatient studies of a variety of treatment modalities, such as psychodynamic/psychoanalytic treatment (Luborsky 1976; Luborsky, Crits-Cristoph, Alexander, Margolis, and Cohen 1983), brief psychotherapy (Harley and Strupp 1983), and behavior therapy (Staples, Sloane, Whipple, Cristol, and Yorkston 1976), have found that a measure of the alliance is predictive of good outcome.

Luborsky's (1976) research defined two types of alliance. What he called a "type 1" alliance was defined as the patient's experience of the therapist being helpful, supportive, and understanding. In other contexts, this has been seen as the "establishment of rapport," a "positive transference," or "viewing the therapist as a good object." Freud (1912) described the use of the patient's attachment to the analyst as a tool of psychoanalysis to induce the patient to perform psychical work, including that of overcoming transference resistances and of analyzing transference conflicts. From our point of view, the type 1 alliance represents the patient's experience of dependent attachment to the therapist or other significant staff member.

Consistent with our model or research, Luborsky (1976) found that, while characteristics of patients or therapists or even the match between therapist and patient characteristics has often not been predictive of outcome, the formation of a type 1 alliance (a dependent attachment) was predictive of improvement in outpatient psychotherapy.

What Luborsky called the "type 2" alliance, by comparison, is based on the collaborative experience of shared purposes and a feeling of mutual work on jointly agreed on tasks. In the psychoanalytic literature, this has been called the "working alliance." It has been advanced by Curtis (1979), Greenson (1967), and Zetzel (1966), who suggest that a distinction can be made between the "real" relationship between two people with a common goal and the transference relationship that is determined by the patient's dynamics. In a critique of the utility of the concept of alliance, Brenner (1979) has argued that all the phenomena that are included within the construct are inseparable from the transference. It is Brenner's belief that patient's experience of resistance or collaboration should be understood and dealt with by the analyst as an aspect of the transference and not seen as a prerequisite for the establishment of a transference neurosis.

In an effort to avoid the inherent difficulties raised by Brenner when the alliance is defined by the patient's feelings, Allen, Tarnoff, and Coyne (1985) focused on a type 2 alliance defined by the patient's level of active collaboration rather than his or her feelings about the therapist. Using an adult inpatient sample, they found that the measurement of the working collaboration at discharge was highly related to improvement ratings, changes in severity of illness, and positive changes in the profile of various ego functions. On the other hand, the level of collaboration at admission was not predictive of these outcome measures and was not correlated with the discharge collaboration scores. These data suggest that the collaboration process is not necessarily present at admission and may evolve over the course of hospitalization in relation to the first phase of changes in the patient.

Studies of the alliance defined as either type 1 or type 2 for inpatient adolescents have not been published. There is, however, evidence that better outcome is associated with the development of relationships within the hospital (Logan, Barnhart, and Gossett 1982) or with higher level of object relations (Masterson and Costello 1980), that are consistent with the underlying principles of the attachment or the capacity to form an alliance.

For the severely disturbed adolescent, the willingness to collaborate with the exploration of one's psychological world is generally not present at the outset of treatment. Mistrust, anger, resistance, and opposition to the work is the usual presentation. The establishment of a type 1 alliance or dependent attachment, therefore, appears to be germane to the understanding of within-hospital improvement during the first stage of treatment. Horowitz (1974) made a similar distinction when he observed that, while psychoanalysis presupposes and assumes a working collaboration between patient and analyst, one basic task of psychotherapy with more disturbed patients is to foster such a collaboration. He felt the formation of a working relationship could itself be an effective agent of change for these patients.

The research is clear that the concept of an attachment or an alliance has been useful in a predictive sense for adult outpatients and inpatients as a way of differentiating those patients who benefit from treatment from those who apparently do not. The intrapychic and interpersonal elements that constitute this construct beyond the phenomenology of the patient's activity remain unexplained. We feel, given the current state of knowledge, that a useful first step in this line of research would be to demonstrate that a relationship exists between the development of an attachment by an adolescent and positive change in his or her clinical course.

This chapter explores the relationships between the adolescent's report of a dependent attachment in the hospital and his or her concurrent decrease in severity of illness and improvement in interpersonal relatedness. The general hypothesis of this study is that, after controlling for severity of illness, those adolescents who form attachments to the program will show greater within hospital improvement than those adolescents who do not.

Methods

SUBJECTS

Subjects for this study came from a pool of consecutively admitted patients to the Adolescent and Child Division of Chestnut Lodge Hospital between the years 1980 and 1986. Sufficient data for this investigation were available on forty-five subjects (twenty-nine male, sixteen female). The adolescents admitted to Chestnut Lodge were predominantly from the upper socioeconomic brackets (Class I and II, Hollingshead and Redlich 1957) and were of normal intelligence ($M = 103$, S.D. $= 13.00$). Age at admission ranged from nine to nineteen years old with a mean age of 14.92. Most patients (70 percent) had at least one previous hospitalization, generally of a short-term nature. DSM-III (American Psychiatric Association 1980) Axis I diagnoses were predominantly dysthymic disorder, conduct disorder, or a combination of the two, with a substantial minority of patients (15 percent) diagnosed as either schizophrenic or schizophreniform disorder.

THE ATTACHMENT SCALE

To assess attachment, we adapted Summers' (1978) Scale of Symbiotic Relatedness. Using this scale, Summers and Walsh (1977) found that the intensity or primitiveness of the parental attachment differentiated among the diagnostic cohorts, with young adult schizophrenic patients significantly more symbiotically attached to their parents than borderline patients and borderline patients more symbiotically attached than normal young adults. This scale was applied to data generated from semistructured interview and projective tests. In the present research, we adapted the Summers scale to assess the attachment between the adolescents and the staff and other patients in the hospital. The scale was then applied to data derived from semistructured interviews.

Forty-five-minute research interviews were audiotaped, following informed consent, at three months and fifteen months after admission and at discharge with the patient and, separately, with a staff member very familiar with the patient. These interviews are semistructured in format and are designed to elicit data on cognitive, affective, and behavioral responses. The interviews are organized around the patient's experiences of a staff person or other patient who is identified as currently significant and meaningful to the patient. Questions about the intensity, quality, and meaning of the relationship are asked. Additional questions are directed at understanding the adolescent's capacity to modulate impulses and to differentiate himself or herself from the others to whom he or she is attached. The study reported here used only patient interview tapes.

As shown in table 1, the scale has seven dimensions: Separation, Possessiveness, Emotional Dependency, Instrumental Dependency, Differentiation, Integration of Hostility, and Modulation of Affects. These dimensions are consistent with the conceptualization of attachment behavior used by Bowlby (1978), Mahler (1979), and others.

Continua have been established in each of these areas with higher scores indicating more developed capacities. The organizing principle for each scale is that, for adolescents, a healthy attachment will involve

TABLE 1
SUBSCALES OF THE CHESTNUT LODGE ATTACHMENT SCALE

1.	Separation	Ability to recognize the importance of the object while maintaining functioning in its absence
2.	Possessiveness	Degree of approval of another person's right to other relationships
3.	Emotional Dependency	Ability to function independently while acknowledging the need for emotional support
4.	Instrumental Dependency ..	Ability to make decisions independently but also seek advice when appropriate
5.	Differentiation	Ability to distinguish one's own emotional state from those of others
6.	Integration of Hostility	Ability to integrate and productively express angry feelings
7.	Modulation of Affects	Ability to modulate the expression of affects in general

elements of dependence and independence. The high end of each subscale describes a quality of relating where the importance of the other is acknowledged and appreciated and where the adolescent is able to use the internalization in the absence of the object to maintain adaptive functioning in the milieu.

Points 1 and 2 of the scale describe autistic or primitive relatedness. This represents an adolescent who is unattached owing to a fragmented and disorganized ego or one for whom relatedness is based on a need-gratifying symbolic relatedness where the patient's functioning is impaired in the absence of the object. The low end of these continua indicate patients who establish intensely overclose ties or inappropriately alienated ways of relating, while patients given high scores (6 or 7) have gained the capacity for appropriately modulating closeness and distance in intimate attachments. The middle levels (3–5) describe two positions. The attachment is a continuation of the lower, symbiotic attachment, but somewhat more integrated. Alternatively, this level defines a denial of attachment needs, where the patient denies the attachment in counterdependent ways that we believe are defensive. It is our assumption that these points constitute an interval scale of the attachment experience. Given this assumption, the subscales sum to yield an overall measure of the adolescent's attachment to the treatment process.

Despite the complexity of the concepts and the clinical nature of the data, with the exception of the Separation scale (intraclass correlation coefficient = .62, Shrout and Fleiss 1979), the scales have been scored with adequate reliability (intraclass correlation coefficients for two raters ranging from .69 to .83 with a mean of .76). This study used the average for the six reliable scales to provide a measure of attachment. Two raters independently rated each tape. An average of these two scores was used in the analysis.

Patients were assigned to "good" or "poor" attachment groups by mean split of all adolescents administered an attachment interview (including those not in this sample because of other missing data). The mean attachment score was 4.10 (S.D. = .80, range = 1–7), suggesting that the data on attachment were normally distributed since 4 is the midpoint of the seven-point scale.

DIAGNOSIS

Since severity of psychopathology has been found to be a useful predictor of outcome, with neurotic and "mild borderline" patients faring better than more severe personality disordered and psychotic patients, the sample was divided into three groups based on severity of illness and level of personality structure as a way to control for this variable. A senior clinician (Goodrich), who was acquainted with the adolescents but blind to the attachment scores, reviewed the admission notes and assigned the patients to the three groups. The first group was labeled "borderline" and included those adolescents for whom a higher-level borderline personality structure was inferred ($N = 28$). A second group ($N = 10$) was called "schizotypal" and included those adolescents who presented with what was essentially a psychotic or severe borderline level of organization to the personality but without recurrent or active psychotic symptoms. These adolescents typically had DSM-III diagnoses of borderline, schizoid, schizotypal, or brief reactive psychoses. A third group, labeled "psychotic," was defined as those adolescents with a chronic psychotic illness. This was a relatively small group ($N = 7$).

Results

The basic design for these analyses was a repeated measures analysis of variance. This design assessed change in level of functioning over time as measured by the Global Assessment Scale (GAS, Endicott,

253

Spitzer, Fleiss, and Cohen 1976) from preadmission (rated from history), three months into treatment, and fifteen months into treatment. This design takes the patients' baseline functioning (i.e., the initial level of psychopathology) into account in assessing the amount of change over time within the hospital.

For the entire sample taken as a whole, there is a significant change from admission to three months ($F = 74.46$, $p < .001$) and a smaller change from three months to fifteen months ($F = 6.89$, $p < .03$) (table 2, fig. 1). These results suggest that, for those adolescents who stay at Chestnut Lodge for fifteen months, improvement is likely.

Previous research had suggested that preadmission and immediate postadmission variables could account for some of the variability in outcome. In our study, these "classic" predictors of improvement—internal locus of control, intelligence level, and age at admission—were associated with neither a higher level of functioning at fifteen months nor change from preadmission to fifteen months for our sample (all Pearson correlations nonsignificant, $p > .10$).

A 2×3 analysis of variance with repeated measures showed that significant differences in within-hospital improvement was an effect of level of psychopathology, attachment, and an interaction between attachment and level of psychopathology. Table 2 provides the mean GAS scores for each time period, subdivided by structural diagnosis and level of attachment.

The classification of adolescents by structural level, as expected, did predict outcome ($F = 10.15$, $p < .001$). Both borderline and schizotypal groups had significantly higher levels of functioning at admission, three months, and fifteen months than the psychotic group ($p < .05$, Duncan range test). The borderline group had significantly higher GAS scores at admission and three months than did the schizotypal group ($p < .05$, Duncan range test), but by fifteen months there were no differences between these two groups. The change lines for all three groups were essentially parallel (fig. 1), suggesting that initial level of functioning is a salient variable for all groups.

The attachment variable—defined as good versus poor attachment through mean split—also predicted which patients made within–hospital improvements. Those adolescents who formed a three-month attachment showed more improvement from admission to fifteen months ($F = 4.37$, $p < .02$, fig. 2) than those who did not. The significant interaction between diagnostic level and attachment

TABLE 2

Mean GAS Scores by Time, Diagnosis, and Level of Attachment

	Admission		3 Months		15 Months	
	Good Attachment	Poor Attachment	Good Attachment	Poor Attachment	Good Attachment	Poor Attachment
Borderline ($M = 51.9$)	41.5	38.7	60.3*	44.0*	63.7*	46.4*
Schizotypal ($M = 47.1$)	37.1	33.0	53.8**	38.0**	58.2	62.4
Psychotic ($M = 31.4$)	30.0	25.6	36.7	38.4	27.7***	45.8***
Mean GAS	37.33		50.93		56.0	

Note.—Contrasts for GAS levels for good attachment *vs.* poor attachment are nonsignificant unless marked with a superscript: * = .001, ** = .009, and *** = .06. For main effects, borderline > schizotypal > psychotic and GAS admission < GAS 3 months < GAS 15 months at $p < .05$.

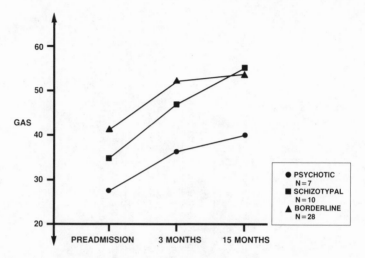

Fɪɢ. 1.—GAS by attachment over time (psychotic)

($F = 5.21$, $p < .001$) suggests that attachment is related to outcome differently for each of the diagnostic groups.

For the borderline group (table 2, fig. 3), there was little difference in functioning at admission for the sample of all borderlines. Those adolescents who formed an attachment made significantly greater

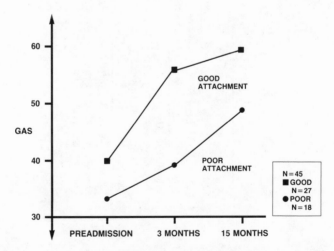

Fɪɢ. 2.—GAS over time: borderline, schizotypal, and psychotic patients

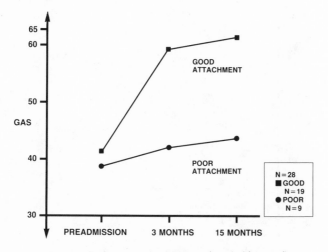

FIG. 3.—GAS by attachment over time (schizotypal)

improvements by three months than did the poor-attachment adolescents and maintained this differential improvement to fifteen months.

For the schizotypal patients (table 2, fig. 4), the quality of the attachment was also significant. Adolescents in this group who made a good attachment showed higher three-month GAS scores than the poor-attachment adolescents did. By fifteen months, however, those who had not made an attachment at three months were functioning at the same level as the good-attachment adolescents.

The data suggest that the good-attachment psychotic adolescent shows no difference in functioning compared to the poor-attachment adolescent at three months. There is actually a trend at fifteen months for the good-attachment adolescents to function less well than the poorly attached psychotic adolescent (table 2, fig. 5). With two adolescents in the good-attachment group, however, it is difficult to interpret these unexpected results with any certainty.

Discussion

These preliminary data suggest that our investigation is headed in the right direction. For adolescents with personality disorders, the formation of a workable, dependent attachment to the major figures in the milieu appears to be a salient variable associated with inhospital symptomatic improvement. This suggests that the model usefully

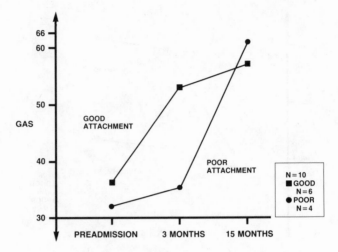

FIG. 4.—GAS by attachment over time (all patients)

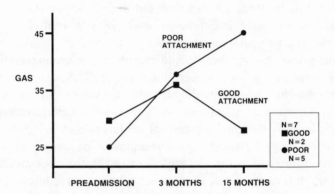

FIG. 5.—GAS by attachment over time (borderline)

highlights an important treatment-process variable. In terms of treatment process, at least for personality-disordered adolescents, the initial task of a long-term residential program may be the formation of this type 1 alliance.

While the attachment can be viewed as another type of admission variable (i.e., a special type of personality variable), the fact that it measures behaviors, attitudes, and feelings directed toward attachment figures within the hospital represents an added dimension. From an empirical standpoint, since the quality of attachment subdivides sub-

258

jects within diagnostic classifications, differential improvement is unlikely to be an expression of simply healthier patients making more improvement. In addition, different change patterns for each of the groups and the fact that change over time was controlled for significantly limit the likelihood that the relation between the attachment process and within-hospital change was simply a function of time in the hospital.

The data on the borderline patients suggest that, for this group, the capacity and/or willingness to form an attachment differentiates between those adolescents who make the most symptomatic progress within the first fifteen months of treatment. The pattern suggests that the potential for either forming an immediate attachment or maintaining a prolonged resistance is present at admission for higher-level borderline patients. The treatment model suggests that it is the patients who have worked through the resistance to engagement with the treatment program who enter the second phase of treatment where transference-based relationships in individual therapy can be used for effecting substantial change. Those who continue to resist the effect of the milieu owing to nonoptimal containment (either too permissive or too restrictive), family resistance, or internal resistance to modifying pathological attachments, as a group, effect much less change. These attachment data, therefore, support this model for understanding differential improvement.

The results for the schizotypal group suggest that, for some of these adolescents, the attachment took longer to make. Improvement from three months to fifteen months may parallel their increased capacity to trust the milieu, the therapist, and the family. The poor-attachment schizotypal group highlights the importance of longer-term treatment for selected adolescents. If discharge would have occurred after only three months in treatment, the functional gains would have been minimal for these adolescents. By fifteen months in the hospital, however, their levels of functioning reached the same level as the good-attachment schizotypal adolescents and the good-attachment borderline adolescents and surpassed the functional level of the borderlines who did not form an attachment.

The psychotic group was puzzling, but, with such a small sample, these results should be seen as hypothesis generating. For the psychotic group as a whole, the attachment during the first three months of hospitalization may be a less significant predictor of level of functioning than other variables, such as the chronicity of the psychosis. It is possible, however, to view the capacity of the psychotic adolescent to resist an early hospital attachment as an expectable resistance rather than a structural weakness and may represent an early effort at differentiation and control over this new social environment. In addition, while not a uniform phenomena, it has been clinically observed that an ego regression frequently accompanies the formation of a therapeutic attachment in our adult and adolescent patients who are psychotic (Pao 1979).

Further clarification is needed to determine the causal relation between formation of attachment and the increase in global functioning among hospitalized adolescents. It is our hypothesis that the formation of an attachment leads to a decrease in symptoms. An increase in global functioning, however, may be a prerequisite for attachment rather than the converse. Furthermore, it is plausible that the relation between attachment and improvement is a function of some third variable that effects each of these dimensions simultaneously.

The containment function of the milieu, for example, is a candidate for this third variable. The milieu may have a differential effect on adolescents with similar levels of disturbance but dissimilar conflict and defense dynamics. For adolescents from traumatic or abusive home environments, for example, the containment may reduce stress and limit regressive tendencies and may permit higher-level capacities to be employed, including the capacity to engage in meaningful relationships with others. For other adolescents at about the same level of symptom expression, the separation from the family may be viewed as traumatic, and the milieu may not attenuate and may even catalyze resistances, with suspiciousness, withdrawal, or oppositionality prevailing. Furthermore, it is entirely possible that for some adolescents, as the data suggest may be the case for psychotic adolescents, resistance to forming an attachment may be a signal of health rather than pathology or resistance. This conundrum speaks to one problem with global measures such as attachment or alliance.

Conclusions

While the constructs have clinical utility and demonstrated empirical predictive power, the intrapsychic elements that constitute a good attachment or a poor attachment for groups of patients with similar levels of psychopathology in general, and for individual patients in particular, have yet to be determined. The constructs themselves do not provide direction on how to facilitate a good attachment, a process that may be quite different for patients with differing needs, conflicts, defenses, and transference propensities. With the addition of measures of intrapsychic functioning such as object relations, reality testing, defenses, and core conflicts that will be included in our future research efforts, we hope to provided further elucidation of these process variables. The ultimate aim of this type of research remains as Gossett et al. (1983) state—to "find a way" of providing effective treatment for these frequently treatment-resistant adolescents.

Despite these limitations, this research demonstrates that attending to hospital change and hypothesized processes can yield interesting results that explain variance associated with hospital treatment above and beyond the variance associated with severity of illness.

NOTE

The authors wish to acknowledge the help and support of many people associated with the research project within the Adolescent and Child Division of Chestnut Lodge: Dexter M. Bullard Jr., medical director; Jaime Buenaventura, clinical director; Mary-Louise Schmidt, director of nursing; Phyllis Stang, nursing coordinator; Maureen Cavanaugh, assistant nursing coordinator; and Ginny Embry, Nancy Mornini, Michael Gleason, Mildred Hamacher-Bennett, and Vivian McCrimon, houseparents. In addition, we would like to thank our colleagues at the Chestnut Lodge Research Institute for their review and support of this project: Thomas McGlashan, director of research; Robert K. Heinssen, research coordinator; David Feinsilver, symposium chairperson; Linda Beth Berman, editorial and research assistant; and Carol Thompson and Patricia Inana, secretaries.

REFERENCES

Allen, J. G.; Tarnoff, G.; and Coyne, L. 1985. Therapeutic alliance and long-term hospital treatment outcome. *Comprehensive Psychiatry* 16(2): 187–194.

American Psychiatric Association. 1980. *Diagnostic and Statistical Manual of the Mental Disorders.* 3d ed. Washington, D.C.: American Psychiatric Press.

Bordin, E. S. 1979. The generalizability of the psychoanalytic concept of the working alliance. *Psychotherapy, Theory, Research, and Practice* 16:252–260.

Bowlby, J. 1978. Attachment theory and its therapeutic implications. *Adolescent Psychiatry* 6:5–33.

Brenner, C. 1979. Working alliance, therapeutic alliance and transference. *Journal of the American Psychoanalytic Association* 27:137–158.

Curtis, H. 1979. The concept of therapeutic alliance: implications for the "widening scope." *Journal of the American Psychoanalytic Association* 27:159–162.

Endicott, J.; Spitzer, R.; Fleiss, J.; and Cohen, J. 1976. The Global Assessment Scale: a procedure for measuring overall severity of psychiatric disturbance. *Archives of General Psychiatry* 33:766–771.

Fineberg, B. L.; Sowards, S. K.; and Kettlewell, P. W. 1980. Adolescent inpatient treatment: a literature review. *Adolescence* 15(60): 913–925.

Freud, S. 1912. The dynamics of transference. *Standard Edition* 12:97–108. London: Hogarth, 1953.

Goodrich, W. G. 1987. Long-term psychoanalytic hospital treatment of adolescents. *Psychiatric Clinics of North America* 10:273–287.

Gossett, J. T.; Lewis, J. M.; and Barnhart, F. D. 1983. *To Find a Way.* New York: Brunner/Mazel.

Greenson, R. R. 1967. *The Technique and Practice of Psychoanalysis.* New York: International Universities Press.

Grob, M. C., and Singer, J. E. 1974. *Adolescent Patients in Transition: Impact and Outcome of Psychiatric Hospitalization.* New York: Behavioral Publications.

Harley, D. E., and Strupp, H. H. 1983. The therapeutic alliance: its relationship to outcome in brief psychotherapy. In J. Masling, ed. *Empirical Studies of Psychoanalytic Theories,* vol. 1. Hillsdale, N.J.: Analytic Press.

Herrera, E. G.; Lifson, B. G.; and Solomon, M. H. 1974. A 10-year follow-up of 55 hospitalized adolescents. *American Journal of Psychiatry* 131:769–774.

Hollingshead, A. B., and Redlich, F. C. 1957. *Social Class and Mental Illness.* New York: Wiley.

Horowitz, L. 1974. *Clinical Prediction in Psychotherapy.* New York: Aronson.

Logan, W. S.; Barnhart, F. D.; and Gossett, J. T. 1982. The prognostic significance of adolescent interpersonal relationships during psychiatric hospitalization. *Adolescent Psychiatry* 10:434–493.

Luborsky, L. 1976. Helping alliances in psychotherapy. In J. L. Clagborn, ed. *Successful Psychotherapy.* New York: Brunner/ Mazel.

Luborsky, L.; Crits-Christoph, P.; Alexander, L.; Margolis, M.; and Cohen, M. 1983. Two helping alliance methods for predicting outcomes of psychotherapy: a counting signs vs. a global rating method. *Journal of Nervous and Mental Disease* 171:480–491.

Mahler, M. S. 1979. *Selected Papers: Separation-Individuation*, vol. 2. New York: Aronson.

Masterson, J. T. 1972. *Treatment of the Borderline Adolescent.* New York: Wiley.

Masterson, J. T., and Costello, J. L. 1980. *From Borderline Adolescent to Functioning Adult.* New York: Brunner/Mazel.

Pao, Ping-Nie. 1979. *Schizophrenic Disorders.* New York: International Universities Press.

Rinsley, D. B. 1980. *Treatment of the Severely Disturbed Adolescent.* New York: Aronson.

Shrout, P. E., and Fleiss, J. L. 1979. Interclass correlations: uses in assessing rater reliability. *Psychological Bulletin* 86:420–428.

Staples, F. R.; Sloane, R. B.; Whipple, K.; Cristol, A. H.; and Yorkston, N. 1976. Process and outcome in psychotherapy and behavior therapy. *Journal of Consulting and Clinical Psychology* 44:340–350.

Summers, F. 1978. Manual for the measurement of symbiosis in the human relationships. *Psychological Reports* 43:663–670.

Summers, F., and Walsh, F. 1977. The nature of the symbiotic bond between mother and schizophrenic. *American Journal of Orthopsychiatry* 47:484–494.

Zetzel, E. R. 1966. The analytic situation. In R. E. Litman, ed. *Psychoanalysis in the Americas.* New York: International Universities Press.

14 THE SIGNIFICANCE OF THE ATTACHMENT PROCESS IN BRAIN-DAMAGED ADOLESCENT PSYCHIATRIC PATIENTS

REBECCA E. RIEGER

In the Chestnut Lodge Adolescent and Child Division, as in other psychiatric inpatient settings (Andrulonis, Glueck, Strobel, et al. 1981), there exists a subgroup of patients with borderline and psychotic diagnoses who began life with discernible biological impairment or whose early development was influenced by biological deficits, abnormalities, or anomalies. These could range from the constellation of early problems in biological regulation manifested by Chess and Thomas's (1984) "difficult" babies, to the diverse problems stemming from prematurity or perinatal complications such as hyperactivity and compromised cognitive and motor development with later school problems, to early onset of neurological abnormalities like the epilepsies, to physical anomalies like undescended testicles or disfiguring aspects of face or body.

If and when such children or adolescents develop severe psychiatric problems at a borderline or psychotic level of functioning and are hospitalized in a psychoanalytically oriented treatment milieu, what treatment responses are likely to occur? In particular, what are the prospects for the initial stage of attachment and for the subsequent formation of a treatment alliance?

Within the borderline and psychotic group of adolescents, among those who often present as more severely ill and disordered, will be patients with impairments in autonomous ego functions whose early object relations may not have been "good enough" to overcome their difficulties but were not malignant. They may be more vulnerable to breakdown as a consequence of their impairment, more limited in their potential for therapeutically induced change, and yet more available for attachment because they have some sense of an internalized good object and, therefore, have some degree of basic trust in a safe dependency. Luborsky (1976) defined a type 1 alliance with a therapist as the patient's experience of the therapist as helpful, supportive, and understanding and a type 2 alliance as the collaborative experience of shared goals and a sense of mutual work on jointly agreed on tasks. For these impaired patients, the type 1 dependent relationship may be facilitated; the capacity for a type 2 more collaborative treatment alliance is likely to depend on the nature and degree of impairment.

The family of an impaired child is subjected to severe emotional, social, and, frequently, financial stresses. From the earliest period, the mother is responsive to the infant's physical and temperamental presentation. Where the infant fails to meet parental hopes and expectations, or where the infant's responses to the mothering one are anxiety provoking or frustrating, the potential for negatively toned affects such as helplessness, depression, disappointment, anger, and guilt can be anticipated in the mothering one, the family, the child, or in all. In the case of a child with a long period of unremitting seizure activity, or in the case of hyperactive children, when the high intensity of internal excitatory states exceeds the child's own regulatory capacity, the mother's availability and competence to soothe and contain become even more critical than in the case of the biologically normal child. Equally, when the child's vulnerability to narcissistic injury is heightened because of unusual physical attributes (such as disfiguring anomalies or abnormal developmental deviations like undescended testicles), the "reflected appraisals" from significant others—the parental capacity to convey loving acceptance but realistic expectations and to demonstrate efforts at appropriate remediation—will greatly influence the self-concept, self-acceptance, and future object relations of the child. The demands on the mothering figure and other caretakers may exceed their resources, but the child may nevertheless experience its object world as concerned and available.

Margaret Mahler (1968), in her work at the New York State Psychiatric Institute in the early 1940s, was struck by the ongoing capacity of the psychiatrically disturbed "organic" child to interact with his human environment: "Against the background of the more usual types of interaction of the organic group of the population of the children's ward (those children displayed a somewhat bizarre, but still, for the most part, clinging, definite, and realistic interaction with the adult), I was able to observe a most striking inability, on the part of the psychotic child, even to see the human object in the outside world, let alone to interact with him as with another separate human entity" (p. 3).

A much later report by Goldfarb, Myers, Florsheim, and Goldfarb (1978) on the treatment of psychotic children at the Ittelson Center included comparisons between the neurologically intact and "organic" children: their familial backgrounds, adaptive capacity (ego resources) at the beginning of treatment, course in treatment, condition at discharge, and follow-up 8.7 years after they returned to their families. Several of the conclusions bear on the hypothesis that the familial environment of the organic child may be more benign than that of the severely disturbed nonorganic child. Goldfarb et al. point out, first, that "organic children come from a broader range of families and more frequently have been reared in average families" (p. 135); second, that "organic psychotic children of early school age responded equally well to treatment in day and residential programs; but that the nonorganic children tended to respond better to the 24 hour program of the residence" (p. 169); and, third, that, although the nonorganic children manifested greater improvement than the organic children at discharge and both groups showed improvements in ego status at follow-up, "the more consistent trend among organic children toward sustaining growth in ego in the period following discharge from residential treatment offset the more successful response of the non-organic children to residential treatment" (p. 138).

The case studies that follow are illustrative of the capacity of some organically impaired adolescents with severe psychiatric symptoms to make the initial attachment to therapist and milieu, but with divergent outcomes. Frank was born full term, weighing five pounds, four ounces, with an initial Apgar of zero, the need to be rescussitated, and a ten-minute cry delay. Prenatal development was abnormal, with delayed intrauterine growth. His mother had taken medications during pregnancy, including antibiotics and phenobarbitol. He spent his first two weeks in a hospital incubator; shortly thereafter, a cogenital heart condition was diagnosed. He was colicky his first year, and his growth rate was slow. With locomotion, he became hyperactive. He had severe temper tantrums by age two, involving head banging, screaming, and destroying objects, and he was sporadically uncontrollable by his depressed mother. In nursery school, he was diagnosed as having an attention deficit disorder with hyperactivity, continued to have severe temper tantrums, then spent nine months in a school for emotionally disturbed children (on medication), and returned home unimproved. There then followed a progression of hospitalizations and special schools, with brief remissions and a variety of diagnoses and medications. He was described as thought disordered and affectively disordered, with mood swings and agitation. He was tried on Haldol, Cogentin, Mellaril, and lithium, among other medications. There were improvements and severe regressions, ambivalence about treatment, and anxiety about discharge. Overall, Frank's IQ remained in the low normal range.

Beginning early in his postnatal development, Frank experienced an inconstant human environment. His affectively unstable mother, ultimately diagnosed bipolar affective disorder, suffered a postpartum depression, and, during her many depressed and manic periods, Frank was cared for in different family households. In addition, he suffered losses of significant objects through divorce (his biological father), through death (his adoptive father), and through separation (from two half siblings), and he was also subjected to his mother's emotional reactions to these events. His half siblings of the same mother but different fathers have been free of psychiatric illness.

On admission to Chestnut Lodge at age sixteen, Frank was a distinctly odd-looking, unusually short adolescent for his age. He and his family regarded the Lodge as a last chance to pull his life together. In the initial process of assigning a therapist, special weight was given to Frank's clearly expressed desire to work with his present therapist both because it was judged wise to assign him to a male and because there had been an immediate feeling of attachment during the admissions interview. This attachment has remained firm and Frank's attitude toward his therapist unambivalent, but idealized, and the social worker, who has a good alliance with Frank's mother, has born the brunt of the split affect.

His therapist's initial optimistic assessment of prognosis included Frank's "remembrance of a good enough experience in the past that has allowed him to move from one developmental phase to another without crippling fixation." Frank was discharged as much improved after eighteen months of inpatient treatment. He has been living in the community with a member of his extended family and working. On a recent visit to Chestnut Lodge, he expressed warm affection for his therapist and appreciation of the hospital's role in helping him to reclaim his life.[1]

Lucy came to the adolescent unit of Chestnut Lodge at the age of seventeen with a diagnosis of schizophrenia, hebephrenic type. Her admitting administrator described her as "one of the sickest people that I have ever seen in my entire life." She was fragmented, hallucinating, and hyperactive and displayed labile affect. Much of the first month was spent in seclusion, as the unit strove to establish a predictable, safe environment. On admission, Lucy attached herself very rapidly to the housemother and then to other staff members. By the second week, she gave staff members names from the past. From about the third week, changes were discernible. She expressed great loneliness and feelings of estrangement. She was allowed to talk to her parents by telephone under supervision, and the contact seemed to have a favorable effect. Within three months of her admission, she had become very attached to her therapist (an older male) and was described as active in the house routines and chores, enjoying many sports, and getting along with her peers in her house and in the other houses.

Lucy, the second of three siblings, was the product of a seven-week premature delivery, weighing two pounds, ten ounces, at birth. Her mother had had German measles at the end of the first trimester and toxemia in the seventh month. Lucy had seizures at five weeks old, and developmental milestones, particularly speech, were slow. She had an eye operation for strabismus at twenty months. At two and a half years old, she was diagnosed as having minimal brain dysfunction, secondary to prematurity.

She was born into a large, wealthy, high-achieving family and during early childhood and latency seemed happy within the structure of the close extended family and the interested, supportive institutions. Her dysarthric speech, which was usually labored and difficult to understand, created a barrier with her peers, and she adjusted best with adults. At age seven, her IQ as measured by the Binet was 95, that is, within the average range, but by the tenth grade her WISC (Wechsler Intelligence Scale for Children) IQ was in the seventies, the impaired range, demonstrating that, despite all the special educational efforts, she fell more and more behind the expanding capacities of her normal peer group.

Her first psychotic break at age sixteen—of one and a half days' duration—was in response to the departure of a teacher with whom she had formed a close relationship, and the psychotic symptoms cleared spontaneously. The second break occurred several days before she was to return from vacation to a special education boarding school where she had roomed with a sexually acting-out girl. Lucy had been witness to some of the activity. During the ensuing ten-week psychotic period, she had a paradoxical response to a large variety of medications before coming to the Lodge, where she was initially taken off medication.

The family has no psychiatric history of either schizophrenia or major affective illness, but the mother did have a period of depression when Lucy was one year old. The mother is described as obsessive, controlling, given to structuring, and very much involved with Lucy. The two siblings (an older brother and a younger sister) show no evidence of psychopathology and have been progressing with their lives.

After coming out of her psychotic state, Lucy remained essentially in remission until about one year after the death of her therapist of three years. She had not openly mourned but had rapidly attached to her new therapist, a young woman. It was on the occasion of the latter's absence on an extended vacation that Lucy began to decompensate and again became psychotic for about eighteen months. During this long period, she maintained the positive attachment to her therapist. Lucy has now been in remission for over two years. Between psychotic periods, she is described as "a sweet, likable girl to meet, and people do gravitate toward her." With her peers, she can be intrusive and naively inappropriate. All who care for her are acutely aware of her vulnerability in the face of separation and moves toward greater autonomy. In Lucy's case, one might address the question that Michael Stone (1980) raised when he suggested that in some organically impaired patients the psychotic symptomatology might be only a "phenocopy" of schizophrenia.

For some patients, with greater biological impairments, the attachment to the therapist may remain quite dependent, but a collaborative attitude toward exploration of feelings, object relations, and behavioral consequences is not precluded, and, therefore, a greater potential for self-regulation exists. Lucy's dependent attachment continues, but she is working on the hospital grounds, and her therapist and the rehabilitation staff are gradually and carefully preparing her for somewhat more autonomous functioning. In the case of less-impaired adolescents like Frank, the initial attachment can move more rapidly into a type 2 therapeutic alliance with greater expectation for stable change and independent functioning.

For the impaired adolescent, the maintenance of a positive transference and a therapeutically supportive position, with flexible expectations regarding the capacity for expressive psychotherapy, is a necessary if not sufficient condition for significant gains in treatment. The issue of potential successful outpatient or residential treatment of organically impaired patients has received little attention because the psychoanalytic community has tended to avoid such patients or, if taken into treatment, to deny the special problems they present. This is particularly so if the impairment itself continues to influence cognition, affect modulation, the attainment of instrumental skills, the course of object relations, and the capacity for autonomous living. Such patients will still have conflicts, disturbed object relations, maladaptive behavior patterns, resistances, and defenses to be analyzed. But, to quote John Gedo (1987), "Insofar as a therapist is either unable or unwilling to assist impaired patients to avoid the deleterious consequences of their insufficient adaptive repertory, this failure to participate in a symbiotic dyad will almost always constitute a repetition within the transference of parental failures to provide the care these individuals required as children."

Conclusions

With the impaired adolescent, it is particularly important to be very clear about differentiating between impairment that would be remediable if he were psychologically available and impairment that could be compensated for, as against fixed and intractable impairment, which would preclude overvalued, narcissistically generated, unrealistic educational and vocational choices and plans.

For the impaired patient, the second phase of treatment—the type 2 alliance—must include not only the collaborative work to gain insight into transferentially based patterns of behavior but also concomitant ongoing ego-strengthening and ego-supportive elements to compensate for, or assist the maturation of, the deficient autonomous ego functions. For these patients, an extended period of "legitimate dependency" may be needed, toward the goal of helping them achieve their optimal sense of well-being and self-worth.

NOTE

1. In the course of a review-of-therapy case conference at Chestnut Lodge, Dr. Wells Goodrich remarked that "those cases where elements of brain damage are present paradoxically often respond more positively to environment. The need for environmental structure is more available and less defended against."

REFERENCES

Andrulonis, P. A.; Glueck, B. C.; Strobel, C. F.; et al. 1981. Organic brain dysfunction and the borderline syndrome. *Psychiatric Clinics of North America* 4:47–66.

Chess, S., and Thomas, A. 1984. *Origins and Evolution of Behavior Disorders.* New York: Brunner/Mazel.

Gedo, J. E. 1987. Character, dyadic enactments, and the need for symbiosis. Paper presented to the Washington School of Psychiatry Symposium on the Interpersonal and the Intrapsychic.

Goldfarb, W.; Meyers, D. I.; Florsheim, J.; and Goldfarb, N. 1978. Psychotic children grown up—a prospective follow-up. *Issues in Child Mental Health* 5(2): 108–172.

Luborsky, L. 1976. Helping alliance in psychotherapy. In J. L. Clagborn, ed. *Successful Psychotherapy.* New York: Brunner/Mazel.

Mahler, M. S. 1968. *On Human Symbiosis and the Vicissitudes of Individuation.* Vol. 1, *Infantile Psychosis.* New York: International Universities Press.

Stone, M. H. 1980. *The Borderline Syndrome.* New York: McGraw-Hill.

15 THE SEX AND EXPERIENCE OF THE THERAPIST AND THEIR EFFECTS ON INTENSIVE PSYCHOTHERAPY OF THE ADOLESCENT INPATIENT

CAROL S. FULLERTON, BRIAN T. YATES, AND WELLS GOODRICH

This chapter explores the effects of matching therapist and patient gender and therapist experience level on psychoanalytic psychotherapy outcome for adolescents hospitalized for an average of thirty-one months. A significant interaction between patient-therapist gender match and therapist experience level was found to affect improvement in severity of illness ($p = .017$) from admission to three months in the hospital. The greatest improvement occurred in same gender matches with therapists who had less than ten years of experience and in mixed gender matches with therapists who had ten years of experience or more. Possible effects of identification and therapist ability to deal with sexual countertransference issues are discussed.

The question of whether an adolescent patient sees a male or a female psychotherapist is a controversial issue with theoretical as well as practical implications for further understanding of psychotherapeutic outcome (Blos 1962; Corday 1967; Godenne 1982; Holmes 1964; Ivey 1960; Kestenberg 1968; Mattsson 1970; Mogul 1982). Experience level of the psychotherapist is also relevant when considering possible correlates to outcome of psychotherapy (Parloff, Waskow, and Wolfe 1978). The current study explores a population of adolescents undergoing psychoanalytic psychotherapy on an adolescent unit within a private psychiatric hospital. The sample of therapists includes therapists who are older and more experienced than those included in previous studies.

In intensive long-term psychoanalytic psychotherapy where structural changes are sought, it is important to study shifts in the transference response and those defensive resistances to attachment or to insight (Goodrich 1984, 1987; Masterson and Costello 1980; Rinsley 1980). The adolescent patient may be especially vulnerable to fearful distrust of the therapist or to an eroticized transference, making it difficult to establish a therapeutic alliance. Although a neutral posture is assumed by the analyst, qualities of the therapist may contribute to the therapeutic alliance and ultimate outcome of psychodynamic psychotherapy.

Method

This study was conducted at Chestnut Lodge Hospital, a private, long-term, psychoanalytically oriented psychiatric hospital located in Rockville, Maryland. In the current study, all patients were seen in psychotherapy for fifty minutes, four times per week. The average length of stay in the hospital was thirty-one months, facilitating exploration of early, middle, and later phases of therapy.

SUBJECTS

Sample size by gender match was as follows: male patient with male therapist, forty-three pairs; female patient with female therapist, sixteen pairs; male patient with female therapist, eleven pairs; and female patient with male therapist, twenty-one pairs. Only patients diagnosed as personality disordered using DSM-III (American Psychiatric Association 1980) were included as subjects in this study. Psychotic patients were eliminated from the study because of the possible confounding effect of diagnosis on psychotherapy outcome. Mean age of the patients on admission was 15.3 years old. All patients were Caucasian and from middle- and upper-class families.

Among the thirty-five therapists (twenty-six male and nine female), there was a mean of 2.6 patients per therapist, and a range of one to eight patients per therapist. Most therapists were psychoanalysts or were in psychoanalytic training. Years of experience since completion of psychiatric residency ranged from 0.5 to 39.5 years of clinical practice, with a mean of 11.2 years experience. The theoretical orientation of all therapists was psychoanalytic, thus making them a rather homogeneous group. The age range of therapists was from twenty-nine to seventy-four years (mean age of forty-three years); the range of therapists' years of experience spanned four decades. Thus, a broader base within which to examine effects of experience was offered than has been reported heretofore.

INSTRUMENTATION

Psychotherapy outcome was measured by change in severity of illness as assessed using the Global Assessment Scale (GAS; Endicott, Spitzer, Fleiss, and Cohen 1976). The scale measured the patient's symptomatic behavior as treatment progressed. Medical records were used to obtain data on patient-therapist match. Independent GAS ratings were carried out concurrently by the clinical administrative psychiatrist and by the head nurse, as they were the only staff with equal exposure to all subjects. Interrater reliability on the GAS was 0.86 (Pearson r) for sixty-three patients. The GAS was measured at admission to the hospital and after three months of treatment.

Results

This study found a significant interaction between gender match and therapist experience that affected improvement in severity of illness. Therapist experience level was divided into two levels (less than ten years and ten years or more of experience) to explore the interaction between patient-therapist gender match and therapist experience level. A significant interaction between gender match and therapist experience level was found that affected improvement in severity of illness (increase in GAS score) from admission to three months in the hospital using a two-way repeated measures analysis of variance, $F(1,62) = 5.98$, $p = .017$ (fig. 1).

This finding was then explored in more detail with therapist experience level divided into three levels (less than five years, five through 9.5 years, and ten years or more of experience). A significant interaction between patient-therapist gender match and therapist experience level was again found that affected improvement in severity of illness from admission to three months in treatment using a two-way repeated

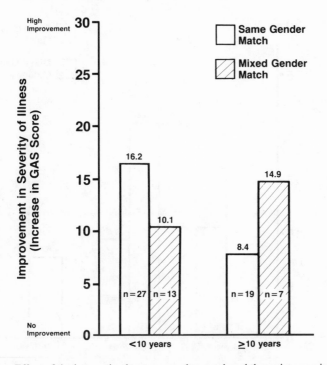

FIG. 1.—Effect of the interaction between gender match and therapist experience level on improvement of severity of illness from admission to three months in the hospital.

measures analysis of variance, $F(2,60) = 3.87, p = .026$. As shown in figure 2, the greatest improvement in severity of illness was found in patients in same gender matches with therapists who had between five and 9.5 years of experience and in mixed gender matches with therapists who had more than ten years of experience.

Discussion

This is the first study examining therapist-patient matching for inpatient psychotherapy of adolescents where the sample included older and more experienced therapists. Two possible dynamics are discussed that may be active in the interaction that was found. The first involves the role of identification between patient and therapist. An aspect that may be relevant to further understanding this dynamic could be the fact that the inexperienced therapist is closer in age to the

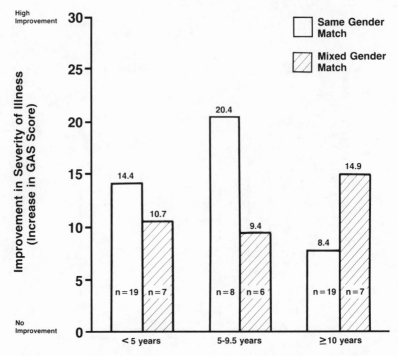

Fig. 2.—Effect of the interaction between gender match and therapist experience level on improvement of severity of illness from admission to three months in the hospital.

patient than the experienced therapist. At three months in treatment, therapists with less than ten years of experience had a mean age of only 35.7 years old, while therapists with ten years or more of experience had a mean age of 51.5 years old. A therapist who is of the same gender and closer in age to the patient could serve as an object of identification because of these gender and age similarities. The second dynamic involves the possibility that the more experienced therapist is better able to deal with countertransference issues of a heterosexual nature in psychotherapy.

Future study should include (*a*) analysis of specific psychological difficulties that may predispose certain patients to respond intensely to the gender of the therapist; (*b*) aspects affecting identification; (*c*) the specific stage of adolescence of the patient; (*d*) the effects of specialized training in child and adolescent psychotherapy; and (*e*) level of completion of the therapist's personal analysis. Although clinical application is a task for the future, this study provides a step in the direction of objective exploration of the process and outcome of individual psychoanalytic psychotherapy with the hospitalized adolescent.

REFERENCES

American Psychiatric Association. 1980. *Diagnostic and Statistical Manual of the Mental Disorders*. 3d ed. Washington, D.C.: American Psychiatric Association.

Blos, P. 1962. Intensive psychotherapy in relation to the various phases of the adolescent period. *American Journal of Orthopsychiatry* 32:901–910.

Corday, R. J. 1967. Limitations of therapy in adolescence. *Journal of the American Academy of Child Psychiatry* 6:526–638.

Endicott, J.; Spitzer, R. L.; Fleiss, J. L.; and Cohen, J. 1976. The global assessment scale: a procedure for measuring overall severity of psychiatric disturbance. *Archives of General Psychiatry* 33:766–771.

Godenne, G. D. 1982. The adolescent girl and her female therapist. *Adolescence* 17:225–242.

Goodrich, W. 1984. Symbiosis and individuation: the integrative process for residential treatment of adolescents. *Current Issues in Psychoanalytic Practice* 1:23–45.

Goodrich, W. 1987. Long-term psychoanalytic hospital treatment of adolescents. *Psychiatric Clinics of North America* 10(2): 273–287.

Holmes, D. 1964. *The Adolescent in Psychotherapy*. Boston: Little, Brown.

Ivey, E. P. 1960. Significance of the sex of the psychiatrist. *Archives of General Psychiatry* 2:622–631.

Kestenberg, J. S. 1968. Phases of adolescence. III. *Journal of the American Academy of Child Psychiatry* 7:108–151.

Masterson, J., and Costello, J. 1980. *From Borderline Adolescent to Functioning Adult*. New York: Brunner/Mazel.

Mattsson, A. 1970. The male therapist and the female adolescent patient. *Journal of the American Academy of Child Psychiatry* 9:702–721.

Mogul, K. M. 1982. Overview: the sex of the therapist. *American Journal of Psychiatry* 139:1–11.

Parloff, M. B.; Waskow, I. E.; and Wolfe, B. E. 1978. Research on therapist variables in relation to process and outcome. In S. Garfield and A. Bergin, eds. *Handbook of Psychotherapy and Behavior Change: An Empirical Analysis.* New York: Wiley.

Rinsley, D. B. 1980. *Treatment of the Severely Disturbed Adolescent.* New York: Aronson.

16 RUNNING AWAY FROM TREATMENT: OBSERVATIONS AND ADMISSION PREDICTORS FOR HOSPITALIZED ADOLESCENTS

LINDA BETH BERMAN AND WELLS GOODRICH

While collecting data for a previous study (Fullerton, Goodrich, and Berman 1986), we found that a substantial number of runaway episodes had occurred during the eleven years since Chestnut Lodge opened the Adolescent and Child Division (ACD). Although case studies have elucidated a variety of concepts that describe individual conflicts and motivations leading patients to run away from the hospital, there has been no agreement as to why this phenomenon is so prevalent; nor has published research often been concerned with adolescent runaways from psychiatric facilities.

The current study was undertaken to review the relevant literature about adolescent runaways, particularly those from hospitals or institutions, and, using hypotheses derived from the literature, to determine how to predict which patients admitted to our hospital might be the ones to run away while undergoing treatment. Since the literature about adolescents running away from hospitals was so sparse, the literature about runaways from home was also examined in detail and is reported here when it appears that the findings might be applicable to hospital runaway behavior. For ease of presentation, most of the literature is presented in four tables (tables 1–4 below) and is summarized in the text.

Running away from psychiatric hospitals is an important phenomenon to study for several reasons, the best statement of which is from Altman, Brown, and Sletten (1972): "It interferes and often hinders treatment; it probably increases the danger of antisocial behavior including suicide; it may influence other patients to act similarly; . . . as a symptom, it may tell us something of importance about the patient's personality, mental illness, and interaction with his environment" (p. 52).

Adolescents and children who run away from home have become a social and developmental problem that has attracted the attention of the press and a few publicly funded foundations, but few researchers. Children who run away from home are often described as having psychological problems or psychiatric syndromes, as having been abused or neglected, and as having families in crisis. Studies have been devoted to defining what a run away episode is, to creating typologies of runaway behavior, to evaluating the treatment of teenage runaways and their families, and to developing theories for the prevention of runaways; however, in the literature, there exists no general consensus about any of these topics or agreement about the meaning of the behaviors involved.

While the adolescents who run away from their homes are perceived to have diagnosable, psychiatric syndromes (often conduct disorders, personality disorders, or dysthymic disorders) in need of treatment, studies of children and adolescents who actually are patients in psychiatric facilities are few. The runaway incidents that occur from these facilities are little studied. Much of the research on hospital runaways (also termed "absconders," "elopers," and "AWOLs") over the past three decades has been about adult patients or has addressed the adolescent runaways from these populations as mere afterthoughts.

Review of the Literature

RUNAWAYS FROM HOSPITALS

Most of the research on hospital runaways from the late 1950s through the 1960s concentrated on the changes in hospital policies from locked to open wards. Many authors theorized that these changes would bring about epidemic proportions of runaways from the hospitals (Antebi 1967; Kernodle 1966; Lewis and Kohl 1962; Meyer,

Martin, and Lange 1967; Muller 1962; Reardon, Butler, and Warshaw 1978; Toolan and Nicklin 1959).

Patients who terminate their treatment by running away from the hospital have often been considered as demonstrating the same behaviors as patients who terminate their treatment "against medical advice" (AMA), signing themselves out of the hospital before their physicians deem them ready. Traditionally, the psychiatric literature has viewed patients who leave AMA as poor risks for a healthy future. The patient who drops out of treatment has most likely dropped out of treatment previously, probably will have multiple psychiatric hospitalizations in his or her future, will become a chronic patient, and may be a treatment failure (Baekeland and Lundwall 1975; Lewis and Kohl 1962).

Several authors have made distinctions between patients signing out of a hospital AMA and patients terminating their treatment by running away from the hospital. Most of these studies are from hospitals for adults or from hospitals that admit children and adolescents in addition to adults. Studies that focus on adolescent and/or child patients who have run away from psychiatric hospitals are small in number. The studies described in further detail in tables 1–4 below that are specifically about children or adolescents are marked. Many of the studies attempted to match runaways to nonrunaways in the same hospital environment, over the same period of time, and with various other criteria that included age, gender, socioeconomic status, race, and so on. These studies are summarized in table 1.

Studies of runaways from hospitals have also concentrated on describing the probable runaway patient. These descriptions range from the patient's age at the time of the runaway, to prior history of runaway episodes, to common precipitants from the treatment situation; findings from several studies are presented in table 2.

While these descriptions are interesting, it must be noted that some of these studies reported only on the sample of patients running away (Altman, Angle, Brown, and Sletten 1972; Benalcazar 1982; Greenberg, Blank, and Argrett 1968; Levy 1972; Lewis and Kohl 1962; Toolan and Nicklin 1959); and in some cases tests of statistical significance were not performed. Several of these researchers also attempted to determine the types of behaviors or environmental factors that might predispose a patient to becoming a runaway or that might precipitate a runaway episode. Table 3 lists factors reported on by more than one study.

281

TABLE 1

SUMMARY OF FINDINGS: STUDIES OF RUNAWAYS FROM HOSPITALS

	N	AWOL	Type of Match	Type of Facility	Termination of AWOL (%)	Significant Findings
Coleman 1966	104	. . .	Gender/time of admission	VA hospital	. . .	Prior AWOLS predicted hospital AWOLS; AWOLS Caucasian > non-Caucasians; AWOLS perceive more family rejection
Kermodle 1966	221	334	None	State hospital	20	Males AWOL > females; divorced-/separated AWOL > single/married; personality disorders AWOL > other diagnoses; psychoneurotic disorders AWOL > other diagnoses; most AWOLS ≤ 3 months in treatment; Adolescents = 2.8 percent of N; 17.2 percent AWOLS; 70.6 percent of all AWOLS one time only
Muller 1962	98	210	None	Public hospital	25	50 percent of all AWOLS one time only
Meyer et al. 1967	280	124	Match 42 AWOL/42 non-AWOL gender/age/race	General hospital	12	Psychotics AWOL > other diagnoses; AWOLS younger than non-AWOLS; AWOLS > time in hospital: female AWOLS > female controls; female AWOLS > male AWOLS
Raynes and Patch 1971	237	. . .	None/compared 25 AWOL/15 AMA/197 WMA discharges	General hospital	10.5	Younger: AMA/AWOLS < WMA; race: black AWO LS > WMA, young/Caucasian AWOLS > WMA/AMA; previous hospitals: AWOLS > WMA; drug abuse: AWOLS > WMA/AMA; hospital stay ≤ 24 hours AMA > AWOL-/WMA

Study	N		Variables controlled	Setting		Findings
Fullerton et al. 1986......	104	...	None	Private hospital	20	Adopted patients AWOL > nonadoptees; adoptees AWOL terminate > nonadoptees
Goodrich and Fullerton 1984..............	60	...	None	Private hospital	28	Peer dependency AWOLs > non-AWOLs
Atkinson 1971	2,529	...	None	University hospital	28	Younger: AWOLs < AMA (most 13–20); adolescents: $N=521$, 40 percent of all AWOLs; 14 percent all AMA; AWOLS > personality disorders; AWOLS > psychoneurotic disorders; time in hospital, AMA < AWOL
Miller et al. 1983..........	200	...	100 AMA vs. 100 AWOL discharges	10 community mental health centers	...	Alcohol/drug abuse, AWOL > AMA; depression, AWOL > AMA; in hospital $\leq$ 8 days, AWOL > AMA
Lubeck and Empey 1968–1969		...	Age (15–19), gender (male)	2 correctional	37 and 39	Previous offenses, AWOLs > non-AWOLs; peer relations, AWOLs < non-AWOLs
Clarke 1980	170	...	Age (12–18)	British training school	N.A.	Delinquency, AWOLs < non-AWOLs; age: older boys AWOL < younger boys; prior AWOLs: AWOLs > non-AWOLs
Edelbrock 1980	2,967	...	Age, gender, SES, race AWOLS vs. non-AWOLs	Outpatient mental health center	N.A.	Based on disturbance level: disturbed 6–11 males AWOL < females, disturbed 12–16 females AWOL < males; females 12–16 AWOLS < non-AWOLs; behavior problems all AWOLs < non-AWOLs

NOTE.—AMA = against medical advice. WMA = with medical advice.

283

TABLE 2

CHARACTERISTICS OF HOSPITAL RUNAWAYS

Category and Variable	Direction of Significance	Study
Demographics:		
Gender	Males are more likely than females to run away	Altman, Angle, Brown, and Sletten (1972), Altman, Brown, and Sletten (1972), Antebi (1967), Benalcazar (1982),* Greenberg, Blank, and Argrett (1967)*
Age.....................	Younger patients are more likely than older patients to run away	Altman, Brown, and Sletten (1972), Antebi (1967)
Race....................	Nonwhites more likely than whites to run away	Altman, Brown, and Sletten (1972)
Religion	Catholics most likely to run away	Altman, Angle, Brown, and Sletten (1972)
Marital status	Unmarried patients more likely to run away than married patients	Altman, Angle, Brown, and Sletten (1972)
Diagnosis:		
Schizophrenia		Altman, Brown, and Sletten (1972), Antebi (1967), Muller (1962), Toolan and Nicklin (1959)*
Personality disorders (including borderline)		Altman, Brown, and Sletten (1972), Goodrich and Fullerton (1984),* Levy (1972)*
Depression		Antebi (1967)
Behavior/character disorders		Toolan and Nicklin (1959)*
Alcoholism/drug addiction ..		Muller 1962
Psychopathic personality ...		Antebi (1967), Muller (1962)
History:		
Previous runaways		Lewis and Kohl (1962), Reardon et al. (1978)*
History of abandonment/ adoption		Levy (1972)*

* Study included only adolescent patients.

TABLE 3
REPORTED PRECIPITANTS AND PREDISPOSITIONS TO RUNAWAY EPISODES

Variable	Study
Predisposition to run away:	
Poor impulse control	Altman, Brown, and Sletten (1972), Lewis and Kohl (1962)
Inability to follow rules/disregard for rules	Altman, Brown, and Sletten (1972)
Poor motivation	Lewis and Kohl (1962)
Acting out/antisocial ideas	Altman, Angle, Brown, and Sletten (1972), Altman, Brown, and Sletten (1972)
Precipitants to runaway episodes:	
Stress	Altman, Brown, and Sletten (1972), Benalcazar (1982),* Levy (1972),* Lewis and Kohl (1962)
Poor interpersonal relationships	Muller (1962)
Family pressure	Benalcazar (1982),* Lewis and Kohl (1962), Muller (1962)
Changes in treatment	Levy (1972),* Muller (1962)
Impending separations/discharges	Benalcazar (1982)*
Poor hospital environment	Muller (1962)
A need to act for the group	Levy (1972)
Psychotic disorganization	Levy (1972)*
Paranoid projections	Lewis and Kohl (1962)
Thoughts of running away	Altman, Angle, Brown, and Sletten (1972)

* Study included only adolescent patients.

Other research on runaways from hospital treatment has concentrated on the outcome of patients after their precipitous discharges. Since the general impression of clinicians has been that patients who discharge themselves AMA or while AWOL are more at risk for continued or chronic mental illness, suicide, and antisocial behavior, several studies of patients' outcome after discharge have been published in the United States and in England (see table 4).

The runaway episode from a hospital has been viewed as a defense mechanism or a treatment resistance (Benalcazar 1982; Fullerton et al. 1986; Goodrich and Fullerton 1984; Levy 1972; Rinsley 1965). Alternately, patients who run away from the hospital have been viewed as communicating with the staff, and the runaway episode can be viewed as a positive action (McNaught and McKamy 1978). Keskiner (1981) explains that "separation often is felt by the patient as rejection or abandonment, a situation that renders him extremely

285

TABLE 4

SUMMARY OF FINDINGS: OUTCOME STUDIES OF RUNAWAY PATIENTS

Study	Subjects, FU Time	Type of Match	Type of Facility	Termination by AWOL (%)	Significant Findings
Milner 1966 ...	$N = 69$ (30 male, 39 female), 22 months	AWOL/AMA, age, gender, time since discharge	Public hospital, England	20	Continuous hospitalization, AWOLs > AMA; suicide attempts, AWOLs > AMA; work, AWOLs < AMA; antisocial acts, AWOLs > AMA;
Pam et al. 1973	$N = 42$, 6 months	21 AWOL/21 WMA at follow-up (95 percent, 62 percent)	State hospital	...	Better social adjustment, WMA > AWOL; time in hospital, WMA > AWOL; younger, AWOL < WMA; race, Puerto Rican, AWOL > WMA
Keskiner 1981	$N = 392$, 10 years	AMA/WMA/transfer	Private hospital	26	Deaths, 23.4% transfer > WMA or AMA; suicides, AMA > transfer/WMA
Glick, Braff, Johnson, and Showstack 1981	$N = 212$, 1 year, 2 years	182 WMA, 30 AMA/AWOL	University hospital	...	Social functioning, AMA/AWOL < WMA at 2 years; global functioning, AMA/AWOL < WMA; schizophrenia, AWOL > AMA/WMA; personality disorders, AMA > AWOL/WMA

NOTE.—WMA = with medical advice.

vulnerable to common life stresses that may contribute to suicide or homicide" (p. 155). These abandonment themes have been discussed at length by Rinsley (1965) and are seen primarily in adolescents diagnosed as borderline personality disorders and/or those who have been adopted or have lived in chaotic families with numerous separations.

Despite the theories that runaway behavior and suicidal behavior are both escapist acts expressed in different ways, the studies on hospital runaways are surprisingly short on reports of suicides or suicidal attempts. Even the reports of follow-up studies for runaway patients have relatively little to say on this matter (Keskiner 1981; Milner 1966), and only one study that focused on adolescents mentioned a group of "suicidal females" (Toolan and Nicklin 1959).

Some reports of runaway patients conclude that they represent a more chronic patient population by virtue of their greater number of previous hospital admissions (Raynes and Patch 1971) or their longer duration of hospitalization (Milner 1966). Yet the argument that terminating treatment early expresses a more chronic illness or a treatment failure has not been well proven. Terminating treatment by running away ranged from low rates of 10–15 percent (Greenberg et al. 1968; Kernodle 1966; Keskiner 1981; Meyer et al. 1967) to high rates of 20–30 percent (Antebi 1967; Fullerton et al. 1986; Goodrich and Fullerton 1984; Milner 1966; Muller 1962; Pam, Rachlin, Bryskin, and Rosenblatt 1973). Few of these studies are about adolescents, and fewer still have attempted to do follow-up studies to determine how patients are faring following discharge and whether the mode of discharge is a discriminant predicting follow-up status.

The literature contains other reports on adolescent runaways from institutions other than hospitals that are worthy of inclusion in this review. In one report, the institution was a training school (Clarke 1980), another studied children who ran away from home but were in treatment at a mental health facility (Edelbrock 1980), and a very recent study reported on runaways from home residing temporarily in a church-sponsored shelter (Hartman, Burgess, and McCormack 1987; Janus, McCormack, Burgess, and Hartman 1987).

RUNAWAYS FROM HOME

To summarize the findings from the literature regarding runaways from home, runaway episodes previous to the episodes studied were reported to range from one to 110 previous runaway episodes, with 33 percent reporting two to four previous runaway episodes in one study (Adams, Gullotta, and Clancy 1985); 92 percent of the male adolescents and 82 percent of the female adolescents in another study reported previous runaway episodes (Shaffer and Caton 1984). In the one and a half years preceding a third study, males ran away an average of 5.5 times and females 6.5 times (Fry 1982). In the most recent study of adolescent runaways, an average of 8.9 previous runaway episodes per adolescent was reported, with 40 percent of the adolescents revealing that they had run away at least three times previously (Hartman et al. 1987; Janus et al. 1987). Brennan, Huizinga, and Elliott (1978) found that 38 percent of the youngest runaways they surveyed, those ten to twelve years old, had run away from home three times or more in the year prior to their study, in contrast to 15 percent of the thirteen- to fifteen-year-old runaways and 10 percent of the runaways sixteen or more years old. When comparisons of socioeconomic status and previous runaway experience were examined, only 5 percent of the adolescents from the highest socioeconomic groups had run away previously, compared to more than 30 percent of adolescent runaways from the lowest socioeconomic group (Brennan et al. 1978).

SUMMARY

Runaways from hospitals have generally been described as younger than nonrunaways. Age ranges for the hospitalized runaway population ranged from eight to eighty years old or older, although most researchers reported that, of the patients who ran away, adolescents contributed most heavily to the overall frequency of runaway episodes. In one study, children eight to nineteen years old constituted only 2.8 percent of the hospital population but 17.2 percent of the runaway population; in another, adolescents in the facility studied were 20 percent of the entire population but were responsible for 40 percent of all the runaway episodes (table 1).

Several studies found that male hospital patients (adult and adolescent) were more likely than females in the same population to run away. One study also found that patients who were nonwhite, unmarried, or Catholic were more likely than white or married patients or patients of other religious affiliations to run away (table 2). Studies of runaways from hospitals have reported that the runaways were diagnosed most frequently as psychotic, particularly with schizophrenia, personality disorders, drug or alcohol abuse, or depressions (table 1).

Hypotheses

This study was undertaken to explore a central question with respect to adolescent patients from the Chestnut Lodge Hospital ACD. Who runs away, and can we determine how to predict who runs away from the hospital?

Findings from the literature on adolescent runaways from home and runaways from hospitals suggested that previous runaway history was predictive of subsequent runaway episodes, that diagnosis was predictive of runaway episodes from hospitals, that severity of illness was predictive of the course of hospital runaways' posthospital course, that gender was predictive in studies of runaways from home and from hospitals, as was age, and that adoptive status was found to be predictive of runaway status in hospitalized adolescents. Therefore, the following hypotheses were identified for study. (1) Adolescents with prior histories of runaway episodes will run away from the hospital more often than patients without prior histories. (2) Adolescents from the most disturbed categories (low Global Assessment Scores [GAS; Endicott, Spitzer, Fleiss, and Cohen 1976]) will not run away while in the hospital. (3) Patients who were adopted into their families will be more likely to run away than nonadopted patients. (4) Age at admission will discriminate the patients who are most likely to run away from the hospital. (5) Gender will discriminate the patients that are most likely to run away from the hospital. (6) Diagnostic classification will help identify those adolescents most likely to run away from the hospital.

Method

SUBJECTS

All patients ($N = 118$) admitted, treated, and discharged from the Chestnut Lodge Hospital ACD between July 1, 1975, and June 30, 1986, were included as subjects of this study. Our hospital provides long-term (average inpatient stay is twenty-two months), psychoanalytically oriented, psychiatric treatment for severely and chronically ill

289

adolescent patients. Patients accepted for admission generally have had previous outpatient treatment and usually have had at least one previous psychiatric hospitalization; approximately three-quarters of all patients are admitted to the ACD as the result of a direct transfer from another facility. Adolescents admitted to Chestnut Lodge have experienced symptoms sufficient to be regarded as dangerous to themselves or others or such that they cannot function appropriately within a less restrictive environment. This resistance to treatment in part is due to the adolescent's intrapsychic disturbances or a combination of these processes and a dysfunctional family system.

All patients resided in one of the four adolescent cottages on the hospital grounds. Homelike in nature, the cottages house from five to eight patients and at least one houseparent and are staffed by psychiatric technicians and nurses. Patients participate in an on-grounds, secondary special education program, which is fully accredited by the state. Participation in four-times-per-week, psychoanalytically oriented, individual psychotherapy as well as family therapy, activity therapy, and milieu therapy are required. Medication is provided if indicated.

The study population was almost evenly divided by gender (see fig. 1) and was relatively homogeneous with respect to social class and race (middle to upper middle class, Hollingshead-Redlich Scale [1957], and Caucasian). Age at admission ranged from 9.2 to 21.3 years old with a mean age of 15.9 years old.

Eighteen percent ($N = 21$) of the total study population had been adopted between the ages of three days old and twelve years old (67 percent adopted under the age of five months old), which contrasts with a rate of approximately 2–5 percent in the general population. Adoptees were equally divided by gender (see fig. 1).

For this study, psychiatric diagnoses were collapsed, and subjects were classified into five diagnostic groups: dysthymic-disordered patients, conduct-disordered patients, psychotic patients, borderline-personality-disordered patients, and patients diagnosed as substance abusers.

Initially, the study population ($N = 118$) was divided into two groups: those patients who never ran away from Chestnut Lodge ($N = 45$) and those who ran away from our hospital at least once prior to discharge ($N = 73$). Univariate tests of significance between groups were performed for all the study variables ($N = 10$) (table 5).

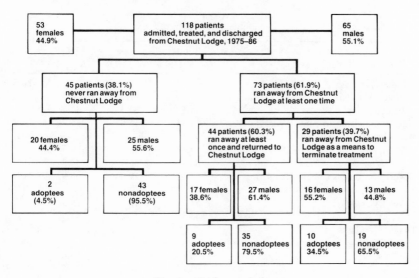

Fɪɢ. 1.—Study population

PROCEDURE

Data for this study were collected from the clinical charts and from weekly hospital census reports. The clinical charts were used to supply the admission note, written by the psychiatric administrator, and the psychosocial history, written by the social workers (on the basis of information supplied from the patients' parents or guardians, previous hospital records, and, in some cases, self-reports). These two documents were screened by research staff for demographic and historical information about each patient. Demographic and historical data collected for the present study were date of birth, gender, date of admission, and adoptive status.

Ratings of the patients' severity of illness using the GAS and any previous history of runaway episodes (frequency and setting) were reliably determined by trained research raters (Pearson $r = .83$ and .89, respectively) from these documents. Research diagnostic groupings were determined by the director of ACD research on the basis of the psychiatric administrator's admission note.

Weekly census reports were used as the record of runaway episodes. From these reports, we were able to collect the date a runaway episode

291

TABLE 5
CHESTNUT LODGE HOSPITAL RUNAWAY EPISODES

Variables	Total (N = 118)	Yes (N = 73)	No (N = 45)	p
Gender (%):				N.S.
Male (N = 65)	55.1	61.5	38.5	
Female (N = 53)	44.9	62.3	37.7	
Age at admission (mean, in years)	15.88	15.95	15.76	N.S.
Adoptive status (%):				.003
Yes (N = 21)	17.8	90.5	9.5	
No (N = 97)	82.2	55.7	44.3	
Severity of illness (mean GAS scores)	39.02	39.04	38.97	N.S.
History of previous AWOLs (%):				.07
Yes (N = 61)	51.7	70.5	29.5	
No (N = 57)	48.3	52.6	47.4	
Diagnosis (%):				
Psychotic:				.06
Yes	6.8	25.0	75.0	
No	93.2	64.5	35.5	
Depressed:				N.S.
Yes	31.4	67.6	32.4	
No	68.6	59.3	40.7	
Conduct disordered:				N.S.
Yes	22.9	66.7	33.3	
No	77.1	60.4	39.6	
Personality disordered:				N.S.
Yes	23.7	64.3	35.7	
No	76.3	61.1	38.9	
Substance abuse:				N.S.
Yes	23.7	67.9	32.1	
No	76.3	60.0	40.0	

began, the duration of each episode, group runaway episode membership, and all instances of termination of treatment by running away.

MEASURES

All 118 subjects' charts were screened and rated.

RUNAWAY EPISODES PRIOR TO HOSPITALIZATION

Reports of patients' previous history of runaway activity were scored if the charts stated clearly that there had been a runaway episode. Reports that the patient had "stayed out all night" or had "not returned home" were considered to be runaway episodes, as were episodes reported to police. The patient's age at the time of each episode was also recorded.

RUNAWAY EPISODES FROM THE HOSPITAL

For the purposes of this study, all unauthorized absences from the hospital that were reported to the census were counted as runaway episodes. Duration of these episodes ranged from several hours to several weeks. For ease of data analysis, any portion of a twenty-four hour-period was considered one day. The number of runaway episodes ranged from none to thirteen per patient.

TERMINATION RUNAWAY EPISODES

Any runaway episode in which the patient did not return to the hospital was counted as a termination runaway episode. These included those patients who refused to return on their own accord as well as patients whose parents decided not to force them to return to treatment.

GLOBAL ASSESSMENT SCALE

As a measure of the patient's global functioning and severity of illness at the time of admission, a 100-point GAS was scored by trained research assistants on the basis of the information contained in the psychiatric administrator's admission note.

Results

The study population as a whole was almost equally divided by gender, and gender did not differentiate runaways from nonrunaways. There was also no significant difference between age at admission to Chestnut Lodge for runaways and nonrunaways: the average age at admission was 15.88 years old (S.D. $\pm$ 1.88 years, range 9.25–21.30 years old). Females were significantly older at admission than males (16.1 vs. 15.7 years old, respectively, $F = 1.91, p = .017$).

Adoptive status was significantly different between the runaway and the nonrunaway groups. While only 17.8 percent of the study population was adopted, 90 percent of the adoptees ran away at least once from Chestnut Lodge. This contrasted with only 55.7 percent of the nonadopted patients ever running away from the hospital (χ^2 = 8.86, df = 1, N = 118, p = .003).

Scores on the GAS ranged from 13 to 52 on a 100-point scale (1 = worst functioning, 100 = best functioning) and were almost identical between runaway and nonrunaway groups, with a mean score of 39.02 for the entire population. These scores represent illnesses in the moderately to severely disturbed range.

Patients studied were as likely to have no previous history of runaway activity prior to admission to Chestnut Lodge as they were to have a history of previous runaway episodes. The frequency ranged from one to eight previous episodes, with an average of 2.4 episodes per patient. The ages for the first reported previous runaway episodes ranged from five to nineteen years old, with an average age at first reported runaway episode of 14.2 years old.

When previous runaway activity was correlated with runaway activity from Chestnut Lodge, it was found that 70.5 percent of the patients with prior histories of running away ran away at least once from the hospital. Interestingly, patients with no previous history of runaways were almost equally divided between the Chestnut Lodge runaway and nonrunaway groups.

History of previous runaway activity did discriminate by age at admission to Chestnut Lodge: patients with previous runaway histories were significantly older on admission than patients with no previous runaway history (16.2 vs. 15.5 years old, F = 2.03, p = .008). Additionally, patients with histories of previous runaway episodes scored significantly higher on the GAS at admission than did patients with no previous runaway history (40.2 vs. 37.8, F = 2.24, p = .002).

The only diagnostic category studied that proved to discriminate runaways from Chestnut Lodge from nonrunaways was the psychotic category: patients diagnosed with psychotic illnesses rarely ran away from the hospital, while almost two-thirds of the patients diagnosed as nonpsychotic ran away from the hospital at least once. This approached significance at a trend level (p = .06). The univariate tests for the patients diagnosed as depressed, conduct disordered, personality disordered, or substance abusers did not show any significant differences among these groups for runaway behavior.

To determine if there is any better way to distinguish between the patients who ran away from the hospital and those patients who did not run away, the ten variables discussed were entered into a discriminant function analysis (Altman, Angle, Brown, and Sletten 1972; Miller, Stone, Beck, Fraps, and Shekin 1983). This procedure allowed us the establishment of statistical criteria to predict group membership. Of the ten variables entered into the linear discriminant function analysis, only three remained in the equation: adoptive status, prior history of runaway activity, and diagnosis other than psychosis. The overall significance rate of the equation was $p = .0021$. These three variables were able to correctly classify the 118 patients into the categories of runaway or nonrunaway 61.86 percent of the time, which was significantly different than classifications occurring by chance alone ($\chi^2 = 4.34$, $N = 118$, df $= 1$, $p = .04$). Table 6 reproduces the classification results.

The decision to divide the patients into three cohorts was based on the literature on runaways from psychiatric hospitalization, which for the most part examined only termination runaway episodes. After the analyses reported, therefore, the study population ($N = 118$) was divided into three cohorts: patients who never ran away from Chestnut Lodge ($N = 45$), patients who ran away from Chestnut Lodge at least once and returned to the hospital ($N = 44$), and patients who ran away at least once and ultimately terminated their hospitalization by running away ($N = 29$). The division of the runaway group was done to determine whether the pattern of running away (those who returned vs. those who used a runaway episode to end hospitalization) might also better discriminate all runaway patients from the patients who never ran away.

TABLE 6

CLASSIFICATION RESULTS: LINEAR DISCRIMINATION FUNCTION ANALYSIS

Actual Group	Cases (N)	Predicted Group Membership (N)	
		Nonrunaway	Runaway
Nonrunaway	45	25 (55.6)	20 (44.4)
Runaway	73	25 (34.2)	48 (65.8)

NOTE.—61.86 percent correctly classified, $\chi^2 = 4.34$, df $= 1$, $p = .04$. Numbers in parentheses are percentages.

The univariate tests of significance for the three-group analysis reported almost identical values as those performed for the initial, two-group (runaways vs. nonrunaways) analysis but reveal how the two patterns of runaway behavior are different and how each contributes to the significance (table 7). The adopted adolescents who ran away from the hospital (90.5 percent of all adoptees) were almost evenly divided between the two runaway groups, while nonadopted adolescents were more evenly divided between the nonrunaway group and runaways who returned to the hospital ($p = .004$; see fig. 2).

TABLE 7
CHESTNUT LODGE HOSPITAL RUNAWAY EPISODES

Variables	Total ($N = 118$)	Never ($N = 45$)	Returned ($N = 44$)	Terminated ($N = 29$)	p
Gender (%):					N.S.
Male ($N = 65$)	55.1	38.5	41.5	20.0	
Female ($N = 53$)	44.9	37.7	32.1	30.2	
Age at admission (mean, in					
years)	15.88	15.76	15.65	16.40	N.S.
Adoptive status (%):					.004
Yes ($N = 21$)	17.8	9.5	42.9	47.6	
No ($N = 97$)	82.2	44.3	36.1	19.6	
Severity of illness (mean GAS					
scores)	39.02	38.97	37.75	41.0	N.S.
History of previous AWOLs					
(%):					.02
Yes ($N = 61$)	51.7	29.5	36.1	34.4	
No ($N = 57$)	48.3	47.4	38.6	14.0	
Diagnosis (%):					
Psychotic:					.08
Yes	6.8	75.0	12.5	12.5	
No	93.2	35.5	39.1	25.5	
Depressed:					N.S.
Yes	31.4	32.3	40.5	27.04	
No	68.6	40.7	35.8	23.5	
Conduct disordered:					N.S.
Yes	22.9	33.2	37.0	29.6	
No	77.1	39.6	37.4	23.1	
Personality disordered:					N.S.
Yes	23.7	35.7	39.3	25.0	
No	76.3	38.9	36.7	24.4	
Substance abuse:					N.S.
Yes	23.7	32.1	28.6	39.3	
No	76.3	40.0	40.0	20.0	

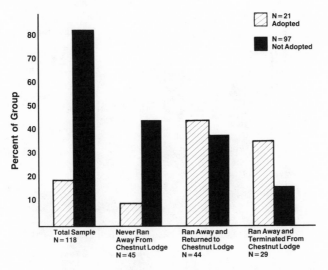

Fɪɢ. 2.—Chestnut Lodge runaways: adoptive status

Differences between the three groups for previous history of runaway episodes were also more distinctive than the two-group analysis. The percentages of patients who had no previous history of runaway episodes and of patients who had histories of previous runaway episodes were almost equal in the "runaway and return" group. Patients in either the "never ran away from Chestnut Lodge" or "ran away and terminated" groups did differ in their patterns of previous runaway histories, with significantly more patients with previous runaway histories terminating treatment by running away from the hospital. Patients with no previous runaway experience displayed significantly more runaway activity while in the hospital (p = .02; see fig. 3).

The diagnostic category of psychosis, when compared over three groups, showed that the small number of psychotic patients who ran away did so in equal numbers in the "runaway and return" and "ran away and terminated" categories. There was a trend toward more nonpsychotic adolescents either never running away or running away and returning to the hospital rather than terminating hospitalization by running away. This difference, however, was still not statistically significant (p = .08).

Nine of the ten variables used in the three-group discriminant function analysis were entered into the equation; these variables

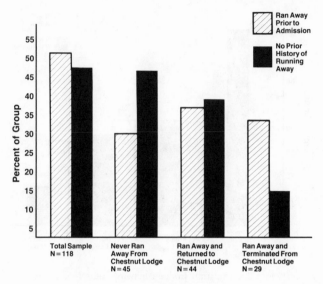

FIG. 3.—Chestnut Lodge runaways: previous runaway history

correctly classified 47.46 percent of the population (χ^2 = 14.03, df = 4, p = .007). The classification table is reproduced in table 8.

Discussion

This study supplements earlier observations from the literature about runaway behavior among adolescents. It provides new information about three predictors of runaway behavior from a long-term psychiatric hospital for severely disturbed adolescents. The literature contrasting adult runaway behavior with runaway behavior among adolescents points out the higher frequency of runaway behavior among adolescents. Our study has observed a particularly high frequency of runaway behavior among early adolescent males or midadolescent females. It seems clear that runaway behavior is an expression of the expectable developmental stage struggle, internally in the adolescent as well as interpersonally between the adolescent and parental figures, or the struggle between childhood dependency needs versus emerging needs for autonomy. The question is why such an extreme behavior that involves alienation is employed rather than the negotiated achievement of adolescent autonomy.

TABLE 8

CLASSIFICATION RESULTS: THREE-WAY LINEAR DISCRIMINANT FUNCTION ANALYSIS

		Predicted Group Membership (N)		
Actual Group	Case (N)	Nonrunaway	Runaway and Return	Runaway and Terminate
Nonrunaway	45	18 (40.0)	16 (35.6)	11 (24.4)
Runaway and return	44	13 (29.5)	22 (50.0)	9 (20.5)
Runaway and terminate ...	29	8 (27.6)	5 (17.2)	16 (55.2)

NOTE.—47.46 percent correctly classified, $\chi^2 = 14.03$, df $= 4$, $p = .007$. Numbers in parentheses are percentages.

Our clinical experience supports the literature in observing the significance of separation or dependency conflicts as precipitants for a runaway episode. Stierlin (1973) observed how parents in conflict can consciously or unconsciously delegate to their adolescent child the task of expressing secret parental wishes to leave home. Within a psychoanalytic hospital program that welcomes the adolescents' transferences, a similar drama may be evoked in situations in which patients project onto staff members to whom they have become attached misperceptions transferentially derived from the earlier parental relationship.

Whereas data from earlier studies, mostly of adults, have suggested that patients who run away from hospitals tend to be male, chronic psychotic patients from minority races, in our population the trend is quite different. Adolescents who are admitted to a private psychiatric hospital unit, as a recent study sponsored by the National Association of Private Psychiatric Hospitals (Miller and PACTE 1988) shows, tend to present with admission symptoms of chronic school failure, self-destructive and violent behavior, and substance abuse. Therefore, our study observations are made on an adolescent population far more chronically and severely disturbed than those admitted to the usual short-term psychiatric unit. If such patients are then found to require over six months' inpatient psychiatric treatment, they are estimated to represent less than 1 percent of the general adolescent population. It is not surprising that such an extreme expression of the dependency-autonomy struggle would appear so commonly among such a depressed, angry, and distrustful group.

We posit that our "group" of adolescent patients may in fact be three groups defined by their three types of runaway patterns. First, there is a small group of patients who are psychotic or severely and perhaps even intellectually damaged and who are basically helpless. They appear to have very little ability to resist the system, may or may not be trusting, and have very low GAS scores. These patients do not run away since they are so damaged that they cannot mobilize a plan of action.

Second, there is a small number of less ill, severely neurotic or less severe borderline adolescents who appear to form early attachments and early good alliances. These patients have mid-level GAS scores (which in our population reflect the highest scores), they are more trusting and able to tolerate dependency than most of our patients, and, if they run away, they do so as a statement to themselves or others and then return to the hospital.

Finally, there is a group of patients who have difficulties with attachments, are not very trusting, and develop negative transferences. These patients have had life experiences that have taught them enforced self-dependence. Their GAS scores fall in the middle of our range, intellectually they are better endowed, and they are resourceful. These patients are always planning to leave and usually run away and return at least once before terminating their treatment by running away. It appears that their stay in the hospital provides them with a strength and maturation to attempt to make a life on their own.

Perhaps the findings in this study that runaways were not psychotic, were often adopted into their families, and were adept at running away support Clarke's (1980) notion that runaway behavior is a learned coping strategy that has been proven especially successful for these adolescents. The prevalence of runaway episodes among nonhospitalized adolescents living in the community also supports this interpretation. Even being contained in a supportive, nurturing, therapeutic environment poses a threat to them since dependence on others has been experienced as always followed by betrayal or rejection. This seems to be the case particularly for the adopted adolescents who appear ready to act out their abandonment fantasies rather than wait for them to come to fruition.

The findings that patients with histories of previous runaway activity had statistically significant, higher scores on the GAS at the time of their admission to Chestnut Lodge than patients with no previous runaway histories and that patients with histories of previous runaway activity were significantly older at admission than patients with no previous runaway histories also support the notion that learned coping strategies may be involved in their behavior. These facts also relate to the finding that patients with psychotic disorders rarely ran away from the hospital. Perhaps their level of disorganization would not allow them to formulate plans to run away. Following these lines of reasoning, it is curious that there were no significant differences in the runaway behavior between the male and the female patients in the Chestnut Lodge cohort, given that the females were significantly older than the males at the time of admission. Perhaps with a larger study population the relations between diagnosis, severity of illness, and gender might tease out an answer for this inconsistency.

Conclusions

Since this was an exploratory study, we cannot offer hard and fast descriptions of the likely candidate for runaway episodes, but we can offer thought-provoking evidence opposing the rather rigidly held beliefs that patients who run away from hospitals tend to be male, psychotic, and from minority races. We hope that this will stimulate further research on adolescent runaway episodes from hospitals so that we may all find some answers. Since our purpose is to treat the patients admitted to our facilities, if they cannot be contained within the hospital, we cannot fulfill that mandate.

NOTE

The authors thank Jaime Buenaventura, M.D.; Mary-Louise Schmidt, R.N., M.A.; Phyllis Stang, R.N., M.A.; and the entire staff of the Adolescent and Child Division of Chestnut Lodge for their participation and cooperation in this project. We also thank Carol Fullerton, Ph.D., Herb Landis, Joan Alden, and Rosalyn Ingall for their assistance in data collection; Richard C. Fritsch, Ph.D., Robert K. Heinssen, Ph.D., Brian T. Yates, Ph.D., and Cheryl Shea Gelernter, Ph.D., for statistical advice; Thomas H. McGlashan, M.D., for incalculable assistance and time to pursue this project; and Pat Inana and Carol Thompson for manuscript preparation.

REFERENCES

Adams, G. R.; Gullotta, T.; and Clancy, M. A. 1985. Homeless adolescents: a descriptive study of similarities and differences between runaways and throwaways. *Adolescence* 20:715–724.

Altman, H.; Angle, H. V.; Brown, M. L.; and Sletten, I. W. 1972. Prediction of unauthorized absence. *American Journal of Psychiatry* 128:1460–1463.

Altman, H.; Brown, M. L.; and Sletten, I. W. 1972. "And . . . silently steal away": a study of elopers. *Diseases of the Nervous System* 33:52–58.

Antebi, R. 1967. Some characteristics of mental hospital absconders. *British Journal of Psychiatry* 113:1087–1090.

Atkinson, R. M. 1971. AMA and AWOL discharges: a six-year comparative study. *Hospital and Community Psychiatry* 22:293–296.

Baekeland, F., and Lundwall, L. 1975. Dropping out of treatment: a critical review. *Psychological Bulletin* 82:738–783.

Benalcazar, B. 1982. Study of fifteen runaway patients. *Adolescence* 17:553–566.

Brennan, T.; Huizinga, D.; and Elliott, D. S. 1978. *The Social Psychology of Runaways*. Lexington, Mass.: Lexington.

Clarke, R. 1980. Absconding from residential institutions for young offenders. In L. Hersov and I. Berg, eds. *Out of School*. London: Wiley.

Coleman, W. B. 1966. Unauthorized departures from mental hospitals. *Mental Hygiene* 50:47–53.

Edelbrock, C. 1980. Running away from home: incidence and correlates among children and youth referred for mental health services. *Journal of Family Issues* 1:210–228.

Endicott, J.; Spitzer, R. L.; Fleiss, J. L.; and Cohen, J. 1976. The Global Assessment Scale: a procedure for measuring overall severity of psychiatric disturbance. *Archives of General Psychiatry* 33:766–771.

Fry, P. S. 1982. Paternal correlates of adolescents' running away behaviors: implications for adolescent development and considerations for intervention and treatment of adolescent runaways. *Journal of Applied Developmental Psychology* 3:347–360.

Fullerton, C. S.; Goodrich, W.; and Berman, L. B. 1986. Adoption predicts psychiatric treatment resistances in hospitalized adolescents. *Journal of the American Academy of Child Psychiatry* 25:542–551.

Glick, I. D.; Braff, D. L.; Johnson, G.; and Showstack, J. A. 1981. Outcome of irregularly discharged psychiatric patients. *American Journal of Psychiatry* 138:1472–1476.

Goodrich, W., and Fullerton, C. 1984. Which borderline patients in residential treatment will run away? *Residential Group Care and Treatment* 2:3–14.

Greenberg, H. R.; Blank, R.; and Argrett, S. 1968. The anatomy of elopement from an acute adolescent service: escape from engagement. *Psychiatric Quarterly* 42:28–47.

Hartman, C. R.; Burgess, A. W.; and McCormack, A. 1987. Pathways and cycles of runaways: a model for understanding repetitive runaway behavior. *Hospital and Community Psychiatry* 38:292–299.

Hollingshead, A. B., and Redlich, F. C. 1957. *Social Class and Mental Illness*. New York: Wiley.

Janus, M. D.; McCormack, A.; Burgess, A. W.; and Hartman, C. R. 1987. *Adolescent Runaways*. Lexington, Mass.: Lexington.

Kernodle, R. W. 1966. Nonmedical leaves from a mental hospital. *Psychiatry* 39:25–41.

Keskiner, A. 1981. Separation can be life threatening. *National Association for Private Psychiatric Hospitals Journal* 12:150–156.

Levy, E. Z. 1972. Some thoughts about patients who ran away from residential treatment and the staff they leave behind. *Psychiatric Quarterly* 46:1–21.

Lewis, A. B., and Kohl, R. N. 1962. The risk and prevention of abscondence from an open psychiatric unit. *Comprehensive Psychiatry* 3:302–308.

Lubeck, S. G., and Empey, L. T. 1968–1969. Mediatory vs. total institution: the case of the runaway. *Journal of Social Problems* 125:1633–1639.

McNaught, T. R., and McKamy, L. R. 1978. Elopement of adolescents: dynamics in the treatment process. *Hospital and Community Psychiatry* 23:303–305.

Meyer, G. G.; Martin, J. B.; and Lange, P. 1967. Elopement from the open psychiatric unit: a two-year study. *Journal of Nervous and Mental Disease* 144:297–304.

Miller, D. J.; Stone, M.; Beck, N. S.; Fraps, C.; and Shekim, W. 1983. Predicting AWOL discharge at a community mental health center: a "split-half" validation. *American Journal of Psychiatry* 140:479–482.

Miller, P., and PACTE (Hospital Coalition for Psychiatric Adolescent and Child Treatment and Education). 1988. Child and adolescent admission profile, 1985 and 1987. Paper presented at the annual meeting of the National Association of Private Psychiatric Hospitals, Phoenix, Arizona, January.

Milner, G. 1966. The absconder. *Comprehensive Psychiatry* 7:147–151.

Muller, D. J. 1962. The "missing" patient: a survey of 210 instances of absconding in a mental hospital. *British Medical Journal* 1:177–179.

Pam, A.; Rachlin, S.; Bryskin, L.; and Rosenblatt, A. 1973. Community adjustment of self-discharged patients. *Psychiatric Quarterly* 47:176–183.

Raynes, A. E., and Patch, V. D. 1971. Distinguishing features of patients who discharge themselves from psychiatric ward. *Comprehensive Psychiatry* 12:473–479.

Reardon, D. F.; Butler, K.; and Warshaw, K. 1978. The effect of an unlocked door on adolescent runaway and aggression. *Journal of the American Academy of Child Psychiatry* 17:372–382.

Rinsley, D. B. 1965. Intensive psychiatric hospital treatment of adolescents: an object-relations view. *Psychiatric Quarterly* 39:405–429.

Shaffer, D., and Caton, C. L. M. 1984. Runaway and homeless youth in New York City: a report to the Ittleson Foundation. Division of Child Psychiatry, New York State Psychiatric Institute and Columbia University College of Physicians and Surgeons. Typescript.

Stierlin, H. 1973. A family perspective on adolescent runaways. *Archives of General Psychiatry* 29:56–62.

Toolan, J. M., and Nicklin, G. 1959. Open door policy on an adolescent service in a psychiatric hospital. *American Journal of Psychiatry* 115:790–792.

17 REFLECTIONS ON THE HOSPITAL TREATMENT OF ADOLESCENTS AT CHESTNUT LODGE

DEXTER M. BULLARD, JR.

Conception of an Adolescent Unit

The design and construction of an adolescent unit at Chestnut Lodge intrigued me because the requirements for hospital treatment seemed somewhat inconsistent with the optimal conditions for adolescent development. When I visited hospitals and residential facilities, I found that severely ill adolescents demanded a substantial emphasis on control of behavior and that issues of safety played a large role in the treatment programs. From painful experience, many facilities had learned that institutional supervision and control of behavior were necessary for the implementation of treatment. I found that spontaneous activity, free time, and voluntary associations with peers and staff were substantially reduced. This compromised the ordinary and expectable experiences that characterize normal adolescent development. For these reasons, many people have felt that optimal treatment takes place in the office or clinic while the patient lives at home. However, as we all know, many disturbed adolescents require hospitalization in order to manage and treat their often life-threatening and destructive behavior. Hospitals, of all institutional treatment settings, have had the most difficulty in resolving the conflict between treatment needs, safety requirements, and the values inherent in ordinary living situations.

The several adolescent psychiatric units that I visited were similar in design to adult units containing fifteen to twenty-five patients cared for by psychiatric nurses and technicians. The treatment and the educational programs were usually provided in the same building. This model of care, while efficient and safe, was far different from the family situations from which patients came to the hospital. The reluctance of many families to permit hospitalization resulted in part from their concerns about the dislocation of their child's life. Over the years, many hospitals have made efforts to address this problem, with only partial success.

I had always felt that treatment must be embedded in ordinary experience and was compromised whenever the therapeutic environment departed from everyday life. The success of adolescent treatment depended on the presence of a familiar, growth-enhancing environment. I wondered whether the requirements of hospital care could be met within another treatment environment, and I found myself attracted to group homes. They seemed to preserve best the relationships, the experiences, the values, and the family structure in which ordinary adolescent development can take place.

With this in mind, I visited several group homes. They contained eight to sixteen adolescent boys or girls and a houseparent couple who were responsible for their care. At times, the houseparents were assisted by others, often volunteers. Professional mental health workers visited regularly for treatment interviews and planning. The adolescents attended school or worked, and they lived in the group home from several weeks to a number of months. Remaining in the home was voluntary, and the problem of adjustment to the home was often solved by the adolescent's running away and subsequent placement elsewhere. Even though group homes were designed for less severely disturbed adolescents than we expected at Chestnut Lodge, the advantages of this type of care were persuasive to me, and I decided to try and adapt the group home model to meet our hospital requirements. As it turned out, many aspects of hospitalization were also altered to accommodate the group home living situation.

This was not a new idea. For years, hospitals had sought to diminish the "institutional" atmosphere of their adolescent units. Yet the demands of efficiency and space and the historical influence of adult hospital programs often blunted this purpose.

Within the group homes, care was based on a family model, which seemed to me to have a number of advantages. It reduced the types of peer group entanglement that characterized much of the behavior of severely disturbed adolescents. A family-oriented approach replicated, to some degree, features of the original home situation and encouraged, or at least allowed, the expression of the symptoms of the illness previously manifested in the adolescent's parental home. From a developmental and psychoanalytic perspective, this model could promote the gradual working through of the process of separation and autonomy by the adolescent in a homelike environment and, it was hoped, avoid a premature dependence on adolescent group formation.

The houseparents are of central importance to the successful operation of any group home. Originally, I thought it might be possible to select talented houseparents who, with supervision, could oversee the home activities morning and evening, leaving their days free while the adolescents attended school. When I described the severity of illness and the size of hospital units to several houseparents, they told me that supervision of such a group would be too great a burden. They said they would need a large number of assistants to support them and to share the responsibilities for twenty-four-hour care, which reminded me of many hospital programs. It occurred to me that the size of each home might have a significant influence on the behavior of its adolescent residents. More severely disturbed adolescents are usually treated in larger groups: group homes cared for eight to sixteen adolescents; hospital units usually treated sixteen or more.

I was reminded of the Tavistock experience and Bion's work, which demonstrated some of the powerful effects of large group interactions on group members (Bion 1974). Large adolescent groups are often difficult to manage because the increased variety of individual interactions decreases the group's stability. In response, adolescents form subgroups and move away from other peers. The resulting isolation and loss of relationships outside the subgroup leads to scapegoating. Institutions, well aware of the difficulties inherent in the psychodynamics of large groups, have usually responded with more clearly articulated rules, more structured daily activities, and more of an emphasis on group treatment. In contrast, smaller groups usually have more individual pairing, less subgroup formation, less frequent scapegoating, and more involvement with outside adults. Smaller groups require a less rigidly structured program and allow more individualized attention to each adolescent and his treatment needs. It seemed to me that smaller group size would benefit our program because of its emphasis on the individual adolescent.

I then wondered how the composition of the adolescent group might influence their behavior. The hospital units that I visited usually contained patients of the same sex and similar age, leading to an inevitable anonymity and loss of individuality. I asked several group home houseparents about including boys and girls in the same home, but most houseparents were concerned about uncontrolled sexual activity. I wondered if social development might be strengthened by not separating boys and girls at this stage in their development. Independent boarding schools for boys that became coeducational have subsequently noted less aggressive behavior among the boys. I hoped the inclusion of boys and girls of different ages in each home might reduce scapegoating and destructive behavior. I finally decided to limit the size of each home to eight boys and girls ranging in age from twelve to eighteen. Houseparents would provide caretaking and supervision assisted by young adult psychiatric technicians.

With this in mind, we built four residential homes situated on a cul-de-sac away from the adult hospital. The homes were ranch style in construction and included a living room, a dining room, a large kitchen, a family room, single and double bedrooms with adjacent baths, a study room, and an apartment for the houseparents. I was surprised to find that, though the homes were unpretentious in design, they were of substantial size. The homes were separated by a short walk from the Clinical Center, which included a school and doctors' offices in an adjacent wing. A play barn for various sports and activities was located nearby.

The first adolescent patients were admitted in the summer of 1975. Within the home, the adolescents participated in cooking, washing the dishes after meals, and cleaning and maintaining their rooms. These chores were distributed by group decision, which differed from home to home. The adolescents decorated their own rooms, reviving the usual debates about the definition of pornography. The television and video equipment was in frequent use, and each home made its own decisions regarding which programs were suitable for younger adolescents. After negotiations with the State of Maryland, pets were allowed, and dogs, cats, and birds have come and gone over the years. I hoped that the homelike living situation would provide the ups and downs of everyday life.

Houseparents, of course, carried multiple responsibilities: they supervised the dress, self-care, and behavior of the adolescents and were also the most important source of support and approval. The psychiatric technicians had less defined roles. They had supervisory responsibilities, but most of their day was spent in mutual tasks or activities with the adolescents. I hoped that the shared chores, games, television watching, and "bull sessions" with members of the nursing staff would be similar to experiences of ordinary adolescence. I realized that no relationships would replace the biological tie to the parents who had legal responsibility for their child. Our goal was to compete directly with current and past peer relationships. A major problem of adolescents who came to our hospital was their disturbed and often self-destructive relationships with peers, most dramatically illustrated in antisocial or antiestablishment gang formation. We found, as had others, that strong relationships with staff diluted peer relationships and reduced pathological group formation and scapegoating. The role modeling that occurred seemed to influence adolescent values as well. Relationships with several staff members allowed each member some respite from the adolescent's sometimes overwhelming demands or needs.

The next task was how best to integrate treatment with the newly constituted family living situation. Our approach to the treatment of adolescents was governed by principles drawn from psychoanalysis and mindful of developmental considerations and the pragmatic requirements of family living. Self-awareness, self-understanding, and the rational direction of behavior remain the primary goals of our treatment. The application of psychoanalytic principles in the hospital setting has meant that all staff interventions to a greater or lesser degree are governed by an awareness of unconscious conflict, transference, and the intimate relationship between emotion and behavior. How much this knowledge is formally and explicitly made a part of the relationship between the patient and members of the treatment team varies greatly depending on the clinical situation. I wondered how different degrees of psychoanalytic sophistication within the staff would influence everyday life experiences in the home situation.

Among the treatment modalities, Chestnut Lodge has always given a special position to intensive individual psychotherapy. My own experience was that significant advantages occurred from more intensive individual treatment of adolescents. The establishment of a stable, nonthreatening, nonjudgmental relationship and the willingness of the psychotherapist to help the adolescent patient come to terms with the conscious manifestations and unconscious origins of his illness seemed most likely to promote normal development. Intensive psychotherapy became a part of every adolescent's treatment plan and took place in the doctor's office, with occasional exceptions.

The interaction of psychotherapy with the home situation was a matter of great interest to me. I wondered if the transference enactments and displacements would prove too intense for the houseparents to manage, given the substantial time they were expected to be in the home. I knew that the intensity of the adolescents' needs and the strength of transference derivatives could re-create, with sometimes frightening realism, the many facets of early parental ties. Further, previous parental relationships had proved unworkable in the family structures from which these adolescents came.

To meet some of these potential difficulties, we drew on the long-established Chestnut Lodge tradition of the therapist-administrator split and our emphasis on clinical consultation and supervision within the nursing service. The term "therapist-administrator split," as it evolved over the years, had become a misnomer and, in fact, referred to the treatment collaboration between the administrative psychiatrist and the psychotherapist. The administrator took medical responsibility for the care of the adolescent, including the management of behavior, the administration of medications, and the level of supervision that was required. The psychotherapist was consulted and participated in discussions of management as needed, but the final decision in such matters was made by the administrative psychiatrist. The psychotherapist did not carry the burden of administrative decisions, and we have found that this freed the patient from modifying his participation in psychotherapy to gain a particular administrative action. The psychotherapist could then explore how the patient felt rather than debate what actions should be taken. The relationship of the patient to the psychotherapist developed with its transference and countertransference aspects unfettered by therapist decisionmaking. The therapist-administrator split had already proved helpful with individual adolescents treated in the adult hospital and seemed a well-suited complement to the individual psychotherapy program.

Supervision of the houseparents and the psychiatric technicians was carried out by supervising nurses assigned to the adolescent program, who, for the most part, acted as consultants in matters of daily living. However, in situations in which more medical-nursing input was required, such as the assessment of suicidal or assaultive potential, the nursing supervisor took responsibility for decisions in the home. If indicated, the psychiatrist-administrator became involved and made such decisions. The layering of responsibility allowed the houseparents to remain focused on their primary role as parental caretakers. I hoped that the division of these responsibilities would replicate to some extent the home situation outside the hospital.

I wondered how the families of our adolescent patients would react to our houseparents and our family-care approach. It seemed likely that the parents of the adolescent patient would respond positively to the less institutional environment. At the same time, I thought the giving up of their child to other caretakers and the potential for competition with the houseparents might become issues in family therapy. Family therapy at our hospital evolved from a traditional social casework approach. The work of family therapy was often limited by the distance the family lived from the hospital and the frequent instability of the home situation. Under these circumstances, it was unclear how our adolescent family therapy program would develop.

Our planning for the Lodge School placed it a short walk from the circle of homes, a geographic separation that I hoped would have the psychological benefit of defining more clearly the distinction between school and home. Leaving the house to go to school did reactivate separation anxieties, school phobia, and truancy in some of our patients. The Lodge School was administratively separated from the clinical supervision of the homes reinforcing the differences between these two realms of adolescent experience. However, the school shared a psychoanalytic orientation with the other elements of the clinical program.

The integration of research and evaluation studies posed difficulties inherent in any research endeavor carried on in a clinical setting. I had seen previously that the introduction of research observers into an ongoing clinical situation created not-so-subtle tensions between the clinical staff and the observers. This limited the willingness of the clinical staff to provide the detailed information that was necessary for our studies. Utilizing the concept of the participant-observer, another tradition at the hospital, the research observer was made a member of the clinical team. The willingness of the observer to help out at times in the care of the adolescents offered something of immediate value to staff members. They, in turn, were quite generous in giving time for structured interviews and recording their observations. The problem of objectivity was met in part by the use of formal rating scales and multiple observations.

The Adolescent Unit at Work

Since the opening of the Adolescent and Child Division in the summer of 1975, succeeding years have given us the opportunity to study and evaluate our initial plans and hypotheses. Experience has led us to change some aspects of the program while confirming the value of this approach for most of the adolescents we have treated.

In general, the plan to have seven or eight patients in each home has worked well, with infrequent subgroup formation or scapegoating within the homes. Scapegoating appears during the initial phase of the treatment of the occasional adolescent who brings to the hospital an unusually chronic pattern of ostracism and rejection by his peers. Relationships among the patients in the home are personal and familiar and subject to the ordinary problems of family living colored by the psychopathology of each patient. Friendships between boys and girls living in the same house have become commonplace. Mixing older and younger patients in each home has increased the variety of individual friendships and reduced rivalrous gang formation. Boys and girls living together on the same unit has provoked occasional sexual acting out, but this more frequently takes place with adolescents from one of the other homes or when the patient is away from the hospital during visits to the family. It has not proved to be a major problem. We speculate that the sharing of meals, evening activities, and close relationships with staff all serve to increase the so-called incest barrier. The associations between adolescents from different homes at school and during afterschool activities leads to multiple, often transient, friendships. I suspect these friendships are benefited substantially by the fact that each evening the adolescent returns to his own home, regulating the intensity of the relationships and their mutual expectations.

Within the division, the adolescents form groups that have an evolving membership and are not isolated generally from the other adolescents. Aggressive group acting out is rare. Substance and alcohol experimentation and abuse has required special attention, and a drug counseling component has been added to the treatment program. Running away is a serious problem and is examined in an initial report by Berman and Goodrich (in this vol.).

Intense romantic entanglement is unusual but is perhaps the most troublesome peer relationship confronting our treatment program. It saps the energy available for investment in psychotherapy and isolates the couple from their peers and staff. We have found these relationships are often resistant to treatment intervention. In this situation, the patient's involvement with staff is a critical factor in modifying these intense but unrealistic romantic attachments.

The houseparent role has changed over the years and continues to evolve. We found that it was very difficult to find both husband and wife who met the requirements of sophistication, maturity, and flexibility necessary in their role as houseparents. We selected couples who were dedicated, caring people. One couple had young children, which occasioned much discussion before we decided to appoint them houseparents. We were concerned about the effect on the houseparents' children of the disturbed adolescent with a history of sibling difficulties. Though the experiment did not work out, it was for other reasons. Despite their dedicated efforts, the couple did not have the requisite energy to manage the adolescents' daily needs and also to provide sufficient care and attention to their own children. The interactions between the adolescents and the younger children were benign.

As we expected, the demands that our patients made were significantly more taxing than the demands made on couples responsible for group homes. Adolescents in group homes could be managed with firm limits, responded more easily to group pressures, and frequently left the group home if they proved unresponsive to these measures. Adolescent patients remained much longer in our program, demonstrated more anxiety and depression, and needed more attention and support than those in group homes. We viewed destructive and self-destructive behavior as a focus of our therapeutic endeavor, not as evidence of unsuitability. Therefore, the natural selection of less troubled patients did not occur.

Over a period of several years, our experience with houseparent couples did not prove to be satisfactory. In response to the adolescents' sadistic or destructive behavior, the houseparents gradually responded with a more punitive approach supported by a more inflexible view of right and wrong. In one instance, houseparents used their strong religious beliefs to influence the personal values of the patients and to improve their conduct. While this approach was successful in part, it depended on a positive response by the adolescents and soon broke down in the face of negativism and anger. These difficulties would have been surmountable had it been easier to educate and supervise the houseparent couples. However, the mutually supportive and autonomous marital relationship, so useful in managing adolescent behavior in family situations, became a serious obstacle to supervision and administrative decision making in our hospital environment. The approach of the houseparent couples eventually came into conflict with our overall treatment strategy of understanding behavior as well as providing controls. We therefore relinquished the requirement that houseparents be couples.

Over the next several years, single adults gradually filled the houseparent positions. Houseparents may now choose to live in the home or in off-grounds living quarters. This has not affected their role as much as I had feared, and both arrangements have worked well.

Our view that treatment is embedded in the living situation is illustrated by our experience with adolescent patients following their admission to the hospital. We found that the most important task was not the immediate implementation of a treatment plan but dealing with the separation of the adolescent from his family and establishing a comfortable place in his new home. This was not an easy task for most of our adolescent patients, many of whom had not had prolonged separations from their families. Prior short-term hospitalizations had ended in early discharge after temporary symptomatic improvements. After admission to our division, some of our patients were overtly homesick, and many were frightened by the implications of long-term treatment. I believe they realized that more was at stake than symptomatic improvement and that their way of life, however compromised, was the object of our treatment efforts.

Their parents suffered the natural reaction to the loss of their child to other caretakers. Relieved of immediate parental responsibilities, the close, though painful, parent-child ties soon became evident. Most families wished for rapid improvement and discharge, a wish not dispelled by extensive discussions prior to admission. Their feelings of responsibility for their child's illness could not be immediately expressed and were externalized initially onto the treatment team, who did not "understand" their child.

Therefore, the initial focus of the treatment team was to help both patients and their families bear the separation, allowing the adolescents to settle in and establish themselves in their new environment. One could say that the first treatment efforts were devoted to an iatrogenic illness caused by the patients' coming to the hospital.

The adolescent community, now numbering twenty-five to thirty patients, is geographically separate from the adult hospital, with little overlap of structured activities. A community store with a snack bar and game room provides an informal meeting place, and we have been surprised at the number of friendships that have been made between the adolescents and younger adult patients. These relationships seem to diffuse the intensity of relationships within the adolescent group.

The separation of therapeutic and administrative responsibility has proved to be an effective means of managing the adolescents' behavior while encouraging the psychotherapeutic exploration of their difficulties. In certain instances, splitting phenomena, the intensely differing and contradictory experiences among staff with a particular adolescent patient, have led to poor treatment coordination, a failure of mutual support, and an undercutting of different aspects of the treatment program. These splitting phenomena have also led to countertransference enactments by the therapist or the treatment staff and have required group discussion to resolve antagonisms aroused among staff members. Episodes of splitting usually have been resolved by one or more meetings with a group of senior staff members. Occasionally, these meetings have resulted in either a shift of therapist or a change of home. In general, two clinicians sharing responsibilities for the care of a single adolescent have offered a broader view of the adolescent's difficulties and reduced extreme staff reactions to the adolescent's behavioral problems.

We regard psychotropic medication, when clinically indicated, to be a valuable component of our treatment program. We often find that, after the living situation is stabilized, medications can be reduced or discontinued with no detrimental effect on the patient's progress.

The Lodge School has gained more importance in the lives of our adolescent patients. Almost every patient attends school, and school extracurricular activities have gradually extended to fill the day. A group therapy program at the school has helped reduce classroom disruptions, confirming the value of group therapy in larger adolescent group situations. A school yearbook was produced for the first time this year, but the goal of a full school activities program similar to an ordinary high school has yet to be reached, owing in part to our school's small size. The faculty remains chiefly concerned with the task of education and remediation of adolescents who have a negative image of themselves as students and who are sometimes several years below their expected grade levels.

We found that approximately half the students did not immediately pursue further education after graduation but sought work instead. This led us to develop a vocational component within the school program, beginning in the ninth grade, that we hope will prepare each student to move comfortably into a job if he or she so chooses.

Several concerns have arisen around the addition of vocational courses. A two-track system, academic and vocational, can lead to the adolescents' perception of themselves as first- or second-class citizens, depending on which track they pursue. We decided to make some vocational training available to every student. Students who wish to pursue vocational training more actively in the latter years of high school can add community-training programs to our curriculum. This has raised other questions. How much should students be encouraged to concentrate on an academic curriculum? Families who have difficulty recognizing the extent to which their child's illness has compromised educational success may be hesitant to support vocational training, fearing that the student's educational future will be ruined. We have learned that pressuring the student in one direction or another conflicts with our efforts to foster autonomy and self-direction—major goals for all our students. Here, success and improved self-esteem take temporary precedence over immediate educational goals. This is in line with the current view of educators that supports time off from school at different points in the educational process. We hope that the students with improved self-images will then continue their education.

We have had a limited but positive experience with preadolescent patients, eleven to thirteen years of age, suggesting that this model of care is appropriate for adolescents in this age range who require hospitalization. The advantages of being a medical facility have been evident in our treatment of adolescents who have physical disabilities or handicaps in addition to their psychiatric problems. This area of psychiatric treatment has been relatively neglected and deserves our further attention.

We have found certain adolescents who are not best served by the full adolescent treatment program. Their illnesses are characterized by rigid and negative behavior patterns, including manipulativeness, deceptiveness, and a disregard for the rights and feelings of others. Peer relationships expectedly have been poor. For such adolescents, the closeness and intimacy of family living provokes intolerable anxiety and an intensification of these defenses. Their peers respond with cruelty and ostracism, thus defeating the initial requirement of treatment, the establishment of a viable home living situation. In such instances, we have found that hospitalizing such adolescents, sixteen or older, on an adult or young adult unit and enrolling them in our school introduces more structured, less dangerous peer experiences and allows a more gradual reinvolvement with ordinary adolescent life.

Further Developments

When I think about the future direction of our work, I am intrigued by the relationships that our adolescent patients have established with their caretakers.

In discussions with former patients, I found that almost all developed intense positive feelings toward particular staff members during the course of treatment. These friendships, as the adolescents described them, were associated with many shared experiences and the development of mutual respect and affection. Our staff members are quite aware of the nature of these relationships but more circumspect in their descriptions because of their investment in their professional role. The chief characteristic of these relationships appears to be the lack of conscious therapeutic intent. Although this quality was greatly appreciated by the adolescents, staff, especially younger staff, were uneasy. They worried about having too much fun or feared they would lose their position of authority. However, these relationships provided the adolescent with expectable, ordinary experiences often sadly lacking in the past. Staff become an important stabilizing influence during periods of personal turmoil and family instability. We know these friendships are not like those the adolescent might have made before coming to the hospital. At that point in their lives and illnesses, they could not make or sustain such relationships.

Many factors color these relationships, such as the varied manifestations of positive transference displacements. The adolescent also seeks refuge in these relationships when he or she is suffering negative transferential feelings toward the psychotherapist. At these points, the patient's need for friendship and support must be integrated with the ongoing psychotherapy. We need to know more about the optimal mix of relationships during different phases of treatment and how the milieu can complement most usefully the formal therapies. The milieu with its multiple, evolving relationships deserves the same deliberate scrutiny we have given to our other therapies.

Another area deserving further study is the effect of development during adolescence on the response to treatment. For many short-term treatment programs, the influence of adolescent development is negligible. In our program, maturation and development become important factors in the progress of our patients. Physical maturation and growth substantially change the adolescent's view of himself or herself. Cognitive development brings an increased capacity for conceptual thinking, which has an effect on the adolescent's understanding of all our therapeutic measures. The intense emotional responsiveness of early adolescence shifts in middle adolescence to more considered reactions to frustration and disappointment. The diminished intensity of negative emotional responses to treatment interventions is a result of successful treatment but also of normal growth. As treatment proceeds, the rigid pathological defenses so prominent in the early phases of treatment give way to the more variable reactions of the developing adolescent. The character of adolescent relationships also change as treatment progresses and maturation occurs. We frequently observe that disturbed adolescents seek friendships with younger children. During treatment, social development resumes, and the adolescent moves toward more age-appropriate peers. These new relationships with peers present a challenge to the treatment process, the successful integration of new capabilities, not just the letting go of maladaptive patterns.

The activities and responsibilities of daily life change dramatically between the ages of thirteen and eighteen. The driver's license, school graduation, the first paid employment, and responsible sexual behavior are some of the milestones that face adolescents emerging from illness. We have found during treatment that the therapeutic focus shifts from the symptom picture and its psychopathological correlates to these developmental issues. Because of the severity of their disorders, almost all our improving adolescent patients remain vulnerable and have difficulty meeting these ordinary demands of growing up. Our successful treatments are increasingly concerned with these developmental steps.

The importance of maturational factors is demonstrated at the time of discharge, when arrangements are made for outpatient treatment. Tempering the adolescent's wish to leave the hospital are the strong relationships that they have built with their peers and with the treatment staff. The adolescents exhibit varying degrees of separation anxiety influenced by their age, stage of development, and remaining vulnerability. As they often comment, they are expected to continue their formal therapies, and they wish to maintain their social friendships as well. Leaving the hospital repeats for many of them the stress of new demands reminiscent of the onset of their illnesses.

For many hospitals, discharge planning involves setting a date, the relinquishing of responsibilities by the hospital, and the move to a new living situation and, often, to a new psychotherapist. Most efforts are devoted to the adequacy of the new treatment plan and the new living situation, which the adolescent sees as further evidence of the finality of his or her departure. Return visits to the hospital are not encouraged, and the relationships established in the hospital are considered a part of the past. The illness has been treated, and the patient resumes life outside the hospital. It is not surprising that therapeutic efforts often falter at this juncture in the patient's treatment program.

At present, we are studying the process of discharge and follow-up outpatient care. Many factors must be considered, chief among them the adolescent's developmental readiness to live independently. Should the adolescent return to the family home, a halfway house, boarding school, college, or an apartment with friends or on his or her own? Should he or she continue in our school or a new school? How should outside employment be related to discharge for the patient no longer in school? These questions face every hospital planning discharge of an adolescent patient. Many of our younger adolescents return to their families. Yet many adolescents and their families agree that returning home may provoke further difficulties, and, therefore, other living arrangements are preferable. Often, our older adolescents establish themselves more independently, living in a dormitory or an apartment with roommates while treatment continues. Ideally, the older adolescent should be able, with guidance, to choose the living situation that most nearly meets his or her needs and sets the stage for further progress. We are developing social networks outside the hospital that will help smooth the transition to independent living. Unfortunately, at present choices are limited, and failure often throws the whole treatment program into jeopardy. I feel that continuity of treatment during this major step toward independence is essential. But what about continued contact with the staff and other patients who remain in the hospital, from the patients' point of view their "friends." Are we to treat this as a regressive dependency, a resistance to be interpreted, or a useful support at a time of transition?

Currently, after discharge from the hospital, we permit visits, limited in scope, feeling that this phase of the treatment is drawing to a close. Concerns about excessive dependency are commonly voiced by parents and by staff who fear an intractable, unrelenting attachment. The conventional view of treatment as having a beginning, a middle, and an end is supportive of this approach. Yet, from a developmental perspective, we know that the separation process during adolescence is filled with progressions and regressions. These shifts in autonomous functioning occur more frequently in our patients, and each discharged adolescent should be scrutinized from this perspective. There should be room for mistakes and a chance to start again in a different direction. With sufficient flexibility, I feel we can be optimistic that time and treatment will produce a satisfactory autonomy.

Conclusions

From the day of admission, developmental considerations are a central part of the treatment program. Individual psychotherapy is a natural arena in which the adolescent's needs and interests can emerge from under the pathological formations that comprise his or her illness. Over time, developmental needs and conflicts and the fear of moving ahead will come to play a major role in the treatment. At this point, the establishment of comfortable age-appropriate activities is a vital part of the treatment process. We know that, at discharge, separation anxieties will stress the adolescent's new found sense of confidence and that neurotic solutions will surface again. Once discharge is comfortably accomplished, developmental issues will return to center stage. Thus, the adolescent and his or her treatment move back and forth between the regressive pull of neurotic solutions and the anxieties raised by the effect of developmental progress.

In the family treatment as well, developmental considerations are emphasized from the time of admission. The parents then come to understand that much more is at stake than the resolution of the symptomatology that brought the adolescent to the hospital. Consolidation of age-appropriate behaviors is as important as the elimination of symptoms, and emotional growth is the best defense against further illness. Parents can and should take vicarious satisfaction in the developmental steps of their adolescent children. They will support the process of treatment only if they take this broader view of their child's difficulties.

As I read this over, I find much that is familiar from the child-care and psychoanalytic literature. Yet the incorporation of what we know into our hospital treatment programs is an evolving process and remains incomplete. I feel fortunate to have had a part in one such hospital program.

REFERENCE

Bion, W. R. 1974. *Experiences in Groups*. New York: Random House.

PART III

DEVELOPMENTAL ISSUES IN ADOLESCENT PSYCHIATRY

EDITOR'S INTRODUCTION

Sheila Hafter Gray, from a psychoanalytic perspective, observes that young adulthood has been a neglected developmental phase. She believes that contemporary society has dispersed young adulthood tasks to adolescence or adulthood proper, where they burden the individual. Gray reviews the process of structuralization and discusses internalization, separation-individuation, and integration of a genital character structure, which she describes as the major developmental task of young adulthood. Other developmental tasks include career development, self-regard, and autonomy formation in self-image development. Pathological disorders of this phase help define the normative state and include pseudoadjustments, identity diffusions, gender confusions, and compromises of integrity. Gray concludes that the most significant developmental achievements are psychosexual genitality and the transformations of narcissism and images of mental representation into mature superego functions.

Joseph Palombo reviews the literature on normal adolescent development, as viewed by self psychologists. While Kohut suggested the general outlines for a developmental sequence, at no time did he propose a systematic progression. Palombo, on the other hand, focuses on the nature of the consolidation that occurs at the conclusion of adolescence and analyzes one aspect of normal adolescent development: late adolescence. He defines the use of self-cohesion and the nuclear self in Kohut's work and further describes the cohesive self, the emergent self, and selfobject experiences. Palombo believes that there is no single path for adolescents to follow; each adolescent must construct a narrative out of past and present experiences; a cohesive on the nature of the consolidation that occurs at the conclusion of adolescence and analyzes one aspect of normal adolescent development: late adolescence. He defines the use of self-cohesion and the nuclear self in Kohut's work and further describes the cohesive self, the emergent self, and selfobject experiences. Palombo believes that there is no single path for adolescents to follow; each adolescent must construct a narrative out of past and present experiences; a cohesive self is a necessary condition for the establishment of a nuclear self. Late adolescent development, a nodal point in the life cycle, occurs with a major reorganization of the self that is described as consolidation of a nuclear self. Further, selfobject functions (grandiose self, idealized parental imago, and alterego) are discussed in the formation of the nuclear self in late adolescence along with modulation of affective intensities and lastly attainment of a value system. The author concludes that the selfobject functions provided by the caregiver result in maintenance of the cohesive self and stabilization of the nuclear self.

Drew Westen, Pamela Ludolph, Kenneth Silk, Alfred Kellam, Laura Gold, and Naomi Lohr present a comparison of groups of patients diagnosed borderline disordered in adolescence and adulthood. Their theory compares multiple dimensions of object relations and development beyond the preoedipal years. The study examines empirically the ways in which the object relations of borderline adolescents resemble, as well as differ from, the object relations of borderline adults. The results corroborate some aspects of the psychoanalytic theory of borderline disorders but challenge the notion that a preoedipal arrest can account for the entirety of borderline object relations in adolescence and adulthood.

Max Sugar describes an indirect approach through questions that provides a group of adolescents an opportunity to explore their feelings in a relatively spontaneous and unstructured fashion. Using an annual rap session at a local general hospital as a vehicle, Sugar describes the methodology that results in two groups of questions: twelve- to fourteen-year-olds and fifteen- to eighteen-year-olds. The author concludes that parents and their teenagers struggle with coincident anxiety but not necessarily psychopathology.

Bernard A. Stein, Harvey Golombek, Peter Marton, and Marshall Korenblum continue their longitudinal study of personality development (see vol. 14). Previous findings supported the view of middle adolescence as a period of stabilization, but those early adolescents with significantly more depression showed the least improvement over time. This chapter presents the research sample as they reach late adolescence. The authors show that both consistency and change are characteristic of personality functioning in adolescents as they grow from middle to late adolescence. Late adolescents demonstrate more dysphoria than do middle adolescents, but in a different context (related to educational and vocational decisions and commitment in personal relationships). On the other hand, a well-functioning teenager does not tend suddenly to develop moodiness during the adolescent years. A relative increase in depressed mood in early adolescence and hatred in middle adolescence is a predictor of personality problems. The authors conclude that these are indications to be taken seriously and not considered vicissitudes of normal adolescent development.

18 DEVELOPMENTAL ISSUES IN YOUNG ADULTHOOD: PSYCHOANALYTIC PERSPECTIVES

SHEILA HAFTER GRAY

Young adulthood has been a neglected developmental phase in our culture and in our science. Increasingly, patients present because they do not complete the developmental tasks of this phase or because they suffer from the residual of the developmental errors that they had committed at this time.

Our contemporary society has dispersed the tasks of young adulthood either to adolescence, where they overburden the young person, or to adulthood proper, where they form inappropriate encumbrances. For example, Austin and Inderbitzin's (1983) paper on brief psychotherapy of late adolescence actually deals with facilitating the transition to young adulthood.

Of the early psychoanalysts, only Jung (1960) paid significant attention to development beyond adolescence. In his outline of the stages of life, he placed youth in the period between postpubescence and adulthood. He described the developmental tasks of this phase as disengagement from childhood aspirations, confrontation with issues of sexuality and self-esteem, and the broadening of one's life perspective. This schema corresponds accurately to the concept of young adulthood as I shall use it.

Erikson (1959) defines young adulthood as the developmental phase that follows adolescence and in which the tasks are to achieve solidarity with one's peers and a capacity for intimacy. The core conflict of this phase is intimacy versus isolation. Following Erikson, we may say that the tasks of young adulthood are socially to develop techniques of cooperation and competition in work and in sex, psychosocially to lose and find oneself in another, and psychosexually to establish genitality. These may be summarized into one concept, integration of a genital character structure (Reich 1929). I propose that this is the major developmental task of young adulthood.

When classical psychoanalysts use the term "development," they usually mean the development of psychic structure, the differentiation of the mind into id, ego, and superego (cf. Freud 1963). Thus, we think about the transformation of libido from oral to anal to phallic to genital as structure formation within the id (Holt 1967). Or we may discuss development or maldevelopment of the ego, as Sigmund Freud did as early as 1911, in the *Two Principles of Mental Functioning* (Freud 1911). Similarly, we read Freud's (1925) comment that in the ideal case the superego becomes the heir of, or the successor to, the Oedipus complex as a statement that psychic structure develops as a result of particular events in the life of an individual.

While Freud's own work concentrated on demonstrating the last point, the roots of adult personality and mental illness in early childhood experience, he indicated that significant development took place later as well. For example, in both 1925 and 1931 he suggested that experiences during adolescence had an important effect on the resolution of the Oedipus complex in women, although he did not develop this idea himself (Gray 1976). Again, when he discussed the formation of the superego, Freud (1923) called attention to its evolution throughout life and to the influence of significant persons besides the parents on its eventual form.

In our own time, structural theory has become more abstract. We now think of the mental apparatus as composed of discrete bits of memory arranged in functional clusters that we call structures. Thus, we speak more precisely of an aggregate of ego functions rather than of a single entity called the ego. This notion helps us conceptualize how with each new experience existing mental structures may be revised or made more elaborate (cf. Loewald 1972). If you can imagine bits of memory arranged and rearranged as if they were mosaic tiles into patterns that are stable but not permanently cemented, you will have the idea. We may then see the formation of psychic structure as the alignment of these bits of memory into those constellations that we call ego or superego.

The formation of psychic structure, or of personality if you take a view from outside, depends in part on the individual's inherent capacity to lay down memory traces of his or her life experience. When we use this concept to understand purely intellectual matters, we call the process learning. When we use this idea to discuss more emotional kinds of learning, we use terms such as "internalization," making someone who was experienced as outside one's self into part of self.

Internalization is the way separation-individuation is achieved. Slowly over the course of development, a normal individual internalizes more and more of his or her interpersonal environment and, therefore, requires the actual presence of the parental figures less and less. Certain minimum standards of internalization must be met before an individual can climb the next rung of the developmental ladder in a healthy, competent way.

One might, for example, think about little children. Many educators, the Montessori group among them, believe that, until somebody is reliably dry, he or she ought not to go to nursery school. This is because the person who is not reliably dry is a person who cannot remember the primary caregiver in a constant meaningful way and, therefore, ought not to be separated. Similarly, an adolescent who cannot perform dependably the activities of daily living and who must rely on parents to protect him or her from the consequences of his absentmindedness ought not to enter a major university. Not having completed the developmental tasks of adolescence effectively, that person will not be able to function on his or her own and is at risk to drop out.

Do note that, besides making a point about the formation of psychic structure, I am comparing age groups that are usually at least ten years apart, the toddler and the young adolescent, the latency child and the young adult. Between toddlerhood and latency and between early adolescence and young adulthood lies the Oedipus complex, the original infantile neurosis and its revival during puberty. The onset of latency and the beginning of young adulthood follow, in ordinary healthy development, the resolution of the Oedipus complex. They are both marked by transformation of id impulses into adaptive ego functions and emergence of new superego functions.

The resolution of the Oedipus complex is also a mourning process. If a process by which the actual parents of childhood are replaced by their mental representations and then by part of the individual's own self, the superego. It eventuates in personal autonomy since the actual presence of parents or their surrogates is no longer required for survival. With the emergence of the superego, learning replaces drive as the prime motivator of human behavior (Hartmann 1960). Psychoanalytic ego psychologists, therefore, defined a fully structured superego as one that functioned autonomously to ensure adherence to moral codes and resisted regressive instinctualization (Hartmann and Loewenstein 1962).

The superego is the third, and ontogenetically the latest, element of the mental apparatus. Superego functions represent parental and, beyond them, societal attitudes. They are usually grouped into two classes, standards and values. These are made part of the individual's self through the processes of internalization, processes that themselves stand in a developmental hierarchy. Thus, while ideals and prohibitions are features of mental life well before the appearance of the infantile neurosis, they are not transformed from simple mental representations of parental attitudes into elements of an individual's psychic structure until the resolution of the Oedipus complex. That transformation may be considered a definition in structural terms of this crucial event.

Outgrowing the initial mother-infant twosome and establishing one's self as a separate individual is the developmental task that begins at birth and culminates in the young adult stage of development. As you recall, development proceeds in order though the oral, anal, and phallic phases, the phallic being the first phase of the Oedipus complex. You will also recall that during adolescence one sees a review in symbolic ways of all these phases, including a grand revival of the oedipal phase. This is expressed in terms of working out the relationships with both parents and working out a sexualized identity. With the optimal resolution of the adolescent Oedipus complex, the close of the adolescent phase of development, one begins the genital phase.

I propose that the integration of a genital character structure is the major developmental task of young adulthood. It is a task at which one must work hard. During young adulthood, a person consolidates the emotional lessons learned during all the earlier phases with those learned from new developmentally appropriate experiences. This leads to the emergence of an autonomous superego that will guide the person in the expression of sexuality and in the formation of a work identity.

Genitality was at one time thought to be an ideal state. Achievement of a solid position in the hysterical, or phallic, phase was deemed healthy enough. Recent developments, particularly in women's psychology, have shown us that we can indeed look forward to more complete emotional growth (cf. Gray 1976).

First, the invention of perfect contraception made it possible to differentiate sexual acts and procreative acts, as Benedek (1960) had done on purely theoretical grounds. Now that artificial insemination permits procreation without a sexual act as such, we can readily discern the two separate developmental lines of adult sexuality, pleasure-seeking sexual activity and parenthood. Psychoanalytic theory now affirms that women experience true orgasm apart from childbirth (cf. Deutsch 1925) and that men wish to facilitate the development of a new human being.

Another important social change has been the women's movement, which may be understood in psychoanalytic terms as the assertion, by both men and women, that the possession of a phallus is not necessary to be a complete individual. There are, rather, two sets of sexual organs, male and female. A women is not an incomplete or defective man but a different person. Appreciating this is a necessary developmental achievement for both men and women. It forms the basis of what is called genitality from a psychoanalytic point of view. The women's movement also reminded us of the rampant phallocentricity of our culture, the endemic arrest of development at the phallic phase. It is particularly evident, as one would expect, when one examines superego functions, our standards and values.

In the 1960s, Lederer (1964) noted that psychoanalysts tended to concentrate on the negative and prohibitive aspects of the superego. Its function was most often seen as one of forcing an individual into compliance with a social order that he or she never made. "The price we pay for our advance in civilization is a loss of happiness through the heightening of the sense of guilt" (Freud 1930, p. 134). Positive, facilitative superego functions were largely overlooked. We tended, instead, to think of pleasure or possessions that had to be renounced in order to live comfortably with the stern, depriving parents who are memorialized in the superego of the phallic phase. Stated a different way, the superego of an individual who is preoccupied with the phallus and with castration is not autonomous. This is very different from the attitude of cheerful, autonomous fulfillment that characterizes the mature masculine or feminine individual.

332

In his classic paper, Erikson (1959) discussed the chief task of adolescence in terms of forming an identity, becoming an individual. During young adulthood, that individual learns to be a partner. The important relationships in this phase are twosomes, one-to-one friendships, sexual partnerships, partners with whom to work together and partners with whom to compete. One makes agreements to disagree according to mutually acceptable rules. This is the time to establish patterns of cooperation and competition that one can use during the rest of one's life. One cultivates modes of differing with coworkers and being amiable with competitors. Splits are healed. Team sports are, for this reason, very popular both in colleges and among blue-collar youths. The participants can take different sides, fight passionately but fairly to win, and remain friends.

Young adulthood is also the period when men and women will, in the course of normal development, begin their careers. It is a time of exploration and of self-discovery. It was once customary for new journeymen, those who had just completed apprenticeship, to travel to several places to work with various master artisans. This helped them gain a broad perspective of their craft, to expand their skills, and then to consolidate a style of their own. It also permitted them a range of new social and sexual experiences before they settled into a permanent position and marriage. Today, young physicians will seek residencies and fellowships in different medical centers for similar reasons.

The behavior of young adults in school or in the workplace will be motivated by and evaluated by superego functions. Here, a lot depends on what, to avoid using the term "narcissism," I like to call self-regard. I prefer it because it precludes confusion with the concept of pathological narcissism. Self-regard is a superego function. If the family or the larger society, or both, emphasizes phallic ideals and attitudes, those are bound to become part of superego and thus to influence the individual's self-image and his or her opinion of appropriate goals (Gray 1985).

Young adulthood is also the period when one must think of oneself as a person who can live alone. Some interesting criteria are, Can you cook your food? Can you iron your shirt? Can you take care of your car? A person who cannot do such things, whose self-image does not include the requirement to do them, is dependent on another person to execute these tasks. Why is this important? It is important because the man who cannot get his housekeeping organized is a person who has not yet outgrown the caregiving mother. He is to a considerable extent susceptible to forming a new dependency with anyone who will just do it for him and, thus, help him recreate the aura of that early, carefree relatedness. With the renewal of social attitudes that encourage people to live alone rather than marry soon out of school, social attitudes that encourage a broad range of work and study experience before settling into a career, we have found that ordinary human beings are, in fact, able to achieve a genital level of development and go on to form relationships that are partnerships of two autonomous persons.

Some of the psychopathology specific to this stage helps us define the normative state. First, in clinical practice, we often see pseudoadjustments, or pathological adjustments, social and behavioral patterns that appear normal but that reflect disturbances of earlier development. A good example is the many young people who marry expecting to accomplish the developmental task of adolescence, to find themselves, in finding one another. Sometimes, I fear, student health officers miss the diagnosis and offer reassurance rather than definitive treatment. We may see these people later in life, when they finally confront their failure to have completed their emotional growth. At this later time, they must do so in the context of complicated relationships with spouse and children. Sometimes they have missed important life opportunities.

One of the easier ways of assessing this process in an individual, I have found, is to examine the superego functions to determine whether they are characteristically phallic or genital. For example, a woman who defines her worth in terms of being a handmaiden to her idealized employer, lover, husband, or children, who glories in, rather than tolerates, the inevitable pain of childbirth, is phallic (Gray 1976). Most examples of the "natural masochism" of women (Blum 1976; Deutsch 1925) or the "natural aggression" of men belong, I believe, to this group of pathological adjustments.

Another kind of pathological adjustment is the triad of ambition, power, and opportunism that Rangell (1975) identified as the hallmark of psychopathology specific to the superego. He named it the syndrome of the compromise of integrity. It is not exclusive to young adulthood, but it seems to surface for the first time in this age group. A contemporary example is an epidemic of outright lawlessness disguised as a quest for prosperity that has sprung up among young members of the business community. They seem to view their behavior as idealistic conformity with the values of their group. Such vulnerability of the superego to peer pressure is, of course, phase normative in adolescence, but it represents a developmental lag when it is found in an older person.

Some of the interesting psychopathology of young adulthood proper can also be found in disorders in which the superego is the mental agency most directly involved. They are related to syndromes of pathological narcissism, but they carry a better prognosis. For example, the task of setting one's career goal is often complicated by excessive self-esteem. In our own culture, the task of coming to terms with who we are is particularly difficult. Children grow up understanding that the little engine could, but sometimes you can say, "Yes, I can! Yes, I can!" all you want, and there are still things you just cannot do. One has to come to terms with these things.

This has become so serious in our own country that it has a proper name, the American Icarus syndrome (Murray 1955). Clinically, it manifests itself as a specific kind of depression. The patients believe that they are wonderful and can do all sorts of amazing things, but they exhaust themselves in activity that gets them nowhere. Our casebook has many entries of young people who have splendid goals, but, while they are thinking about writing the great American novel, they lack the capacity to earn a living as a file clerk. They are not organized. Such people may not be very sick or maldeveloped. They may have had and profited from emotional advantages in their early lives, including secure homes and loving parents who repeatedly told them, "You're a wonderful kid!" Unfortunately, their enhanced self-esteem may interfere with their perception of the reality of where they stand in the larger society. Bright people, especially, may have failed to develop adequate study skills because they continue to believe that success can be achieved simply by asserting one's will.

The therapeutic task in dealing with the American Icarus syndrome is to help the patient balance self-image against actual experiences with others, primarily friends and teachers, and to form a more realistic ego ideal. Some psychotherapists work toward this goal by focusing on the patient's narcissism. Making an effort to transform that narcissism into mature superego functions may, however, make for a briefer and more successful treatment (cf. Gray 1978).

Conclusions

I have tried to share some of my ideas about the developmental tasks of young adulthood. Significant among them are the achievement of psychosexual genitality and the transformations of both narcissism and the mental representation of significant relationships into mature superego functions. These permit the consolidation of a genital character structure. I hope I have also demonstrated that classical psychoanalysis offers useful ways of thinking about new problems.

NOTE

An earlier version of this chapter was presented to the American Society for Adolescent Psychiatry, Chicago, May 8, 1987.

REFERENCES

Austin, L., and Inderbitzin, L. 1983. Brief psychotherapy of late adolescence. *American Journal of Psychotherapy* 37:202–209.

Benedek, T. 1960. The organization of the reproductive drive. *International Journal of Psycho-Analysis* 41:1–15.

Blum, H. P. 1976. Masochism, the ego ideal, and the psychology of women. *Journal of the American Psychoanalytic Association* 24S:157–191.

Deutsch, H. 1925. The psychology of woman in relation to the functions of reproduction. In R. Fleiss, ed. *The Psychoanalytic Reader*. London: Hogarth, 1950.

Erikson, E. 1959. Growth and crises of the healthy personality. In *Identity and the Life Cycle: Selected Papers: Psychological Issues* 1(1): 50–100.

Freud, A. 1963. The concept of developmental lines. *Psychoanalytic Study of the Child* 18:245–265.

Freud, S. 1911. Formulations on the two principles of mental functioning. *Standard Edition* 12:213–226. London: Hogarth, 1961.

Freud, S. 1923. The ego and the id. *Standard Edition* 19:13–63. London: Hogarth, 1961.

Freud, S. 1925. Some psychical consequences of the anatomical distinction between the sexes. *Standard Edition* 19:248–258. London: Hogarth, 1961.

Freud, S. 1930. Civilization and its discontents. *Standard Edition* 21:64–145. London: Hogarth, 1961.

Freud, S. 1931. Femininity. *Standard Edition* 22:112–135. London: Hogarth, 1961.

Gray, S. H. 1976. The resolution of the Oedipus complex in women. *Journal of the Philadelphia Association for Psychoanalysis* 3:103–111.

Gray, S. H. 1978. Brief psychotherapy: a developmental approach. *Journal of the Philadelphia Association for Psychoanalysis* 5:29–40.

Gray, S. H. 1985. Women's experience of their intellectual life. Paper presented to the Michigan Psychoanalytic Society, Dearborn, Mich., November 2, 1985.

Hartmann, H. 1960. *Psychoanalysis and Moral Values*. New York: International Universities Press.

Hartmann, H., and Loewenstein, R. M. 1962. Notes on the superego. *Psychoanalytic Study of the Child* 17:42–81.

Holt, R. 1967. The development of the primary process: a structural view. *Psychological Issues Monograph* 5(2): 343–383.

Jung, C. 1960. *The Collected Works*. New York: Pantheon.

Lederer, W. 1964. Dragons, delinquents, and destiny: an essay on positive superego functions. *Psychological Issues* 4(3): 3–76.

Loewald, H. 1972. Perspectives on memory. In *Papers on Psychoanalysis*. New Haven, Conn.: Yale University Press, 1980.

Murray, H. A. 1955. American Icarus. In A. Burton and E. Harris, eds. *Clinical Studies of Personality*. New York: Harper.

Rangell, L. 1975. A psychoanalytic perspective leading currently to the syndrome of the compromise of integrity. *International Journal of Psycho-Analysis* 55:3–12.

Reich, W. 1929. The genital character and the neurotic character. In R. Fleiss, ed. *The Psychoanalytic Reader*. London: Hogarth, 1950.

19 THE COHESIVE SELF, THE NUCLEAR SELF, AND DEVELOPMENT IN LATE ADOLESCENCE

JOSEPH PALOMBO

The literature on normal adolescent development as viewed by self psychologists is sparse indeed. Although Kohut makes scattered references to adolescence in his work, his only contribution (Kohut 1972) was the discussion of a paper by Wolf, Gedo, and Terman (1972). The posthumously published *The Kohut Seminars* (Elson 1987) deals with patients who might be considered to be addressing issues of late adolescence. However, since those seminars took place during the early 1970s, they reflect the thinking to be found in *The Analysis of the Self* (Kohut 1971) rather than Kohut's more mature later reflections on the development of the self. The essays on courage, leadership, and idealization of cultural selfobjects, also published posthumously (Kohut 1985a, 1985b), have some direct bearing on adolescent issues but do not discuss developmental trends directly.

Other contributors include Basch (1980), who discusses the treatment of a young adult and elaborates on the specific selfobject dynamics that the patient confronts. Wolf (1982) outlines some of the selfobject needs of adolescents and discusses these within the framework of needs for selfobjects within the life cycle. Marohn (1977, 1980, 1981, 1982, 1984) has written extensively on delinquency and on adolescents with severe acting-out problems. Buffington (1984, 1985), Burch (1985), Goldberg (1978, 1984a), and Wolf (1984) have also contributed to the literature.

In order to place adolescent development within the broader context of all development, it must first be noted that, originally, Kohut appears to have accepted without question the principle that development could be reconstructed from pathological and regressive states. In *The Analysis of the Self*, Kohut (1971) suggested the general outlines for a developmental sequence based on the reconstruction made in the analyses of narcissistic personality disorders. Later, he seems to have shifted his position without rejecting the principle entirely (Kohut 1978), but at no time did he propose a systematic developmental progression.

There is, at present, a consensus that theories of development should not be devised solely from the reconstructions of the lives of pathological individuals but must also be complemented by observations of a normal population (Lichtenberg 1983; Stern 1985). However, since no systematic observations of normal adolescents by self psychologically informed observers have been made, and since, strictly speaking, we can say that at present no theory of normal adolescent development from that perspective exists, I believe that it is beneficial to begin the task of outlining some of the issues that adolescents confront. The data on which this chapter is based come from a group of adolescent patients who were seen in psychotherapy over a period of years. Furthermore, since it would be too large a task to undertake the conceptualization of the entire phase, I have chosen to focus on one aspect of that phase: the subphase of late adolescence. This subphase presents some challenging conceptual problems, one of which will be focused on in this discussion: the problems of the nature of the consolidation that occur at the conclusion of adolescence.

Among many of the adolescents that I have seen for long-term psychotherapy, I have noted that, at around age seventeen, a remarkable shift occurs. The shift in adolescents' attitudes includes a lessened resistance to the therapeutic process, a less confrontive attitude toward parents, a greater sense of responsibility for their own actions and the consequences of these actions, and a more active involvement in planning for their future. This shift seems not only to reflect the benefits derived from the therapeutic process but also to be the result of a stabilization in the adolescents' sense of self. They exhibit a qualitatively different internal balance than that present in the more tumultous prior years. Clinically, a demarcation appears to exist between the sense of cohesion with which they entered adolescence and the sense of cohesion present toward the end of that phase.

These observations led to the search for a conceptual explanation for what was occurring and to the attempt to frame the explanation in terms of the concept of self-cohesion and the "cohesive self." However, in retracing Kohut's use of the term, I discovered that the use Kohut made of the concept changed over time. In his later writings, the concept of the "nuclear self" was consistently substituted for that of the "cohesive self." The reason for the shift, while never addressed directly by Kohut, can be inferred from the context in which it occurred. By taking the distinction implicit in these references, a solution to the problems involved in understanding this aspect of adolescent development can be found.

The aim of this chapter, then, is to address one aspect of normal adolescent development: late adolescence. This subphase of adolescence is of special interest because of the consolidation that occurs in the sense of self and also because it represents a coalescing in the sense of self unlike that of any other phase of development. In order to undertake this discussion, it will first be necessary to address some specific issues related to the definitions of the "cohesive self" and the "nuclear self." I shall then turn to a systematic presentation of a self psychologically informed view of normal development in late adolescence. This schema is based on clinical data, although it will obviously not be possible to present the supporting material here.

The Definitions of Self-Cohesion and the Nuclear Self in Kohut's Work

In this section, I review the history of Kohut's usage of the concepts of the "cohesive self" and the "nuclear self" to highlight an interpretation that makes possible the retention of both concepts in the service of making an important distinction that I believe to be inherent in his work, a distinction that will be critical to this conceptualization of late adolescence.

The distinction between the concepts of the "cohesive self" and the "nuclear self" that seems implicit in Kohut's work is that the former concept accounts for the inborn factors that contribute to the formation of the self and the latter for the accretions to the structure of the cohesive self that result from selfobject experiences. I argue that it would be useful for us to retain both concepts and that, while the concept of the "cohesive self" serves to describe the structures present at birth, the concept of the "nuclear self" may serve to characterize the kind of consolidation and reorganization of the self that occurs at the end of adolescence.

Controversy exists among self psychologists regarding Kohut's use of the concepts of the "cohesive self" and the "nuclear self." One interpretation is that by "nuclear self" Kohut meant the unchangeable, innate patterns that unfold during development and that "cohesion" represents a consolidation at eighteen months when the infant attains the capacity to use the personal pronoun "I." It is, therefore, an achievement rather than an innate pattern. Another interpretation is that the infant is born in a prestructural, prepsychological state in which no cohesion is possible. The "nuclear self" is attained at the age of eighteen months when consolidation of the two poles of the self is achieved and some structural solidity occurs. According to this interpretation, "cohesion" is a quality of the nuclear self that reflects its functional status.

A careful review of Kohut's work reveals that the terms "cohesive self" and "nuclear self" underwent a historical evolution that requires clarification. While the concept of the "cohesive self" appears central to Kohut's thinking in his earlier work, the concept of the "nuclear self" does not even appear in the index of *The Analysis of the Self*, a fact that Kohut himself noted in a letter written in 1972 (Ornstein 1978, 2:866). As the concept of the "nuclear self" became more central to his thinking in later works, it began to be featured more prominently, and the concept of the "cohesive self" seemed to recede into the background (Kohut 1984).

Furthermore, a clear distinction must be made between the usage of the concept of the "cohesive self" and that of "self cohesion." The latter concept is often used by Kohut in conjunction with other descriptors to indicate a state of the self such as firmness, vigor, vitality, and harmony. The former concept is clearly a structural concept that indicates either an inborn given, a developmental achievement, or the reestablishment of a structural stability following an experience of fragmentation. The focus in this discussion is on the structural concept.

In his early work, and utilizing a developmental perspective, Kohut began with the hypothesis (derived from reconstructions) that the self develops out of body self-nuclei, which coalesce to form the cohesive self. This progression follows from the movement of the libidinal drives that cathect body parts at first, during the phase of autoerotism, to cathecting the mental self as the shift to narcissism occurs (Kohut 1971, pp. 214–217). The occurrence of this shift is marked by "the mother's exultant response to the total child" (p. 118).

For Kohut, the fact that some patients appear to survive terrible deprivations in infancy and are healthier than the facts of their histories would warrant is an indication of the operation of innate factors in the maintenance of self-cohesion. Furthermore, he suggests that it is possible at times for innate factors actively to interfere with the coalescing that should occur: "The psychopathology associated with the schizophrenics and of borderlines stem from their proneness to protracted states of fragmentation that is due to innate factors. In contrast, the narcissistic personality disorders suffer from structures that are either insufficiently cathected or if cathected or hyper-cathected are not integrated into the rest of the personality" (Kohut 1971, p. 19).

This view, which is highly colored by the drive psychology within which it developed, was subsequently modified in important ways. During what appears to have been a transitional period, Kohut seems to have substituted the "nuclear self" for what he had previously denoted as the "cohesive self" (Kohut 1978, p. 741). Here, he uses the "nuclear self" where previously he had used "cohesive self." In this seminal paper on development, Kohut rejects the notion that the cohesive self results from the coalescing of the body nuclei. By rejecting the language and the premises of drive psychology, he also rejected the implications that arose from hypothesizing a movement from a phase of autoerotism to that of primary narcissism. However, he was careful to point out that this rejection did not imply that he did not think that there was no evidence for the hypothesis that the nuclear self may be derived from prior experiences in which the totality of the self was not existent as a whole (p. 749).

The distinction that begins to appear seems to be around the old formulation of the progression of cathexis that led to the coalescing of the cohesive self and the new formulation that was centered around the formation of the nuclear self. The nuclear self encompasses the psychological structures associated with the two poles of the self, the nuclear ambitions and ideals. This would suggest that it resulted from developmental factors related to the selfobject functions rather than from strictly innate factors. "On the basis of certain genetic reconstructions . . . I arrived at the hypothesis that the rudiments of the nuclear self are laid down by the simultaneously or consecutively occurring processes of selective inclusion and exclusion of psychological structures. And, furthermore, I came to hold the view that the sense of abiding sameness along the time axis—a distinguishing attribute of the healthy self—is laid down early as the result of the abiding action-promoting tension gradient between the two major constituents of the nuclear self" (Kohut 1977, p. 183).

However, we also read the following: "The self arises thus as the result of the interplay between the new-born's innate equipment and the selective response of the selfobjects through which certain potentialities are encouraged or are even discouraged. Out of this selective process there emerges, probably during the second year of life, a nuclear self which, as stated earlier, is currently conceptualized as a bipolar structure; archaic nuclear ambitions form one pole, archaic nuclear ideals the other" (Kohut and Wolf 1978, pp. 416–417). While it is understandable that the interplay between the innate factors and the environment might play a role in the formation of the nuclear self, what is unclear is why it should occur at the age of two. Kohut had much to say about the realization of nuclear ambitions and ideals as part of the actualization of the program of the nuclear self. He implied that this program is laid down very early, that in some fashion the course of one's life is set by the time this event occurs. I find it difficult to give any credence to the concept of ambitions and ideals as laid down by the second year of life. While it is, of course, obvious that particular selfobject functions have accrued to the developing child by that age, these cannot by any measure be viewed as resembling the later accretions that do in fact propel a young adult into the world. I would suggest that it makes more sense to think of such a consolidation as occurring toward the conclusion of the adolescent process. The broader issues of the effect of early childhood experiences on later development and of the relation between self-experience and the internalization of selfobject functions, prior to adolescence, are complex and deserve much greater discussion than is possible in this chapter.

In order to justify maintaining the distinctions between the "cohesive self" and the "nuclear self," other facts must be adduced to support the contention. It may be possible to retain both concepts and to elaborate on their definitions if the findings of infancy researchers are interpreted in a way that suggests that infants are generally born with a cohesive self. It may then be maintained that those infants who do not possess a cohesive self at birth would be thought of as suffering from serious emotional illnesses such as schizophrenia, autism, or the severe borderline disturbances. Lichtenberg's (1983) and Stern's (1985) work suggests that such an interpretation is sound, even though their definitions of the concept of "self" differs from that of Kohut.

The task, for developmental theorists, would then be that of spelling out what it means to have a "cohesive self." The articulation of the meaning of "cohesion" would be critical to this view of development. The "nuclear self" would then be understood to come about from the consolidation of the sense of self that results from the internalization of selfobject functions. The timing of the occurance of this consolidation would then be subject to empirical verification. My data lead me to believe that it occurs following the resolution of the processes of adolescence. Such an interpretation need not preclude that an ongoing developmental progression in the acquisition of selfobject functions also occurs; it posits only a qualitative difference in the form of the consolidation as it occurs in late adolescence.

It now becomes possible to turn our attention to a brief discussion of the meaning of self-cohesion within the context of this understanding of the nature of a cohesive self; this will be followed by a discussion of the concept of the "nuclear self" as it relates to late adolescent development.

The Cohesive Self

The concept of self-cohesion may be used phenomenologically to describe a state of self-consolidation (Stolorow, Brandchaft, and Atwood 1987, p. 90). The sense of coherence reflects the stability and integrity of a set of meanings that have organized the person's experiences into meaning systems (Saari 1986a, 1986b) or scripts and narratives.

From a structural perspective the conditions necessary for the establishment of a cohesive self are to be found in the innate givens with which each person is endowed. These givens may be described in a variety of ways: from a neurological perspective or from a more psychological perspective (Palombo 1983, 1987b; Palombo and Feigon

1984). Some of the components that may be included within the structure of the cohesive self are those described by Stern (1985) as forming part of the domain of the emergent self. Again, while Stern's concept of "self" is quite different from that being used in this context, the functions and processes that he lists are the same.

If structure represents a set of enduring functions, then psychic functions may be conceived of as a set of symbols that remain stable over time and become imbricated into the self through redundant usage (Demos 1988). Thus, action patterns that contain not only the infant's activity but also the associated affects and the caregiver's responses and that have been experienced a multitude of times (cf. Stern's concept of "RIGs," or representation of internalizations generalized) form self-object functions. The totality of these functions lend the unique quality that characterizes each person as an individual. Eventually, the hierarchies of meanings associated with these functions acquire a coherence that defines the personality. This coherence is experienced as a sense of cohesion that is reflective of the sense of intactness, of wholeness, and vitality. The cohesive self is the structure that is constituted of the set of coherent meanings that have arisen during the course of development. It is the product of endowment in tandem with the self-object experiences that facilitate the integration of affective experience. It is the center of a person's organization.

From an introspective perspective, meanings are attained through shared experiences with others and through the particular imprint that a person's innate givens lends to what is experienced. Since meanings arise through discourse, the dialogue is fundamental to the acquisition of a set of meanings. In this sense, the dialogue plays a fundamental role in the structuralization of self-experience and of relationships. The dialogue between caregivers and infant is the fundamental and critical component in the development of a sense of coherence.

Self-cohesion is not a static state but a dynamic force that represents the organizing capacities that are at play to synthesize and integrate self-experiences. During the life cycle, the sense of cohesion is maintained as a result of the successful attempts at synthesizing new experiences into old ones, at reworking old experiences and reinterpreting them in the light of new ones, and at maintaining a level of selfobject experience in which functions are provided at a level that is appropriate to the person's capacity to integrate life experiences. Self-cohesion does not represent an attempt at reaching a stable homeostatic or nirvana-like state. Rather, it is a dynamic, active expression of the continual movement from destabilization to restabilization.

The Cohesive Self in Adolescent Development

Adolescents arrive at this phase with specific developmental needs for particular responses from their caregivers. The nature of the self-object functions required at this stage is different from those of prior phases. The caregivers, who are the vehicles through whom these selfobject functions are performed, are required to play a different role from that played in former phases. Their ability to be responsive to the adolescent's needs are determined not only by the relationship that they have had to their child prior to that phase but also by the issues that are activated within them by the adolescent. The issues of their own adolescence may become entwined with their responses to the adolescent.

While adolescents may bring with them unresolved issues or selfobject deficits from prior developmental phases, these serve to render more complex the task of the traversal of this phase. These deficits, or the regressions to prior modes of functioning, do not constitute the essence of the phase-appropriate struggle. Rather, the complementing of the self by new selfobject functions is central to the negotiation of this phase.

There is also no single path through which all adolescents must travel for them to be considered as having had a model adolescent phase. Rather, different adolescents will address issues differently and will resolve them in accordance with their endowments and the availability of selfobjects to complement them or to compensate for possible deficits. There is no set script, narrative, or myth that guides the adolescent developmental process. Each adolescent must construct a narrative out of past and present experiences.

In adolescence a number of factors may either threaten or bring an imbalance in the sense of cohesion. First are the biological changes brought about by puberty. While these have been discussed extensively in the literature from an object relations or an ego psychological perspective, they have not been dealt with from an empathic perspective. Other factors related to innate givens, which also have significant consequences, may be mentioned. These are the possible presence of neurocognitive deficits (i.e., learning disabilities; Palombo 1979, 1983, 1985, 1987b), the emergence of affective disorders or panic disorders, the presence of attention-deficit disorders, or the onset of a thought disorder that heralds a potential for a schizophrenic process.

It is important to note that a phase-appropriate loosening of the sense of coherence may result in experiences of temporary fragmentation. These adolescent processes may lead to a diffuseness in the cohesiveness of the self that challenges the adolescent's level of integration to reach a sense of reequilibration. The restoration of a new balance would represent the reassessment of the meanings of prior experiences and their integration into a new set of meanings. The capacity for formal operational thought may facilitate the process. Thus, while temporary regressions to older modes of behaving and relating may manifest themselves, these are in sharp contrast to the highly mature symbolic forms of thinking that may also be present.

What may then be concluded is that a cohesive self is a necessary condition for the establishment of a nuclear self. An adolescent whose sense of cohesion is either tenuous or nonexistent will be unable to negotiate the tasks of adolescence successfully.

The Nuclear Self in Late Adolescent Development

Reorganizations of a person's system of meanings occur at nodal points in the life cycle. Some of these reorganizations result from specific developmental processes, such as the emergence of language in infancy, while others result from life experiences, whether traumatic or momentous in their significance. To the extent that the concept of phasic development is applicable to the evolving personality, the emergence of a phase may be said to occur when such a major reorganization takes place. One way to conceive of such a reorganization is to think of it as consisting of the emergence of a new edition of an old narrative.

During late adolescence, clinical observation reveals a number of shifts in the adolescent's sense of self. The painful self-consciousness that was previously noticeable begins to dissipate. The egocentrism and sense of uniqueness give way to more empathic attitudes toward others. Self-regulation becomes more possible and is less dependent on others for reinforcement. Affect states are less labile, and mood swings decrease, a greater modulation of these states being evident. Greater

347

self-confidence and self-assurance are manifested. The capacity to be assertive without having to be hostile is also observable. Regressions are less frequent and less severe when they do occur. There is less need to experiment with fringe activities, such as substance abuse or delinquency, because of peer pressures. Fantasy appears more in the service of creativity or for trial action than for defensive purposes.

A number of factors appear to contribute to the processes underlying these changes. First, the past is reassessed through the eyes of the present. In some measure, past events are reinterpreted and reintegrated within a different set of meanings than previously existed. As a result, the adolescent views his childhood in a different light and, depending on his or her introspective capacities, places a distance between those events and the present that results in a new perspective. Second, the increased capacity for selfobject experiences at a symbolic rather than a concrete level leads to a shift in the meanings that others have, or have had, for the adolescent. The adolescent begins to look beyond the narrow circle of family and peers for selfobject experiences. While seeking avenues for self-actualization, the adolescent searches for values and ideals that are consonant with the rest of his or her experiences, focusing less on the person as the embodiment of the function and more on the content associated with the function.

Third, the integration of gender role and sexuality into the rest of self-experience acquires an urgency that was not present before. The meanings of femaleness or of maleness, of sexual expression or of its inhibition, become a focal preoccupation. Fourth, the advent of formal operational thought at the onset of adolescence plays an important role in the transformation in the adolescent's meaning system. Kohlberg and Gilligan (1972) describe the cognitive stages that occur at that time as follows: "Inferences through local operations upon propositions or 'operations upon operations.' Reasoning about reasoning. Construction of systems of all possible relations or implications. Hypothetico-deductive isolation of variables and testing of hypotheses" (p. 34).

The capacity for formal operational thought cannot be considered a necessary condition for the development of a nuclear self. It is a competence that an adolescent may use in the struggles with the revaluations of the meanings of past attitudes and experiences.

As a result of these processes, the adolescent will begin to construct a coherent narrative that attempts to encompass the totality of self-experiences. If the attempt is successful, a unification and consolidation in the sense of coherence will emerge that may be described as a different configuration of the self than previously existed. This new configuration may be described as the emergence of a nuclear self. The adolescent is then able to select an avenue through which to express the acquired values, ambitions, and ideals. The adolescent's inner resources may be mobilized to move forward in the direction of the attainment of a life goal (Kohut 1972). For the adolescent who successfully completes this phase, a new narrative emerges. It is at this point that it may make sense to speak of an inner program that the person is propelled to actualize. While this process may be thought to be akin to Erikson's (1959) notion of the consolidation of identity, it is different because of the perspective from which adolescent processes are being viewed. The nuclear self is not formed in response to the need for adaptation; rather, it occurs irrespective of the adaptive consequences of the adolescent's behavior. Thus, the "unrealistic" attitudes of some youths, which to some adults appear foolish and impractical and represent perennial generational struggles, result from the tension between the older generations' exhortations to adolescents to adapt and the adolescents' rebelliousness, which insists on the modification of reality to suit their internal needs—needs that are defined by the nuclear self.

The attainment of a nuclear self does not foreclose the possibility of continual growth in the course of the life cycle. Neither does it guarantee that destabilizations will not occur. Significant life events may lead to the amendment, or the revision, of a person's guiding narrative. The achievement of the consolidation of the nuclear self may also be culture bound. In cultures in which the opportunities for the exercise of formal operational thought is either not valued or not made possible, a nuclear self may still evolve, although the timing of its emergence and the form it would take may be quite different from that of the middle-class Western culture.

It is interesting to note that, in summarizing the psychoanalytic perspective on late adolescence, Kaplan (1980) states, "In the final stages of adolescence, Jacobson finds a hierarchical reorganization and final integration of value concepts, arising from both ego and superego into a new coherent structure and functional unit, the ego ideal. Ritvo states that the ego ideal as a structuralized institution of the mind is a development of adolescence. Blos holds that the structuralization of the ego ideal renders it qualitatively different from antecedent developmental stages and determines the end phase of the adolescent process" (p. 391). The authors cited attribute to the ego ideal the consolidation that is reflected in the observed changes that adolescents manifest. The perspective presented here argues that the reorganization of the cohesive self results in a structural change that might best be described as the consolidation of a nuclear self.

Selfobject Functions and the Formation of the Nuclear Self in Late Adolescence

Among the functions of the self, which are organized through the available selfobject experiences, are the functions of the grandiose self, the idealized parental imago, and the alterego. While there is a consensus that these functions constitute a subset of a larger, but undefined, set of functions and that they characterize culturally determined experiences, the value of these concepts in organizing clinical data and in hypothesizing the presence of parallel developmental issues has been amply demonstrated in work with adults and, to a much lesser extent, in clinical work with children and adolescents. Direct observations of a population of normal children and adolescents will still be required to complement clinical inferences.

Only the specific experiences associated with three sets of selfobjects functions will be discussed here, and their bearing on the development of the nuclear self will be focused on. These functions are as follows: (1) for the idealizing functions, the experience of attributing power and the capacity for protectiveness as represented by the feelings of safety and trust in a relationship, the experience of being capable of modulating and regulating intense affects that permits their integration into self experience, and the sense of conviction that results from the adherence to a set of values and ideals; (2) for the mirroring functions; the experiences of firmness, harmony, and vitality of the sense of self as well as the feeling of worthiness; and (3) for the alterego functions; the experience of a common bond to others as human beings and the feelings of being like others in the possession of competencies and capacities for effectiveness.

The relation between selfobject functions and the emergent nuclear self requires clarification. Kohut assumed that selfobject experiences follow a developmental path from less mature to more mature forms of selfobject experiences. He also posited the concept of "transmuting internalization" to explain this process. However, it has been pointed out (Goldberg 1984b) that there are difficulties with this spatial metaphor (Palombo 1987a). It is possible to substitute the explanatory metaphor of maturation through a progression from the more concrete, global expression of the need for the experience to the more symbolic, abstract expression of the need without introducing any other major theoretical changes (cf. Werner and Kaplan 1963). If this substitution is accepted, then it is possible to specify a developmental phase when a transition occurs to the expression of selfobject experiences, which are enacted symbolically rather than concretely. I suggest that such a process begins to occur in the course of adolescence and may, in fact, extend to the rest of the life cycle.

At some point toward the conclusion of adolescence, the clinical data indicate, not only are most selfobject experiences integrated into the sense of self at a symbolic level, but the interrelations among the various selfobject experiences are also appraised. This process is undertaken mostly unconsciously; it is, however, at times a conscious one that has as its goal the unification of self-experiences into a coherent whole, which constitutes the nuclear self.

The Idealizing Functions and the Nuclear Self

Preadolescents enter the phase of the idealizing functions and the nuclear self experiencing their parents as globally embodying the functions of protectors, modulators of intense affects, and standard-bearers of all values. In the child's mind, the person of the adult is not distinguished from the function itself; for example, omnipotence may be concretistically attributed to the parents. With the onset of the capacity for formal operational thought and the increased capacity to process the meanings of these experiences, a reevaluation of the parents' capacities and functions occurs. The functions may become disassociated from the person performing them.

Some adolescents, for example, experience their parents' efforts at protection as intrusive and infantalizing. These experiences are often based on the adolescent's inability to integrate his own infantile desires into the rest of his self-experience. The result is that the parents' interventions are interpreted as negating their more mature strivings. This may result in the denigration and deidealization of the parents,

351

who are now perceived very differently. If a massive disillusionment ensues, the adolescent may become depressed and enraged. The injury to the self leads to a conviction that the parents intentionally misled or deceived the adolescent.

The parents' actual response will in part determine the developmental outcome. Parents whose own needs for their child's admiration and adulation are great become incapable of tolerating these assaults. They will compound the problems by their inability to respond to the experience the adolescent desires. Their angry or defensive responses are experienced as further confirmation of the adolescent's perception. If, on the other hand, parents can good-naturedly accept the reassessment and shift to a more symbolic expression of the function sought by the adolescent, a different outcome becomes possible. The adolescent can retain a selfobject tie at the level of admiration and respect for the adult while at the same time gaining a measure of pride and self-respect. It is the integration of the latter experiences, which are more abstract and symbolic, that contributes to the consolidation of the nuclear self.

The second set of idealizing functions relates to the modulation of affective intensities and to self-regulation. The reliance of preadolescents on parental selfobjects for these functions has been ongoing up to this point. During latency, children acquire a modicum of self-control and self-discipline, although these require the reinforcing presence of adults, whose interventions are necessary to provide stable utilization of the functions. The pubertal changes bring shifts in mood states and fluctuations in affect, which result in a destabilization of the self. Since the parents are often seen as unreliable in providing modulating influences, or since, at times, adolescents reject those functions when they are offered, adolescents feel that they are left to their own devices. What emerges are wide fluctuations in both mood and behavior. Disorganization appears to be the order of the day. The indulgence in excesses seems to alternate with periods of quiescence.

Parents are presented with a dilemma that is not easily resolved. If their efforts at regulating their child's distress are ill timed or off the mark, the adolescent feels either infantilized or free to defy rational limits. If the parents themselves are vulnerable in these areas and are unable to regulate themselves or unable to modulate their own intense feelings, then their responses will be perceived as unempathic, ineffectual, or arbitrary. The injured adolescent will then respond with rageful defiance, passive compliance, or withdrawal.

In late adolescence, some of these issues become ritualized. The ritualization is achieved through the available social channels that sanction "parties" at which it is permissible to get drunk, to shoplift, to trash the house or yard of a member of the out group, or to engage in the initiation rites of a fraternity or sorority. By the time the late adolescent is a freshman in college, these rituals alternate with periods of intense study (e.g., for exams) or concentration on a physical activity that requires hours of practice for mastery. What permits this transformation to take place is the beginning integration by the adolescent of the meaning of self-control and self-regulation. These qualities are no longer experienced as emanating from outside sources; rather, they become an integral part of the adolescent.

The last set of idealizing functions is the acquisition of a value system. In latency and early adolescence, the parents have been the providers of a set of moral, social, and cultural values that the child has accepted unquestioningly. Obedience out of a desire to please or fear of disapproval or punishment linked the acceptance of those values with compliance and conformity. In peer relations, the acceptance of group norms is motivated more out of considerations of fairness than out of a sense of justice. The reassessment of the values is driven at first by the desire to challenge parental authority rather than by disbelief in the values themselves. The selfobject functions associated with authority figures who require conformity are rejected. Paralleling the reevaluation of parental authority is a reevaluation of the content of that authority, that is, the precepts and teachings.

The void creates a challenge that may lead either to a reconcretization of more archaic values, that is, to the fuller acceptance of the "traditional" values, or to turning to a new set of values. The phenomenon of adolescents embracing either religious or social beliefs that represent even greater conformity than their parents had demanded reflects the former outcome. Adolescents who turn to peer groups as substitute idealized selfobjects (i.e., gangs, cults, or fraternities, who come to represent alternatives to parental values) are examples of the latter phenomenon. For the adolescents, the motive for joining a counterculture group is not always the desire to rebel against parental values; it may also be that they are attempting to find an ideology that is concordant with a life-style that they are developing and that particular group is the vehicle through which they can attain that goal. In either case, the selfobject functions have undergone a

353

transformation that leaves a permanent mark on the lives of adolescents.

The extent to which values carried over from latency will be rejected, retained, or revised and integrated within a broader set of values to be included within a nuclear self is determined by a number of factors. Among these are the nature of the selfobject experiences to which the adolescent is exposed, the stability and coherence of the latency value system, the effect of the shifts in attachment from parents to others who are idealized, the blossoming of a particular talent that expands in importance in the adolescent's world, or some accidental factors such as the death of a close friend, the influence of a boyfriend or girlfriend, or an encounter with a charismatic teacher.

The Mirroring Functions and the Nuclear Self

Two sets of selfobject functions are associated with mirroring: the wish to be affirmed and the wish to be valued and esteemed. The egocentrism that is typical of the early adolescent combines with exhibitionistic longings to make the yearnings for mirroring exceed any possibility of satisfaction. These feelings are compounded by the physical changes brought on by puberty, the considerable self-consciousness, and the awareness of the body self in the adolescent. The preoccupation with appearances, whether it be in the direction of obsessive slovenliness or of studied casual "preppiness," is not only dictated by group norms but also driven by the desires to be distinguishable from others and, hence, to be recognized. To be perceived is to have one's existence acknowledged. Not to have one's existence acknowledged is equivalent to having one's sense of self negated. The latter can lead to feelings of dissolution or fragmentation. The adolescent feels caught between the embarrassment of openly desiring direct praise and the fear of being flooded by those longings.

For most adolescents, parental responses appear to be of relatively little importance in this regard. What is of greater importance is the peer group's responses. Within the group, praise can take the form of teasing or ridicule, both of which bring satisfaction of the longings while avoiding embarrassment. At one time, the desire to be valued might have been satisfied through the parents' expression of pride and joy in their child's achievements. In adolescence, however, such expressions would bring forth unbearable embarrassment. They would be seen as touching only on appearances rather than on substance, the desire for experiences that penetrate to the core of their being and truly permit them to feel worthwhile.

The Alterego Functions and the Nuclear Self

This set of functions relates to the desire for experiences of kinship to others as human beings. The wish to belong to a group of like-minded others, the desire to minimize differences in appearances and ways of thinking from those of others, the easy contagion that permits becoming engulfed in mass activities, the exquisite sensitivity to the suffering of those who belong to the group concomitant with harsh cruelty to others who do not belong—all these experiences provide the rich fabric of a subculture to which adolescents feel bound.

Opposite feelings are directed at outsiders who are considered to be "nerds," "geeks," "spooks," "greasers," and so on, all being beyond the pale and considered as utterly inhuman. The bigotry, the fanaticism, the elitism, that characterizes some adolescent groups may have its roots in the desire to strengthen a vulnerable sense of self. Since difference is often equated with deficiency, the very presence of others who are different becomes a reminder of inner experiences of being deficient.

This set of functions is also greatly affected by experiences of physical or psychological intactness. If an adolescent suffers from a physical handicap, the sense of difference and of alienation from others may be felt acutely regardless of how much mirroring the adolescent may receive. If, as in the case of learning-disabled adolescents, the handicap is not "visible," the experience of the sense of difference leads to the conviction of being defective or repulsive.

Ultimately, the feelings of true kinship with others, the comfortable acceptance of differences from others, and the respect of the values and ideals of others are based on the integration into the adolescent's meaning system of a view of human beings within a social, cultural, and political context that is in harmony with his or her own sense of history and the narrative that has been constructed to bring a sense of coherence. The achievement of self-confidence, self-assurance, and self-respect comes as a result of the consolidation of the nuclear self in the context of the attainment of achievements that are the fulfillment of the destiny that the adolescent has chosen for himself or herself.

Conclusions

The sense of self-cohesion has been defined as the experience that results in the establishment of a coherent personal or shared set of meanings. It is constituted of the totality of the person's experiences, both conscious and unconscious. It is enduring in its stability. It is reflected by the sense of firmness, intactness, wholeness, and vitality. The cohesive self is the structure that is constituted from the set of meanings that have arisen in the course of development. It is the product of one's endowment in tandem with the selfobject's experiences that facilitates the integration of affective experience and leads to the structuralization of meaning. It is the center of a person's organization. Among the functions of the self and organized around a set of meanings are the grandiose self, the idealized parent imago, and the alterego. These functions result from the integration of experiences and affect states as facilitated by self objects.

The late adolescent recursively reworks old experiences leading to the formation of the nuclear self. The nuclear sense of self is the set of meanings that have accrued to the person, through which life goals are defined, through which the means for their attainment are examined, and through which the plans for their pursuit are established. This consolidation is the culmination of the increased symbolization of specific selfobject functions. The integration of the cognitive strides with affective experiences takes place within the context of the self/selfobject milieu. The selfobject functions provided by the caregiver represent the context and the means through which cohesion is maintained and the nuclear self is stabilized.

REFERENCES

Basch, M. F. 1980. *Doing Psychotherapy.* New York: Basic.
Burch, C. 1985. Identity foreclosure in early adolescence: a problem of narcissistic equilibrium. *Adolescent Psychiatry* 12:145–161.
Buffington, J. 1984. Emerging values in a university community. In D. Brochman, ed. *Late Adolescence: Psychoanalytic Studies.* New York: International Universities Press.
Buffington, J. 1985. A reconsideration of the therapeutic process in short term therapy from the vantage point of the self psychologist.

Paper presented at the Western Regional Adolescent Psychiatry Conference, Phoenix, Arizona.

Demos, E. V. 1988. Affect and the development of the self: a new frontier. In A. Goldberg, ed. *Frontiers in Self Psychology,* vol 3. Hillsdale, N.J.: Analytic.

Elson, M., ed. 1987. *The Kohut Seminars on Self Psychology and Psychotherapy with Adolescents and Young Adults.* New York: Norton.

Erikson, E. H. 1959. Identity and the life cycle. In *Psychological Issues,* vol. 1. New York: International Universities Press.

Goldberg, A. 1978. A shift in emphasis: adolescent psychotherapy and the psychology of the self. *Journal of Youth and Adolescence* 7(2): 119–132.

Goldberg, A. 1984a. Depression and the unstimulated self. In D. Brochman, ed. *Late Adolescence: Psychoanalytic Studies.* New York: International Universities Press.

Goldberg, A. 1984b. One theory or more. *Emotions and Behavior Monograph* 1(2): 626–638.

Kaplan, E. H. 1980. Adolescents, age fifteen to eighteen: a psychoanalytic developmental view. In S. I. Greenspan and G. H. Pollack, eds. *The Course of Life.* Vol. 2, *Latency, Adolescence and Youth.* Washington, D.C.: U.S. Department of Health and Human Services, U.S. Government Printing Office.

Kohlberg, L., and Gilligan, C. 1972. The adolescent as a philosopher. In J. Kagan and R. Coles, eds. *Twelve to Sixteen: Early Adolescence.* New York: Norton.

Kohut, H. 1971. *The Analysis of the Self.* New York: International Universities Press.

Kohut, H. 1972. Discussion of "On the adolescent process as a transformation of the self" by Ernest S. Wolf, John E. Gedo, and David Terman. In P. H. Ornstein, ed. *The Search for the Self: Selected Writings of Heinz Kohut, 1950–78.* New York: International Universities Press.

Kohut, H. 1977. *The Restoration of the Self.* New York: International Universities Press.

Kohut, H. 1978. Remarks about the formation of the self—letter to a student regarding some principles of psychoanalytic research. In P. H. Ornstein, ed. *The Search for the Self: Selected Writings of Heinz Kohut, 1950–78.* New York: International Universities Press.

Kohut, H. 1984. *How Does Analysis Cure?* Edited by A. Goldberg. Chicago: University of Chicago Press.

Kohut, H. 1985a. On courage (early 1970s). In *Self Psychology and the Humanities: Reflections on a New Psychoanalytic Approach.* New York: Norton.

Kohut, H. 1985b. On leadership (1969–70). In *Self Psychology and the Humanities: Reflections on a New Psychoanalytic Approach.* New York: Norton.

Kohut, H., and Wolf, E. S. 1978. The disorders of the self and their treatment: an outline. *International Journal of Psycho-Analysis* 59:413–425.

Lichtenberg, J. D. 1983. *Psychoanalysis and Infant Research.* Hillsdale, N.J.: Analytic.

Marohn, R. C. 1977. The juvenile imposter: some thoughts on narcissism and the delinquent. *Adolescent Psychiatry* 5:162–212.

Marohn, R. C. 1980. Adolescent rebellion and the task of separation. *Adolescent Psychiatry* 8:173–183.

Marohn, R. C. 1981. The negative transference in the treatment of juvenile delinquents. *Annual of Psychoanalysis* 9:21–42.

Marohn, R. C. 1982. Juvenile delinquents and violent death. *Adolescent Psychiatry* 10:186–212.

Marohn, R. C. 1984. Disappointing and deviant youth and the rage of the elders. *Children and Youth Review* 6:367–373.

Ornstein, P. H., ed. 1978. *The Search for the Self: Selected Writings of Heinz Kohut, 1950–78.* New York: International Universities Press.

Palombo, J. 1979. Perceptual deficits and self-esteem in adolescence. *Clinical Social Work* 7(1): 34–61.

Palombo, J. 1983. Borderline conditions: a perspective from self psychology. *Clinical Social Work* 11(4): 323–338.

Palombo, J. 1985. The treatment of borderline neurocognitively impaired children: a perspective from self psychology. *Clinical Social Work* 13(2): 117–128.

Palombo, J. 1987a. Critique of Schamess' concept of boundaries. *Clinical Social Work* 17(3): 184–293.

Palombo, J. 1987b. Selfobject transferences in the treatment of borderline neurocognitively impaired children. In J. S. Grotstein, M. F. Solomon, and J. A. Lang, eds. *The Borderline Patient.* Hillsdale, N.J.: Analytic.

Palombo, J., and Feigon, J. 1984. Borderline personality in childhood and its relationship to neurocognitive deficits. *Child and Adolescent Social Work Journal* 1(1): 18–33.

Saari, C. 1986a. *Clinical Social Work Treatment: How Does It Work?* New York: Gardner.

Saari, C. 1986b. The use of metaphor in therapeutic communication with young adolescents. *Child and Adolescent Social Work Journal* 3(1): 15–25.

Stern, D. N. 1985. *The Interpersonal World of the Infant.* New York: Basic.

Stolorow, R. D.; Brandchaft, B.; and Atwood, G. 1987. *Psychoanalytic Treatment: An Intersubjective Approach.* Hillsdale, N.J.: Analytic.

Werner, H., and Kaplan, B. 1963. *Symbol Formation: An Organismic-Developmental Approach to Language and the Expression of Thought.* New York: Wiley.

Wolf, E. S. 1982. Adolescence: psychology of the self and selfobjects. *Adolescent Psychiatry* 10:171–181.

Wolf, E. S. 1984. Freud's adolescent creativity in the light of the psychology of the self. In D. Brockman, ed. *Late Adolescence: Psychoanalytic Studies.* New York: International Universities Press.

Wolf, E. S.; Gedo, J. E.; and Terman, D. M. 1972. On the adolescent process as a transformation of the self. *Journal of Youth and Adolescence* 1:257–272.

20 OBJECT RELATIONS IN BORDERLINE ADOLESCENTS AND ADULTS: DEVELOPMENTAL DIFFERENCES

DREW WESTEN, PAMELA LUDOLPH, KENNETH SILK, ALFRED KELLAM, LAURA GOLD, AND NAOMI LOHR

Theories of borderline psychopathology, and particularly borderline object relations, have typically stressed the continuity of adolescent and adult borderline phenomena and have argued for similar etiologies in both age groups. Kernberg (1978) suggests that, although the diagnosis is much more difficult to make in adolescence, borderline pathology is essentially the same in adolescents as in adults. According to Kernberg (1975, 1978), the roots of borderline object relations in both adolescence and adulthood lie in a developmental failure in the preoedipal years to integrate positive and negative representations of the self and of others. The consequent failure to achieve libidinal object constancy, that is, the ability to love someone even when he or she is not currently gratifying, leads to many of the manifest interpersonal difficulties of the borderline patient.

Like Kernberg, Masterson (1972, 1976, 1980) views adolescent and adult borderline psychopathology as fundamentally the same (Masterson 1978). Masterson locates the origins of borderline disorders in a developmental arrest at Mahler's (Mahler, Pine, and Bergman 1975) rapprochement stage of separation-individuation. In this stage, the toddler has come to recognize the separateness of self and other and is tremendously conflicted between desires for autonomy and the continued need for security and dependence. According to Masterson, borderline psychopathology typically arises because the mother has so much difficulty with separation-individuation herself that she uses her child as an extension of self or as an object for self-soothing; consequently, she cannot allow the child to individuate. The result is that the child splits off two object-relational part units. The first is a withdrawing object-relational unit (WORU), which includes a representation of a malevolent mother abandoning the child for attempts at individuation and an affective component of abandonment depression and rage. The second is a rewarding object-relational unit (RORU), which includes a representation of a gratifying mother and a dependent, compliant self who must sacrifice autonomy to maintain maternal supplies. For both Kernberg and Masterson, who locate the origins of borderline pathology at the same developmental juncture, adolescence becomes a likely period for the emergence of borderline disorders. In part, this is because of the consolidation of personality structure that should occur during that time. Adolescence is also a key period because of the salience of concerns about identity and the resurgence of conflicts around separation-individuation.

The aim of the present study is to examine empirically the ways in which the object relations of borderline adolescents resemble, as well as differ from, the object relations of borderline adults. Although the theoretical accounts of Kernberg, Masterson, and other object-relations theorists have been crucial to the evolving understanding of these patients, three aspects of these theories, which bear on the relation between adult and adolescent borderline psychopathology, require reconsideration (see Westen 1989). First, object-relations theories imply that "object relations" refers to a unitary phenomenon and, thus, that a patient's object relations can be diagnosed as fixated as a whole at a particular level. While in the broadest sense this hypothesis is clinically useful because it allows one to distinguish patients at different levels of character organization (Kernberg 1975, 1984), the assumption of the unity of object relations as a construct may now limit our understanding as much as enhance it. The term "object relations" refers less to a single property than to a set of interdependent cognitive and affective structures and processes. These include representations of self and others organized in various ways along networks of association; representations of social interaction and relationships; ways of understanding or attributing the causes of people's thoughts, feelings, and actions; capacity to take the perspective of others; moral development; empathy; interpersonal wishes,

361

affects, and conflicts; and extent to which relationships are expected to be relatively hostile or enriching. These represent interdependent but distinct phenomena and developmental lines, and they differ in their maturity and quality across individuals as well as within a single individual at any given time (Westen, in press). For example, many mildly mentally retarded individuals have object representations that are cognitively "primitive" but an object world that is affectively benign.

Because of the assumption in psychoanalytic theory that a continuum of pathology is identical with a continuum of development (see Peterfreund 1978), theorists of borderline disorders tend to view all aspects of these patients' pathology as representing a preoedipal arrest at a normal stage of development. If "object relations" is a unitary construct, then all aspects of object relations must be fixated at the same point. For Kernberg, the critical indicator of the point of fixation is whether the patient relies on splitting or on repression; for Masterson, the critical indicator is whether the patient is dominated by separation fears and abandonment depression. An alternative hypothesis is that some elements of borderline pathology may, indeed, reflect fixations or regressions to preoedipal levels of functioning whereas others may reflect developmental arrests in the latency or adolescent years. Still others may reflect deviant development off the beaten track of normal development. The chronic expectations of malevolence in the object world of the borderline may reflect less a fixation at a paranoid or schizoid position, hypothesized to be normative in infancy (Klein 1948), than an unfortunate object-relational and attributional bias produced through an interaction of constitutional aggressivity (Kernberg 1975), difficulty self-soothing or regulating affects, and pathogenic child-caregiver interaction. Further, probably no living human being could think, feel, and behave like a borderline all the time. Borderline patients have a tendency to regress to primitive forms of thinking and to activate malevolent representations under certain conditions, but at other times they are clearly able to produce representations that may have considerable subtlety and complexity and can in no way be considered preoedipal.

A second problematic aspect of these theories is the implicit suggestion that fixation or developmental disturbance in the preoedipal years prevents continued object-relational development after age three. A corollary of this is the assumption that the development of object relations is essentially completed with the attainment of "whole objects" during or directly preceding the oedipal period and that, once one has passed through the critical period of object-relations development in the first three to four years, one may safely move on to psychosexual tasks (e.g., Balint 1968; Kohut 1971). The problem with this position is that considerable evidence from developmental psychology suggests that many of the capacities and processes that are critical to the development of object relations develop considerably throughout the adolescent years and probably beyond. These include the increasing complexity of representations of self and others, the developing capacity to take others' perspectives, the growth of self-reflection, the movement from need-gratifying to more mature patterns of emotional investment in relationships and values, and the developing capacity to understand why people act, think, and feel as they do (see Selman 1980; Shantz 1983; Westen 1989). One must, therefore, address the ways in which early disturbances could affect these developmental lines and consider the possibility that aspects of object relations may continue to develop both in neurotics and in borderlines throughout adolescence and beyond. If development proceeds beyond the preoedipal years, this should lead to discernible differences between the object relations of borderline adolescents and those of adults.

A third issue for reconsideration is the predominant assumption that the effect of pathogenic environmental influences lies strictly or largely in the rapprochement period, or, more generally, in the preoedipal years. From an empirical point of view, it is difficult to know precisely when a disorder was set in motion by pathological parenting or parent-child interactions when the same child and the same parents may interact for the entirety of the patient's childhood and beyond. Current theories lead us to focus on a particular developmental period for the etiology of borderline disorders, largely because these disorders are seen as more severe than neuroses and less severe than psychoses. In psychoanalytic theory, psychoses have been linked to infantile disturbance, whereas neuroses have been linked to oedipal disturbance, leaving borderline disorders by default to the preoedipal years. Even setting aside the question of whether infantile experience is really a useful model for psychosis (and vice versa), it is unclear to what extent an incipient borderline disorder could be headed off by a mother learning to control her dependency needs and her tendency to treat her child as a self-object as the child enters adolescence, even in the face of a structural defect established during the child's preoedipal years.

Observations of the families of borderline disorders (Berkowitz 1981; Berkowitz, Shapiro, Zinner, and Shapiro 1974; Shapiro 1978) suggest that these families tend to split the object world and project univalent properties onto specific family members as well as hindering the developing individuation of the adolescent. If this were avoided, would a borderline disorder be avoided in the adolescent? Mahler and Kaplan (1977) have, in fact, suggested that the identification of a specific developmental period, namely, rapprochement, may be inaccurate in etiological theories of borderline disorders, as has Gunderson (1984). Shay (1987) has examined the way in which clinicians and theoreticians stretch the time frames of their theory to fit the specifics of a particular case while refusing to abandon the theory that the developmental disturbance must occur at a particular point. "It is not 'cricket,'" he asserts, "to argue that the borderline is born in the heart of Boston and then to call a suburb the heart when you realize you were wrong" (p. 713).

The present study compares the object relations of a sample of borderline adolescents with a similar sample of borderline adults. It was hypothesized that, if one separates specific dimensions of object relations, one will find areas of developmental difference as well as dimensions in which the two groups appear the same. Quality of object relations was coded from responses to the Thematic Apperception Test (TAT), a projective test in which subjects make up stories about cards depicting ambiguous social scenes. The TAT responses of reliably diagnosed borderline adolescent and adult inpatients were compared on the following four dimensions: complexity of representations of people (the extent to which the subject attributes complex dispositions to characters whose perspectives are clearly differentiated); affect tone of relationship paradigms (the affective quality of the object world, from malevolent to benevolent); capacity for emotional investment in relationships and moral standards (the extent to which the person transcends a need-gratifying interpersonal orientation); and understanding of social causality (the extent to which attributions of causality in the social realm are accurate, complex, and psychologically minded).

Recently completed research with a normal adolescent sample (Westin, Klepser, Silverman, Ruffins, Boekamp, and Lifton 1989), using both the TAT measure (Westen, Silk, Lohr, and Kerber 1985) and an analogous interview measure (Westen, Barends, Leigh, Mendel, and Silbert 1988) for object relations, found, as predicted, that three of these dimensions develop throughout adolescence whereas one, affect tone of relationship paradigms, does not. This latter dimension was hypothesized to be a nondevelopmental, stylistic difference in object relations that probably is relatively stable from early childhood. Consequently, we hypothesized that, on the three developmental dimensions of object relations, borderline adults would show significantly higher levels of object relations than borderline adolescents whereas the two groups would be indistinguishable in the degree of malevolence of their object world, a dimension that has been shown to distinguish borderline patients (Lerner and St. Peter 1984; Spear and Sugarman 1984; Stuart, Westen, Lohr, Silk, and Benjamin, in press; Westen, Lohr, Silk, Gold, and Kerber 1988). Borderline adults have already been shown to have significantly lower scores on all four scales than major depressives and normals in recently completed research, and borderline adolescents were found to have lower scores than both psychiatric controls and normals on all scales except complexity of representations (Westen, Ludolph, Lerner, Ruffins, and Wiss, in press).

Methods

SUBJECTS

This study represents a liaison between two independent ongoing research projects, one studying borderline personality disorder (BPD) in adults and the other studying BPD in adolescents. The first author is an investigator in both projects, ensuring some comparability of methods. Potential subjects for the study were drawn from the inpatient adult unit and the inpatient adolescent unit at the University of Michigan Medical Center and the inpatient adolescent unit at Wyandotte General Hospital. Exclusion criteria for both adult and adolescent samples included chronic psychosis, clear evidence of neuropathology (such as documented epilepsy or severe head injury), IQ below seventy, or medical problems that would complicate diagnosis or psychological testing results.

365

Potential adult subjects (including adult psychiatric controls, who are not included in the present study) met at least two criteria for DSM-III BPD or schizotypal personality disorder or three criteria for DSM-III major depressive episode on admission. Ninety-one percent of eligible subjects consented. While consenting subjects were drug free, they were administered the Diagnostic Interview for Borderlines (DIB; Gunderson, Kolb, and Austin 1981), a well-validated instrument that has been shown to predict DSM-III diagnosis of BPD with sensitivity and specificity typically above .8. Interviewers achieved interrater reliability of .80 (kappa; see Cornell, Silk, Ludolph, and Lohr 1983), and reliability has been maintained through periodic retraining and assessment. Patients were defined as meeting criteria for BPD by obtaining a DIB score greater than or equal to 7.

Borderline adolescent subjects were also defined by a score of greater than or equal to 7 on the DIB and were obtained as follows. During 1983 and 1984, consecutive patients were administered the DIB by interviewers who had achieved interrater reliability (kappa = .80) on diagnosis. In order to fill the borderline cell and to obtain appropriate adolescent controls, from 1985 to 1987 potential subjects were targeted who met at least four DSM-III criteria for BPD, criteria for anorexia nervosa, or two criteria for major depressive disorder or dysthymic disorder on admission. Two of the DIB interviewers had established reliability with the adult project and trained the remaining interviewers, who achieved perfect agreement on DIB diagnosis on a sample of consecutive taped interviews and fell within one scaled point of criterion coder from the adult project on every section and final score. The DIB was modified slightly for use with adolescents (see Block, Westen, and Jackson 1988).

PROCEDURES

Adult subjects were administered a variety of biological and psychological tests and interviews as part of a larger project on the relation between BPD and affective disorder. Psychological tests included standardized administration of a battery of projective tests, the Wechsler Adult Intelligence Scale—Revised (WAIS-R), and a series of self-report measures of psychiatric symptoms, depression, and social adjustment. A series of cards from the TAT was administered in standard sequence with standardized administration, including order of presentation of cards.

Adolescent subjects were administered a variety of biological and psychological tests, including a battery of projectives and a series of self-report measures. During the first phase of data collection, before the present study was conceived, order of presentation of TAT cards was not standardized; during the second, order of cards was standardized. Adolescent and adult subjects were given similar instructions on the TAT to tell a story, including what was happening in the picture, what led up to it, the outcome, and what the characters were thinking and feeling. If a subject provided an incomplete response (omitting or minimally elaborating any of the elements of the story), testers inquired about missing elements. This inquiry was done both to minimize biases of verbal productivity or motivation and to elicit adequate material for scoring and for clinical use. The present study examined responses to six cards that were used in over 90 percent of all protocols and that were included in the standardized sequence for both adult and adolescent subjects: cards 1, 2, 3BM, 4, 13MF, and 15.

MEASURES

The six TAT cards were coded using a multidimensional measure of object relations for use with the TAT (Westen et al. 1985) that assesses four aspects of object relations: complexity and differentiation of representations of people, affect tone of relationship paradigms, capacity for emotional investment in relationships and morals, and understanding of social causality. Each scale has five levels, level 1 representing the lowest-level response and level 5 the highest. The TAT measures were derived from psychoanalytic clinical experience, object-relations theory and research (for reviews, see Blatt and Lerner 1983; Greenberg and Mitchell 1983; and Urist 1980), and research in developmental social cognition (Bogen 1982; Damon 1977; Selman 1980; Shantz 1983; Thompson 1981).

The TAT is an excellent source of data for assessing object relations because subjects are asked to draw on their internal object representations to construct characters and interactions in response to an ambiguous interpersonal situation depicted on the card. Recently completed research (see Westen et al., in press) has begun validating the measures with both normal and clinical populations, establishing

367

correlations with similar measures designed for use with interview data and early memories, and demonstrating their capacity to predict clinician ratings of interpersonal functioning, scores on measures of various related constructs, and self-reported social adjustment on Weissman and Bothwell's (1976) Social Adjustment Scale. The measures have also been able to discriminate in theoretically predicted ways among adolescent borderlines, psychiatric controls, and normals and among adult borderlines, major depressives, and normals. The four scales are described below. A brief description of the levels of each scale is provided in table 1.

COMPLEXITY OF REPRESENTATIONS OF PEOPLE

Although object-relations theorists vary widely in their particular models of the development of self- and object representations, they are largely in agreement about three developmental phenomena (see, e.g., Greenberg and Mitchell 1983; Jacobson 1964; and Kernberg 1976). First, development of representations is characterized by increasing differentiation, in which the subjective experience and points of view of self and others become more clearly distinguished. A second feature of the psychoanalytic account is that object representations gradually become more complex and integrated as children mature. Third, whereas young children tend to split their representations of people by affective valence, that is, have difficulty integrating representations of people that include both positive and negative attributes, both children and adults are able to integrate more complex, ambivalent representations.

While challenging some of the developmental timetables, research in developmental psychology has by and large documented these developmental processes (Harter 1986; Shantz 1983; Westen 1989, in press). The present measure assesses the extent to which the person processes information about people using complex, differentiated object representations. At the lowest level of the scale, subjects have difficulty differentiating their own perspective from the perspectives of others. At slightly higher levels, they provide simple, unidimensional portraits of people who are clearly differentiated from each other. At the highest levels, subjects manifest a complex understanding of the nature, expression, and context of personality and subjective experience.

AFFECT TONE OF RELATIONSHIP PARADIGMS

A critical dimension of the representations underlying interpersonal functioning is the affect tone of relationship paradigms or of the object world. The empirical study of this dimension has involved measurement of affective qualities of human figures on projective tests (Krohn and Mayman 1974; Mayman 1967, 1968; Urist 1977). Blatt, Brenneis, Schimek, and Glick (1976) have developed a system for coding the malevolence of representations from Rorschach human figures. As noted earlier, borderline subjects have been found to have significantly more malevolent responses on the Rorschach than various control groups. The measure of affect tone of relationship paradigms for use with the TAT was designed to assess the extent to which the person expects relationships to be destructive and threatening or safe and enriching. At the lowest level of the scale, subjects manifest an expectation of relationships as profoundly hostile or malevolent, whereas, at the higher end of the scale, subjects have a broad range of affective expectations but generally expect relationships to be benign and enriching.

CAPACITY FOR EMOTIONAL INVESTMENT IN RELATIONSHIPS AND MORALS

Although object-relations theorists diverge in their particular accounts of development, they all posit a developmental movement from a need-gratifying pattern of emotional investment in people toward mature object relations based on mutual love, respect, and concern for others, who are valued for their specific attributes (e.g., Fairbairn 1952). Research in developmental psychology on the development of children's conceptions of friendship, justice, convention, and authority tends to support this view. Once again, however, these bodies of literature document a much longer maturational process than suggested by psychoanalytic theory, which proposes that need-gratifying object relations are transcended by the end of the oedipal period (see Damon 1977; Selman 1980; Shantz 1983; Westen 1989, in press).

Research on moral development has also extensively documented the developmental shift away from need-gratifying object relations (see Kohlberg and Kramer 1969; Rest 1983). It posits a movement from preconventional moral reasoning in which the child views good and bad

TABLE 1
BRIEF SYNOPSIS OF MEASURES OF OBJECT RELATIONS

	Complexity of Representations of People	Affect Tone of Relationship Paradigms	Capacity for Emotional Investment	Understanding of Social Causality
Principle	Scale measures the extent to which the subject clearly differentiates the perspectives of self and others; sees the self and others as having stable, enduring, multidimensional dispositions; and sees the self and others as psychological beings with complex motives and subjective experience	Scale measures affective quality of representations of people and relationships. It attempts to assess the extent to which the person expects from the world, and particularly the world of people, profound malevolence or overwhelming pain or views social interaction as basically benign and enriching	Scale measures the extent to which others are treated as ends rather than means, events are regarded in terms other than need gratification, and moral standards are developed and considered	Scale measures the extent to which attributions about the causes of people's actions, thoughts, and feelings are logical, accurate, complex, and psychologically minded
Level 1	People are not clearly differentiated; confusion of points of view	Malevolent representations; gratuitous violence or gross negligence by significant others	Need-gratifying orientation; profound self-preoccupation	Noncausal or grossly illogical depictions of psychological and interpersonal events
Level 2	Simple, unidimensional representations; focus on actions; traits are global and univalent	Representation of relationships as hostile, empty, or capricious but not profoundly malevolent; profound loneliness or disappointment in relationships	Limited investment in people, relationships, and moral standards; conflicting interests recognized, but gratification remains primary aim; moral standards primitive and unintegrated or	Rudimentary understanding of social causality; minor logic errors or unexplained transitions; simple stimulus-response causality

Level 3	Minor elaboration of mental life or personality dispositions	Mixed representations with mildly negative tone	Conventional investment in people and moral standards; stereotypic compassion, mutuality, or helping orientation; guilt at moral transgressions	Complex, accurate situational causality and rudimentary understanding of the role of thoughts and feelings in mediating action
Level 4	Expanded appreciation of complexity of subjective experience and personality dispositions; absence of representations integrating life history, complex subjectivity, and personality processes	Mixed representations with neutral or balanced tone	Mature, committed investment in relationships and values; mutual empathy and concern; commitment to abstract values	Expanded appreciation of the role of mental processes in generating thoughts, feelings, behaviors, and interpersonal interactions
Level 5	Complex representations, indicating understanding of interaction of enduring and momentary psychological experience; understanding of personality as system of processes interacting with each other and the environment	Predominantly positive representations; benign and enriching interactions	Autonomous selfhood in the context of committed relationships; recognition of conventional nature of moral rules in the context of carefully considered standards or concern for concrete people or relationships	Complex appreciation of the role of mental processes in generating thoughts, feelings, behaviors, and interpersonal interactions; understand

in terms of the hedonistic implications of action (rewards or punishments) toward conventional moral reasoning in which the child seeks the approval of authorities and internalizes moral standards that are viewed as right and legitimate. A small percentage of adults progress to post conventional moral reasoning, in which the person considers moral questions in more abstract, less culture-bound terms by formulating and applying general principles rather than specific, learned rules. Gilligan (1982) has recently amended Kohlberg's theory, arguing that high-level moral development in women frequently takes the form of a greater concern for responsibility in relationships and for the needs and feelings of others in a more immediate way.

The TAT measure for assessing capacity for emotional investment used in this study reflects a three-stage developmental model aimed at integrating developmental research with object-relations theory and clinical observation (Westen 1985). In the first stage, to the extent that others are clearly differentiated from the self they are viewed primarily as instruments of gratification, security, and comfort. In the second stage, people, relationships, and ideals come to be valued as ends in themselves. Moral values at this stage reflect an emotional investment in the ideals, values, and prohibitions of idealized and respected authorities, as understood by the child. Failure to meet these standards leads to guilt, shame, and lowered self-esteem. In the third stage, the person is capable of forming deep, committed relationships in which the other is valued for his or her unique qualities. He or she attempts to achieve autonomous selfhood within the context of real involvement and investment in others and may reconsider conventional social rules that regulate relationships. The five-level TAT measure adds transitional levels between the three broad stages.

UNDERSTANDING OF SOCIAL CAUSALITY

Clinical experience with patients with BPD suggests that these patients tend to make highly idiosyncratic, illogical, and inaccurate attributions of people's intentions. Extensive research in the development of understanding of social causality in children (Chandler, Paget, and Koch 1978; Donaldson and Westerman 1986; Piaget 1926; Shantz 1983) suggests a number of developmental shifts in the way children infer causality in the social realm, including increased complexity, abstractness, accuracy, internality (i.e., focus on internal psychological processes rather than surface-level, observable behavioral causes), and understanding of unconscious processes. The measure of understanding of social causality for use with TAT responses was designed to assess the logic, complexity, and accuracy of social causality as manifest in subjects' descriptions of interpersonal events. At the lowest levels, causality is illogical or alogical, with confused, inappropriate, highly unlikely, or absent attributions of interpersonal phenomena. At the middle levels, subjects make accurate attributions that are relatively simple. At the highest levels, subjects manifest an understanding of the way complex psychological processes are involved in the generation of thoughts, feelings, and actions.

CODING AND INTERRATER RELIABILITY

The TAT responses were coded by two advanced graduate students in clinical psychology and three B.A. research assistants. All cards were double-coded independently by two raters. Each story was provided to coders on a separate page presented in random order so that rating of multiple stories in the same protocol would be entirely independent. Reliability was computed using Pearson's R, with Spearman-Brown correction for double-coding. Uncorrected pairwise reliabilities ranged from .83 to .95 for affect tone, from .79 to .92 for complexity of representations, from .73 to .89 for capacity for emotional investment, and from .90 to .92 for social causality. Corrected reliability coefficients for each scale were as follows: affect tone, .93; complexity of representations, .91; capacity for emotional investment, .87; and social causality, .95. Coders met at regular intervals to discuss independently scored responses in order to prevent coder drift and to reach consensus scores.

Data were analyzed by repeated-measures analysis of variance and by one-tailed t-tests in which directional hypotheses were tested on mean data. A discriminant-function analysis was performed to determine whether pattern of object-relations scores could discriminate the adult from the adolescent borderlines.

Results

Subject characteristics are reported in table 2. As can be seen from the table, both samples were primarily female, reflecting the sex ratio of the disorder. The IQ of the adult borderlines was less than one standard deviation higher, with the difference accounted for by significantly higher verbal intelligence.

Table 3 reports object-relations scores for the adolescent and adult borderlines. The table shows mean scores for the adolescent and adult samples as well as *F*-statistics and significance values for repeated-measures analysis of variance. As can be seen from the table, all four main hypotheses were supported: the one dimension of object relations that was hypothesized not to be developmental, and hence was not expected to yield any developmental differences, showed no differences between the adults and the adolescents (affect tone of relationship paradigms). The other three scales (complexity of representations of people, capacity for emotional investment, and understanding of social causality) all showed developmental differences between the adolescents and the adults, with complexity and emotional investment both highly significant and social causality approaching significance at $p = .06$.

In further analyses, we attempted to determine precisely where developmental differences between the two groups emerged. The first analysis separated the TAT cards by their affective quality. A team of

TABLE 2
SUBJECT CHARACTERISTICS

	N	Sex (% Females)	Age	IQ	Verbal IQ	Performance IQ
Adolescents	36	86.0	15.6	100.8	96.0	104.1
Adults	37	73.7	27.0*	107.0*	107.9*	104.9

* Significantly greater at $p < .05$.

TABLE 3
MEAN OBJECT-RELATIONS SCORES FOR ADOLESCENT
AND ADULT BORDERLINES

	Adolescents	Adults	*F*-Statistic	Significance
Affect tone	2.42	2.58	1.75	N.S.
Complexity	2.54	2.83	8.74	.004
Emotional investment	1.98	2.21	4.62	.035
Social causality	2.18	2.53	3.66	.06

NOTE.—Data analyzed by repeated-measures analysis of variance, $df = 1,71$.

clinicians familiar with the TAT independently rated each of the six cards used in the study as "relatively neutral" or "relatively evocative of negative affect." All seven raters placed three of the cards (cards 1, 2, and 4) in the neutral category and the other three (cards 3BM, 13MF, and 15) in the negative category. Table 4 reveals the analysis of object relations scores for the two samples divided by affective quality of the card. Affect tone, as in the previous analysis, showed no developmental differences on either neutral or negative cards. The patterns for the remaining three scales, however, are of note. On complexity of representations, developmental differences emerged on both neutral and negative cards, although the differences were much more significant on the neutral cards. On capacity for emotional investment, only the neutral cards distinguished the two groups. On the negative cards, both groups tended to have low scores (relative to controls described in other studies). On social causality, in contrast, the neutral cards showed no differences between the groups, but, on the negative cards, the adults had significantly higher scores than the adolescents ($p < .0001$).

Previous studies with both adult and adolescent borderlines (Westen et al. 1988; Westen et al., in press), in comparison with controls, found that the percentage of pure pathological responses, scored as level 1 on each scale, distinguishes borderlines from other psychiatric patients and from normals. Thus, we compared the percentage of pathological scores on each scale in the two groups. In general, we expected to find a greater percentage of pathological scores in the adolescents because lower scores are normative in adolescents in general on these measures, except on complexity of representations, on which a level 1 (poor self-other differentiation or profound egocentrism) score is reflective of a level of functioning not typically found in normal adolescents or adults. The data were analyzed by paired t-tests with arc-sine transformation to equalize variance.

As can be seen from table 5, significant differences emerged on affect tone of relationship paradigms and capacity for emotional investment. Table 6 reports percentage of high-level scores (scored level 4 or 5) in the two groups. We did not expect to find any developmental changes in affect tone of relationship paradigms, which is not viewed as a developmental dimension. We did, however, expect to find developmental differences in complexity of representations, emotional investment, and social causality, a pattern that did in fact emerge in the data, as can be seen from the table.

375

TABLE 4
MEAN OBJECT-RELATIONS SCORES BY AFFECTIVE QUALITY OF STIMULUS
(Card × Group Effect)

	Group		Group Effect		Card Effect	
	Adolescents	Adults	F-Statistic	Significance	F-Statistic	Significance
Affect tone:						
Neutral cards	2.84	3.04	1.47	N.S.	4.79	.01
Negative cards ...	2.07	2.20	1.10	N.S.	5.98	.004
Complexity:						
Neutral cards	2.59	2.98	8.08	.006	.98	N.S.
Negative cards ...	2.47	2.78	4.80	.03	.34	N.S.
Emotional investment:						
Neutral cards	2.05	2.37	6.40	.014	5.93	.004
Negative cards ...	1.95	2.10	1.38	N.S.	11.54	.0001
Social causality:						
Neutral cards	2.31	2.23	.29	N.S.	19.39	.0001
Negative cards ...	2.10	2.57	14.42	.0003	.28	N.S.

NOTE.—Data analyzed by repeated-measures analysis of variance, $df = 1,71$.

TABLE 5
PERCENT OF PATHOLOGICAL SCORES (Level 1) for Adolescent
and Adult Borderlines

	Adolescents	Adults	t-Statistic	Significance
Affect tone	25	15	3.50	.016
Complexity	4	6	−.84	N.S.
Emotional investment ..	34	21	2.14	.018
Social causality	14	9	.90	N.S.

NOTE.—Data analyzed by paired t-tests (one tailed), $df = 71$.

TABLE 6
PERCENTAGE OF HIGH-LEVEL SCORES (Level 4 or 5) FOR ADOLESCENT
AND ADULT BORDERLINES

	Adolescents	Adults	t-Statistic	Significance
Affect tone	18	21	.51	N.S.
Complexity	15	24	1.54	.064
Emotional investment	2	8	2.20	.015
Social causality	7	23	3.04	.002

NOTE.—Data analyzed by paired t-tests (one-tailed), $df = 71$.

Finally, a discriminant-function analysis was performed using all scores on the six TAT cards as independent variables and adolescent or adult status as the dependent variable. The discriminant function correctly classified 92.8 percent of subjects as either adolescent or adult borderlines on the basis of a linear combination of scores.

Discussion

Within the limitations of the present methodology, the results of this study support the following conclusions. First, the data suggest the importance of delineating multiple dimensions of object relations rather than referring to object relations as a unitary phenomenon. Whereas three of the dimensions examined in this study did show developmental differences between the groups, one did not, as predicted. A theory of object relations that does not differentiate multiple processes would have difficulty explaining these findings.

Second, object-relations development continues beyond the preoedipal years in borderline patients. Previous research (Westin et al. 1989) demonstrated developmental differences on the same three dimensions of object relations between eighth and twelfth graders in a

377

normal sample. This suggests that object relations mature throughout adolescence in normal development. What the present findings suggest is that borderline adolescents are also different from borderline adults in their object relations. The difference lies in their greater immaturity: their representations are less complex; their capacity to invest emotionally in others is less developed; and their understanding of social causality is less mature than adult borderlines. This has significant theoretical implications, not only because object-relations theories have typically described the development of object relations in only the first five years, but also because theories of borderline object relations have suggested that borderline adults and adolescents share the same preoedipal developmental arrest. If that were true, there would be no developmental differences between the two samples in this study.

Interactions of age and affective quality of the stimulus suggest that the differences between the adolescents and the adults on complexity of representations are larger on the neutral cards. One possible explanation of this for the adults is that, when strong affects are not aroused, object representations may be relatively mature. Under conditions of affective arousal, however, both the adolescents and the adults drop in their level of complexity of representations. The adolescents, of course, do not have as far to drop since normal adolescents between the ages of thirteen and eighteen do not have very complex representations (although, of course, there are considerable individual differences; Shantz 1983). The same pattern was true for capacity for emotional investment, although the differences between the neutral and the negative cards were more significant. On the negative cards, there were no differences between the two groups, whereas there were significant differences on the neutral cards. The opposite pattern strongly emerged on understanding of social causality: neutral cards did not distinguish the two groups, but the negative cards did significantly. It may be that a capacity to regulate distorted attributional processes does not emerge in borderlines until adulthood. These attributional distortions are most likely to arise under conditions of negative affective arousal.

Analysis of the percentage of pathological scores for the two groups suggests that, by adulthood, borderlines may have learned to regulate or modify some of their malevolent object representations and have developed a greater capacity for emotional investment in relationships and morals. The analysis of percentage of high-level scores suggests that much of the difference between the adolescent and the adult borderlines lies in a normal developmental process, namely, the movement from a predominance of scores of levels 1, 2, and 3 to an emergence of scores of levels 4 and 5 on each of the developmental scales (although scores of predominantly levels 4 and 5 are not even normative in adulthood).

To summarize, the major conclusion of these findings is that object relations in borderlines continue to develop beyond adolescence, producing developmental differences in dimensions of object relations between adult and adolescent borderline patients. Thus, if borderline pathology represents a preoedipal fixation or developmental arrest, this cannot explain the entirety of borderline object relations. A more comprehensive theory will need to account for the ways that object relations change throughout childhood and adulthood, even in patients with object-relational pathology.

The reader may object that we are attacking a straw man, that no theorist literally believes that borderline patients are like toddlers in all aspects of their object relations. Careful examination of basic writings in object-relations theory from Klein (1948) to Kernberg (1975), Kohut (1971), and Masterson (1976) suggests, however, that metaphor, factual assertation, and explanation are rarely carefully distinguished. When borderlines act like Mahler's rapproachment toddlers, clinicians and theorists routinely nod their heads, confirmed in their belief that they are witnessing infantile functioning. The many ways in which border-line patients do not seem like toddlers in their object relations may be observed clinically but are not explained theoretically. Further, as noted earlier, for both Kernberg and Masterson, a single index defines a patient's overall level of object-relational functioning as either oedipal or preoedipal. Theory and observation are dialectically related: the aim of theory is to enhance observation, and, when observation begins to move beyond and be encumbered by theory, theoretical change is once again in order.

Before concluding, it is important to note the limitations of the present study. First, the research involves a cross-sectional rather than a longitudinal design, which means that we can confidently speak only of age differences and not of age changes in the dimensions studied here. A more definitive study would follow up the adolescent patients as adults and hence be able to address changes in object relations over time directly. One could argue that the differences found here reflect differences in the two samples, such as greater pathology in the adolescent sample leading to early hospitalization. This alternative hypothesis seems less likely, however, because most of the adult subjects, who themselves were typically young (mean age twenty-seven), had multiple previous hospitalizations. It would clearly be useful to know, however, how many had been hospitalized in adolescence and to what extent different age of hospitalization reflected a meaningful difference between the two samples.

Another limitation stems from the fact that this study represents a liaison between two projects with slightly different methodologies. By definition, in order to assess adolescent borderline pathology validly and reliably, the DIB was slightly modified with the adolescent sample so that one could argue for subtle differences in diagnosis. The only change that had any effect, however, was quite minor (questioning adolescent subjects about several of their relationships rather than simply their most intimate relationship in the Interpersonal Relations section of the DIB since few had developed long-term love relationships). Screening criteria for consideration for the study also differed between the adults and the adolescents, which could potentially have led to some sampling biases. However, criteria for inclusion in the borderline cohort in both samples was uniform, namely a score of 7 or greater on the DIB, assuring comparability of the two samples.

In addition, the two interviewers who trained DIB interviewers for the adolescent study were both interviewers for the adult study, again leading to comparability of samples. Finally, within the adolescent sample, diagnosis was defined by DIB score and was thus reliable and standardized; however, different criteria were used to screen potential subjects, different interviewers administered the DIB at different points in the study, and subjects were obtained from two hospitals, which could have introduced variability in the sample. Paired *t*-tests comparing TAT scores from the two hospital samples and from the two phases of data collection, however, found no significant differences, and similar comparisons on thirty-five DIB item and section scores found only one significant difference between the two hospital samples (psychosis section score), less than expected by chance.

Conclusions

Despite these limitations, the present study represents a first systematic empirical comparison of the object relations of patients diagnosed with borderline disorders in adolescence and adulthood. The data suggest the need for a more comprehensive account of differences in object relations between these two groups based on a theory that focuses on multiple dimensions of object relations and on development beyond the preoedipal years.

REFERENCES

Balint, M. 1968. *The Basic Fault*. London: Tavistock.

Berkowitz, D. A. 1981. The borderline adolescent and the family. In M. Lansky, ed. *Family Treatment of Major Psychopathology*. New York: Grune & Stratton.

Berkowitz, D. A.; Shapiro, R. L.; Zinner, J.; and Shapiro, E. R. 1974. Family contributions to narcissistic disturbances in adolescents. *International Review of Psycho-Analysis* 1:353–362.

Blatt, S.; Brenneis, C. B.; Schimek, J. G.; and Glick, M. 1976. Structural dimensions of object relations on the Rorschach. Yale University. Typescript.

Blatt, S. J., and Lerner, H. 1983. Investigations in the psychoanalytic theory of object relations and object representations. In J. Masling, ed. *Empirical Studies of Psychoanalytic Theories*, vol. 1. Hillsdale, N.J.: Erlbaum.

Block, M. J.; Westen, D.; and Ludolph, P. 1989. Distinguishing borderline adolescents from their normal and psychiatrically disturbed peers. Paper presented at the annual convention of the American Psychological Association, Atlanta, August.

Bogen, T. M. 1982. Patterns of developmental change in formal characteristics of stories children tell. Ph.D. diss., University of Michigan.

Chandler, M. J.; Page, K. F.; and Koch, D. A. 1978. The child's demystification of psychological defense mechanisms: a structural and developmental analysis. *Developmental Psychology* 14:197–205.

Cornell, D.; Silk, K.; Ludolph, P.; and Lohr, N. 1983. Test-retest reliability of the diagnostic interview for borderlines. *Archives of General Psychiatry* 40:1307–1310.

Damon, W. 1977. *The Social World of the Child*. San Francisco: Jossey-Bass.

381

Donaldson, S. K., and Westerman, M. A. 1986. Development of children's understanding of ambivalence and causal theories of emotion. *Developmental Psychology* 22:655–662.

Fairbairn, W. R. D. 1952. *Psychoanalytic Studies of Personality.* London: Routledge & Kegan Paul.

Gilligan, C. 1982. *In a Different Voice.* Cambridge, Mass.: Harvard University Press.

Greenberg, J. R., and Mitchell, S. A. 1983. *Object Relations in Psychoanalytic Theory.* Cambridge, Mass.: Harvard University Press.

Gunderson, J. 1984. *Borderline Personality Disorder.* Washington, D.C.: American Psychiatric Press.

Gunderson, J. G.; Kolb, J. E.; and Austin, V. 1981. The diagnostic interview for borderline patients. *American Journal of Psychiatry* 138:896–903.

Harter, S. 1986. Cognitive-developmental processes in the integration of concepts about emotions and the self. *Social Cognition* 4:119–151.

Jacobson, E. 1964. *The Self and the Object World.* New York: International Universities Press.

Kernberg, O. 1975. *Borderline Conditions and Pathological Narcissism.* New York: Aronson.

Kernberg, O. 1976. *Object Relations Theory and Clinical Psychoanalysis.* New York: Aronson.

Kernberg, O. 1978. The diagnosis of borderline conditions in adolescence. *Adolescent Psychiatry* 6:298–319.

Kernberg, O. 1984. *Severe Personality Disorders.* New Haven, Conn.: Yale University Press.

Klein, M. 1948. *Contributions to Psycho-Analysis, 1921–1945.* London: Hogarth.

Kohlberg, L., and Kramer, R. 1969. Continuities and discontinuities in childhood and adult moral development. *Human Development* 12:93-120.

Kohut, H. 1971. *The Analysis of the Self: A Systematic Approach to the Treatment of Narcissistic Personality Disorders.* New York: International Universities Press.

Krohn, A., and Mayman, M. 1974. Object representations in dreams and projective tests. *Bulletin of the Menniger Clinic* 38:445–466.

Lerner, H. D., and St. Peter, S. 1984. Patterns of object relations in neurotic, borderline, and schizophrenic patients. *Psychiatry* 47:77–92.

Ludolph, P.; Westen, D.; Misle, B.; Jackson, A.; Wixom, J.; and Wiss, F. C. 1988. The borderline diagnosis in adolescence: developmental histories and symptomatology. Ann Arbor: Department of Psychology, University of Michigan. Typescript.

Mahler, M. S., and Kaplan, L. 1977. Developmental aspects in the assessment of narcissistic and so-called borderline personalities. In P. Hartocollis, ed. *Borderline Personality Disorders*. New York: International Universities Press.

Mahler, M.; Pine, F.; and Bergman, A. 1975. *The Psychological Birth of the Human Infant: Symbiosis and Individuation*. New York: Basic.

Masterson, J. 1972. *Treatment of the Borderline Adolescent: A Developmental Approach*. New York: Wiley.

Masterson, J. 1976. *Psychotherapy of the Borderline Adult*. New York: Brunner/Mazel.

Masterson, J. 1978. The borderline adolescent: an object relations view. *Adolescent Psychiatry* 6:344–359.

Masterson, J. 1980. *From Borderline Adolescent to Functioning Adult: The Test of Time*. New York: Brunner/Mazel.

Mayman, M. 1967. Object-representations and object-relationships in Rorschach responses. *Journal of Projective Techniques and Personality Assessment* 31:17–24.

Mayman, M. 1968. Early memories and character structure. *Journal of Projective Techniques and Personality Assessment* 32:303–316.

Peterfreund, I. 1978. Some critical comments on psychoanalytic conceptualizations of infancy. *International Journal of Psycho-Analysis* 59:427–441.

Piaget, J. 1926. *The Language and Thought of the Child*. New York: Humanities, 1951.

Rest, J. R. 1983. Morality. In J. H. Flavell and E. M. Markman, eds. *Cognitive Development*. Vol. 3 of P. H. Mussen, series ed. *Handbook of Child Psychology*. New York: Wiley.

Selman, R. L. 1980. *The Growth of Interpersonal Understanding: Developmental and Clinical Analyses*. New York: Academic.

Shantz, C. U. 1983. Social cognition. In J. H. Flavell and E. M. Markman, eds. *Cognitive Development*. Vol. 3 of P. H. Mussen, series ed. *Handbook of Child Psychology*. New York: Wiley.

Shapiro, E. R. 1978. Research on family dynamics: clinical implications for the family of the borderline adolescent. *Adolescent Psychiatry* 6:360–376.

383

Shay, J. J. 1987. The wish to do psychotherapy with borderline adolescents—and other common errors. *Psychotherapy* 24:712–719.

Spear, W. E., and Sugarman, A. 1984. Dimensions of internalized object relations in borderline and schizophrenic patients. *Psychoanalytic Psychology* 1:113–129.

Stuart, J.; Westen, D.; Lohr, N.; Benjamin, J.; Becker, S.; Vorns, N.; and Silk, K. In press. Object relations in borderlines, major depressives, and normals: analysis of Rorschach human figure responses. *Journal of Personality Assessment*.

Thompson, A. E. 1981. The theory of affect development and maturity: applications to the TAT. Ph.D. diss., University of Michigan.

Urist, J. 1977. The Rorschach Test and the assessment of object relations. *Journal of Personality Assessment* 41:3–9.

Urist, J. 1980. Object relations. In R. W. Woody, ed. *Encyclopedia of Clinical Assessment*, vol. 2. San Francisco: Jossey-Bass.

Weissman, M., and Bothwell, S. 1976. Self-report version of the Social Adjustment Scale. *Archives of General Psychiatry* 33:1111–1115.

Westen, D. 1985. *Self and Society: Narcissism, Collectivism, and the Development of Morals*. New York: Cambridge University Press.

Westen, D. 1989. Are "primitive" object relations really preoedipal? *American Journal of Orthopsychiatry* 59:331–345.

Westen, D. In press. The relations among narcissism, egocentrism, self-concept, and self-esteem. *Psychoanalysis and Contemporary Thought*.

Westen, D.; Barends, A.; Leigh, J.; Mendel, M.; and Silbert, D. 1988. Manual for assessing dimensions of object relations and social cognition using interview data. University of Michigan. Typescript.

Westen, D.; Klepser, J.; Silverman, M.; Ruffins, S.; Boekamp, J.; and Lifton, N. O. 1989. Object relations in the elementary and high school years: the development of working representations. Department of Psychology, University of Michigan. Typescript.

Westen, D.; Lohr, N.; Silk, K.; Gold, L.; and Kerber, K. 1988. Object relations in borderlines, major depressives, and normals: TAT study. Department of Psychology, University of Michigan. Typescript.

Westen, D.; Ludolph, P.; Lerner, H.; Ruffins, S.; and Wiss, C. In press. Object relations in borderline adolescents. *Journal of the American Academy of Child and Adolescent Psychiatry*.

Westen, D.; Silk, K.; Lohr, N.; and Kerber, K. 1985. Measuring object relations and social cognition using the TAT: scoring manual. University of Michigan. Typescript.

21 DEVELOPMENTAL ANXIETIES IN ADOLESCENCE

MAX SUGAR

Adults often seem envious of the adolescent's apparently fun-filled days, while some professionals still feel that all adolescents have a stormy time. Is adolescence pleasurable or painful? We assume that questions about these issues may be an avenue for indirect communication about anxieties and concerns that may be normative and developmentally appropriate or signals of pathology.

Although theories abound about adolescent emotional development (Erikson 1950; Freud 1958), there is a question about how well they apply to the nonpatient population at large since most of the literature is about patients. The studies by Block (1971), Offer (1969), and Vaillant and McArthur (1972) are among the few of nonpatient adolescents.

By presenting questions from nonpatient teenagers who are presumed to be normal, although among them 15 percent may have emotional illnesses (*Report of the President's Commission on Mental Health* 1978), an attempt is made to present aspects that seem related to adolescent development. This provides an indirect approach to their feelings about themselves in a relatively spontaneous and unstructured fashion. This chapter also seeks to clarify how well our theories apply to youths in regard to sexuality and other developmental issues.

Adolescent Developmental Tasks

The adolescent has developmental tasks that consist of adapting to physical growth and hormonal changes; emotionally separating and individuating from parents (Blos 1962; Sugar 1968); further cognitive development, with the attainment of the adult level of intelligence and abstract thinking ability (Piaget and Inhelder 1958); developing a sexual identity; achieving intimacy (Erikson 1950); attaining heterosexual relationships; further development of the ego, superego, and ego-ideal; and preparing to take on a vocational role. We theorize that the youngsters' questions reflect elements of uncertainty and anxiety about various areas of development, change, conflicts of the past and present, as well as curiosity about themselves and their changing physical, sexual, emotional, social, and cognitive identities. These involve a major set of issues in the development of the youngster through adolescence into adulthood.

Adult Developmental Tasks

Parents often ask physicians to tell them how to get along with their teenage offspring by requesting information about the youngster's thinking or prominent interests. If the parents were to take a few minutes to recall their own adolescent years, they might remember their own burning issues of a generation or two ago, including their anxiety about sexuality and fears about their parents learning about their preoccupation. However, many adults repress or suppress those memories and face their youngsters with a blank memory bank.

Parents of adolescents are usually in their middle years and have a different set of tasks. Their foci are dealing with changing sexuality (theirs is declining, while the adolescent's is increasing); changing physical status; generativity versus stagnation (Erikson 1950); maintaining stability; and having their ego and superego hold up in the face of various changes, restrictions, and adversities that may occur in the course of life. Parents have questions about the adolescents and about themselves as parents and as adults in mid-life. Therefore, parents' questions about their adolescents should also give us ideas about general parental concerns, which also reflect specific developmental tasks of mid-life that might affect their approach to their offspring.

Methodology

Since 1979, a local general hospital, with a great interest in community affairs and problems, has hosted and supported rap sessions for teenagers and their parents. The discussion sessions are free. They are advertised in the hospital newsletter and in various community publications. It is assumed that the youngsters attend on their parents' suggestion.

These annual rap sessions begin each year in September, with a series of three meetings at monthly intervals with the parents. In January, monthly rap sessions for the adolescents begin, alternating between the twelve- to fifteen-year-olds and the fifteen- to eighteen-year-olds until the end of the academic year (i.e., two sessions with each age group, for a total of four). The youngsters attend the sessions only after presenting written parental permission. About 95 percent of the youngsters attending are white middle class, with a few low socioeconomic, black, or Hispanic teenagers among them. Thus, there are two stages of adolescence available for scrutiny through the questions: the early and the midadolescent.

Sessions were conducted by panelists interested and experienced in dealing with adolescents: a pediatrician, one or two psychiatrists, an obstetrician-gynecologist, a juvenile court judge, and a social worker. The composition of the panel varies at times, but essentially the same disciplines are represented quite regularly on the panel. The first hour is taken up with presentations of about ten to fifteen minutes by each of the panelists on aspects of adolescence from a normative viewpoint and situations from their respective disciplines and experience. These include physical, emotional, cognitive, sexual, and family alterations as part of adolescent development.

After a break for refreshments, the youngsters can speak from the floor and ask or turn in written questions. The youngster or the chair of the panel selects the panelist to answer, unless one of the panelists volunteers because he or she feels particularly interested in and qualified to discuss that point. The impression remains that about 95 percent of the questions are written. Over the years, the questions have been collected at the end of the evening, which is the source of the material presented here. The questions varied remarkably little over the years (1979–1984) reviewed. Perhaps 40–50 percent of the youngsters submitted questions. The written questions were much more detailed and explicit than the oral.

Parents also meet at the hospital for rap sessions with the same panelists and format. However, with them the introductory remarks are focused on normative issues of adolescents and their parents.

Possible (but not to be considered exclusive) motivations for the teens' attendance are anxieties, fear of pregnancy, need for support, social and sexual interests, and a search for validation, to find similar others, or to feel less strange. For the parents, the need for support and reassurance, as well as social and validating needs, seems prominent.

In the first six years, from fall 1979 through spring 1984, usually 75–150 youngsters or parents attended each of the sessions, for a total of about 2,000 youngsters and 1,500 parents. These sessions for teens and parents continue, but data for the chapter were limited to 1979–1984, the years during which I was actively involved.

Questions from Twelve- to Fourteen-Year-Olds

Of the questions asked by the twelve- to fourteen-year-olds (see table 1), 59 percent were about sex: sexual behavior, anatomy, physiology, and reproduction. They also included such things as menses, pregnancy, venereal disease, homosexuality, masturbation, contraception, abortion, and rape. In the next largest category, 15 percent of the questions were related to drugs, alcohol, and parents' or youngsters' abuse thereof.

Ten percent of the questions were about relationships with parents and other authorities. Personality issues about themselves, their shyness, and how to talk with people constituted 2 percent of the questions. Eight percent were related to issues about petting and dating. These could be considered under the topic of sex—which would then represent about 66 percent of the questions. Questions about peer relations constituted 6 percent of the questions.

TABLE 1

QUESTIONS FROM TWELVE- TO FOURTEEN-YEAR-OLDS

Topic	Percentage of Questions
Sex—(physiology, anatomy, behavior, reproduction, venereal disease)	59
Drug abuse	15
Relations with adults, including parents ..	10
Dating	8
Personality and relationships............	2
Peers................................	6

Questions from Fifteen- to Eighteen-Year-Olds

As shown in table 2, among the fifteen- to eighteen-year-olds sex and sex-related issues constituted 55 percent of the questions. These included such items as pregnancy, contraception, incest, venereal disease, and abortion. There were fewer questions related to anatomy and physiology in this age group and more questions about the various developments in relationships that might go awry. Drugs and alcohol were the topic of 26 percent of the questions. Nine percent concerned issues relating to parents.

Five percent dealt with peer relations, problems that they might have, and how they might be helped. There was a new set of questions —2 percent— about their future in a vocational field. Questions about dating and relationships made up another 2 percent. Issues of discipline and authority conflicts such as curfew, telling parents their whereabouts and whom they were with, and so on, totaled 3 percent of the questions.

Typical Questions in Early Adolescence

The early adolescent boys asked questions about female anatomy. They projected a great deal onto the girls, and many theories were evident in their use of slang and understanding of reproduction. Their braggadocio and macho behavior was clearly a cover-up for their ignorance and anxiety.

The early adolescent females asked questions about the boys' use of slang terms designating anatomical references as well as anatomical questions about boys. The girls seemed to be completely awash in trying to

TABLE 2
QUESTIONS FROM FIFTEEN- TO EIGHTEEN-YEAR-OLDS

Topic	Percentage of Questions
Sex	55
Drugs	26
Parents	9
Peers	5
Authority issues	3
Vocations	2

understand these terms. This seemed to involve repression, denial, and ignorance of many things about themselves and boys. But each sex was curious about the other. Questions from the early adolescents included,

> What is the G spot?
> What is the vagina?
> What is gynecology?
> What would you give to a person if they fell back in their grades?
> What is VD?
> What are wet dreams?
> What are periods?
> Is there a way to break up with a girl without hurting her?
> What does "making out" mean?
> What is semen?
> What is a penis?
> What are testicles?
> What are the ways to arrange contraception?
> What is the pill?
> Should a girl swim when she is on her period?
> What do you do about VD?
> Should a girl smoke when having her period?
> Is there anything wrong with teenagers having sex?
> What's the difference between alcohol and pot?
> What is the best method of birth control?
> How old do you have to be to have a baby?
> What are your recommendations for the period? Tampons?
> Can a boy tell if you're having your period?
> What is Spanish Fly?
> What is a cherry?
> What should you do if you think you hear your parents making love?
> How often does a married couple have sex?

Typical Questions in Midadolescence

The midadolescents were not asking the same kinds of questions, but they were also very anxious and curious. They were more interested in intercourse, in heterosexuality, and in relationship aspects of sexuality rather than anatomy and physiology. Among the questions of the fifteen- to eighteen-year-olds were the following:

I go to an all-girls school; I don't know how to act around boys. How should I?

I think I act too babyfied. There is a boy that I really like who is trying to talk me into having sex with him. I really don't want to have sex with him, but if I don't, I know I will lose him. I really love him. What should I do?

What do you do when a boy that you just met asks you to make out, but you like him too?

How old is too young for a girl to get sexually involved?

I am pregnant; I haven't told my mom yet. He, the guy, told me to have an abortion. What should I do?

Why have most men and boys changed from being gentlemen to wild beasts who love to touch whatever they see?

My life circles around this one man, but I know I'll never have him because he's already married to a girl because he got her pregnant. I'll never be able to tell him how I feel about him because he lives far away from here, and I have no address or phone number. I've faced reality and I'm willing to let him go, but I have some very sad and painful feelings about this. How can I cope?

Tell me about female reproduction.

Does sex hurt?

Last week one of my very best friends and I got into a big argument. Now the whole school knows about it and they know the story wrong. Everyone thinks it's my fault, and three-quarters of the school hate me. They are constantly talking about me; what should I do?

My mom hasn't yet told me about the birds and the bees at all, and I think I should know. Signed, Helpless.

What do you do when your parents say be in by ten, when all of your other friends stay out until 11:00 and you are responsible?

What if you don't have your period until you're sixteen; what is wrong with you?

My mom and dad are divorced and every time he comes to get me, all they do is yell at each other. My dad was at fault, and I feel sorry because I don't have a dad hardly any more. I wish they wouldn't fight, but they do anyway. I love both of them.

My mother is always yelling at me and I have to do a lot of work around the house and sometimes I hate her, and I want to run away.

But I also love her and I can't run away. What shall I do? P. S. I am too scared to talk to her about it for I will get slapped in the face.

When I tell my mom I love a certain boy, she says I'm too young to love and leave him alone. She treats me like a baby.

What would a girl say to a boy if she has never talked to this boy before and she thinks he's cute; what would be a first line?

What do you do when someone you really like is a newcomer to the school? Everyone hates her because she is so different but you really like her. Your friends don't like her, and you do. If you like her, everyone will hate you. What should you do?

I have heard of these words at school, but I don't know what they mean: blow job and masturbate.

What do you do when you have a brother that beats you up and a girlfriend that is two-timing you?

What do girls' breasts have to do with sex?

Why do girls take Spanish Fly to make them want to have sex?

Why or how do you become a homosexual?

Why do homosexuals have sex?

What is a transvestite?

What do you do when you want to meet a guy but he ignores you?

What do you do at a toga party?

What do you do when you're pregnant and your boyfriend wants nothing to do with you or your baby?

How old do you think a girl should be to go on a car date and to make your parents understand that the guy is not after one thing?

All my parents think is that I'm going to get pregnant at seventeen to nineteen if I start dating at fourteen, but I know I won't.

How do you go about meeting a girl?

Should my mom get mad at me if I don't listen to her so good?

Yesterday some people were making fun of me and they were my friends. What should I do?

If you like a boy and he likes another girl, how can you get him to like you, not in a forceful way?

Parents' Questions

In tabulating the parents' questions (see table 3), 14 percent turned out to be about adolescent sex, while 16 percent were about alcohol and other drugs. School problems of the youngsters constituted twelve

TABLE 3
PARENTS' QUESTIONS ABOUT ADOLESCENTS

Topic	Percentage of Questions
Adolescent sex........................	14
Drugs...............................	16
School	12
Disciplinary privileges	39
Youngsters' self-esteem	10
Single-parented youngsters	8
Emotional disturbances	1

percent of the questions. Discipline, privileges, communication problems, dating, peers, and curfew made up 39 percent.

Questions about the youngsters' self-esteem made up 10 percent. Questions about raising a young adult in a single-parent family totaled 8 percent. Considerations about the young adult's disturbed emotional state—depression, anxiety, suicide potential, and so on—were 1 percent of the questions.

Discussion

It should be understood that this is not a controlled study with rigorous methodological requirements, but the data do provide some measure of validity and utility since the questions were spontaneously offered and collected immediately, though tabulated later; the youngsters were there voluntarily and not as part of an experimental group with its inherent issues of being observed; and there was consistency in the type and phrasing of questions over the years. The population was self-selected and assumed normative since it was not a patient population.

Whether the rap program helped the youngsters or parents in the long or short run is unknown. The youngsters learned some things about sexual anatomy, physiology, and social function, while the parents may have gained some knowledge and understanding about adolescence from the sessions. A research study of a similar program (Benson, Perlman, and Sciarra 1986) indicated a 32 percent improvement in knowledge with excellent retention of sex education material by seventh and eighth graders.

393

The rap sessions may have helped many youngsters feel more positive and comfortable about the changes they were negotiating in their bodies, with peer groups, and with their parents by reducing their feelings of loneliness and strangeness. The parents seemed to feel some increased measure of comfort by sharing with us and the other parents. They then seemed to feel less isolated and anxious and also that their concerns were normal. That both the adolescents and the parents seemed to derive some benefit from the sessions was attested to by their repeat attendance—some for several years—and their spontaneous, enthusiastic comments to various panelists when they met long after the rap sessions. This seems to indicate a need for more and better sex and family education for both generations.

Although many of the youngsters may have needed (or been in) psychiatric treatment, this was an unknown quantity. If we assume that perhaps 15 percent of the youngsters were emotionally disturbed to some degree, the other 85 percent still provide a significant group from which to gather insight into the sexual and other anxieties of normal adolescents. Perhaps their questions reflect something that might help us both in approaching them and in checking the validity of our theory building against nonpatient youngsters' questions.

It is possible that some of the questions were stimulated or suggested by the panelists' introductory remarks, and this is difficult to discount as an influence. However, these remarks were general, nontechnical, and devoted to normative aspects of adolescence. In addition, the questions were uniquely those of the registrants and were not paraphrases of the panelists since the issues or questions concerned (e.g., "blow job," "cherry," divorced parents, drug-using parents, homosexuality, etc.) were not brought up in the introductory remarks. Since AIDS did not become a public health issue until after the period under scrutiny here, there were no questions about the disease.

It was obvious that the early adolescent boys were much more anxious and less socialized and showed less controls, courtesy, and ordinary good manners than the girls. They were more prone to become a gang with very little stimulus in that direction. The girls were better behaved and more sociable. These items may reflect the fact that, in latency and early adolescence, girls are advanced and more mature physically and socially by about two years than the boys.

Sixty-six and fifty-five percent of the questions of the early and the mid-teens, respectively, are focused on questions of sexuality: intercourse, physiology of reproduction, and anatomy of the sexes and their differences. Thus, a major issue was the physical changes in the body to which they are accommodating. Their concerns about changes in the body were in reference to their earlier and future physical status, the opposite sex, and the hormonal rearrangements that added to their questions about physical and sexual identity. These reflect the normal body narcissism of early adolescents as well as the anxiety about changes in their body. Along with increases in weight in both sexes, girls have three dimensions, while boys have only height and width, to worry about.

The ego of the adolescent is undergoing changes, and these are due partly to the physical changes. Since the ego is to begin with a body ego, any physical changes will cause some anxiety, to which the ego reacts. The analogy of getting comfortable with adjustments to postextraction changes in the oral cavity may be usefully applied in thinking of the adolescent's anxious response to unfamiliarity with his body, even as a result of small changes.

Adolescent boys and girls normally check, test, and parade their bodies like two-year-olds: "Look, see what I am, see what I can do." For the male, this occurs mostly as performance in athletics. For the girl, the approach is along affiliative lines as she parades her beauty, and she may also engage in athletics.

In the muscle-flexing and epidermal display is the need to prove oneself not weak, not small, and not unattractive for the purpose of validating that the body changes have led to improvement and not the monstrous alteration they fear. Since their image or performance is hard to objectify by themselves, consensual validation from peers is most important.

The display and validation needs are significant for confirmation of physical ability, as an expression of anxiety about bodily changes, as a body check and a need for reassurance (as for a two-year-old— "You're OK"), as a representative of one's sex, and as being attractive to the opposite sex. For girls, this often begins in late latency under the tutelage of their mothers. It becomes more intense thereafter for boys and girls throughout adolescence and continues less intensely in adulthood. It connotes a need for acceptance by the peer group via hair style, music, clothes, speech, and so forth. It also increases and fosters socialization into the wider world.

For youngsters with emotional, physical, or sensory deficits, display and validation may or may not be available as an avenue for reinforcing self-acceptability. For example, the blind obviously have the most difficulty; the retardate or the deaf may have similar problems; and the eating disordered have difficulties that are due to distorted ideas about their body size.

In their display, some youngsters present themselves as if they are more mature than they actually are. They then get the appellation of "boy crazy" or "girl crazy" when they may not have yet experienced any heterosexual activity but are simply excessively anxious and covering up with a lot of braggadocio or excess flirting. This was amply demonstrated by some youngsters in the rap sessions whose behavior, questions, and comments indicated sexual abstinence and a lack of basic knowledge.

There were questions about functioning with their fellow humans and getting along with peers, adults, rules, and their own concepts about right and wrong. This reflects their cognitive and abstract ability developing variably to a higher level than before. The questions also indicate ego and superego functions at differing levels as well as identity and personality development, dependency needs, and shifts away from parents.

Early adolescence is initiated by physical changes and the capacity for the normal mourning process (Sugar 1968). Although puberty begins sometime from eleven to fifteen (Tanner 1978), with some girls pubertal changes start as early as eight or as late as sixteen or so. For males in early adolescence, the ability to ejaculate brings masturbation, with its attendant anxieties and guilt, into the direct focus of their sexuality. For early adolescent girls, the onset of menses may bring a positive sense of femaleness, but it is mostly negative and increases the sense of ambivalence about their genitals (Offer and Simon 1975).

Female sexuality involves feelings and moods more than male sexuality does. Before any sexual act occurs in adolescence, the girl may already have become frightened by mood alterations unrelated to external situations, alterations that are due to hormonal level variations of which she may or may not be aware, even dimly. These premenstrual, menstrual, and postmenstrual changes may make her feel out of control, confused, and needing someone to watch out for and comfort her. This creates a special problem for the girl in her strivings for autonomy since such swings make her feel less ready to be self-sufficient than her male counterpart. This strain may help her stay attached to infantile objects longer than otherwise.

For the adolescent, the premenstrual syndrome (PMS) may indeed be a formidable barrier to feeling more self-control, to trusting herself to be less dependent on parents, or even to trusting age-mates, female or male. The additional problem of irregular, anovulatory menses for several years after menarche, followed by ovulatory menses with cramps and altered moods, further confuses and compounds the girl's sense of stability about her body and emotions. The mood swings may not be a hindrance, however, if they are satisfactorily explained to her and especially if she has a suitable age-mate support system.

By becoming more attuned to her emotional variations, the girl becomes more aware of her moods, their effect on others, and their use socially as an all-inclusive face-saving device and as an apology. When a girl says, "Sorry, I'm in a bad mood," other girls know what she means. Boys are confused by this. They may blame themselves or harangue the girl to explain further since boys' awareness or understanding of their own or others' feelings is much less developed than girls' at this age and is based on a concrete approach regardless of their abstract ability.

Normal adolescent mourning (Sugar 1968) involves giving up infantile objects, with separation-protest as the first phase. This is characterized by disequilibrium, with angry, rebellious actions aimed at restoring the lost objects alternating with separation efforts. This, as part of the second separation-individuation (Blos 1962), leads to less emotional dependence on the parents, with more autonomy in thinking, feeling, and planning with its inherent anxieties. The problem for the youngster in thinking and coping independently involves questioning parental attitudes, doing the opposite, possibly giving up some parental ideas, or putting them on the shelf while trying out new ones and developing new heroes or heroines to replace the parents. In early adolescence, the fears of fusion with the same-sex parent and of closeness with the opposite-sex parent lead to more closeness among same-sex peers as an anxiety-reducing device.

These early adolescent tasks and feelings are involved in the development of the adolescents' identity, their sexual identity, and their ego and superego capacities and also with ego-ideal changes. These tasks and feelings are very clearly reflected in the topics listed in the tables. Thus, it would seem that their questions reflect anxiety about various areas of their development having to do with the developmental tasks outlined earlier.

Disorganization, the second phase of normal adolescent mourning (Sugar 1968), usually occurs in midadolescence, following the unconscious acceptance by the youngster of the futility of reunion with the infantile objects. Now the youngster may feel inadequate, worthless, and empty, with the potential (due to increased muscular ability and motility) to manage unpleasant or conflicted feelings by impulsive behavior. This may be based on sexual guilt or guilt about actions to parents.

For males at this time, the commitment to masturbation continues, as does further detachment from adult supervision (Offer and Simon 1975). Their social activities are still influenced by same-sex attachments, although there is a greater degree of heterosexual activity in the lower socioeconomic class than in the middle class. The relatively brief interval of a relationship before intercourse begins may reflect their inability to manage their emotional requirements (Offer and Simon 1975) and impulsivity.

For the midadolescent, further development may occur in IQ or abstract thinking, as may more involvement with the opposite sex. Educational concerns leading to plans for and a commensurate shift in vocational choices become more prominent in this age group.

The midadolescents' questions reflected concerns about pregnancy, parenthood, and fidelity as well as choices and preparations for a vocation. This means further separation from the parents, becoming more responsible and more autonomous as they approach late adolescence and adulthood. This is in keeping with Erikson's (1950) psychosocial stages.

The adolescent female and male have similar normative sources of anxiety but some significant differences throughout their development. For the boy, performance needs and vocational choices become paramount in the late adolescent stage, although fidelity and object choice are important. For the girl, in this stage, her affiliative needs are in the ascendancy, and she has to concern herself with choices and anxieties about career versus family planning. Vocational pursuits and plans are part of the separation from dependence on parents and promote their own set of anxieties (Scharff 1980).

To turn now to the parents' questions, only 14 percent were about adolescent sexuality in comparison to the 55 and 66 percent of adolescents' questions on that topic. Almost 40 percent of the parents' questions had to do with authority issues: how to set limits, communication problems, and discipline. There was some concern about the youngsters being troubled emotionally— how to recognize and prevent further escalation of problems and what to do about them. There were some important socioemotional questions having to do with the single-parent family and self-esteem development for the youngsters. These questions reflect a different set of developmental issues for these parents compared to those of younger children. These include responsibility for their charges along with anxieties about them, themselves, and their self-assessment as parents.

It should be noted and clearly understood that the two generations are not exactly in line with each other since they should not and could not be. The adolescent is a marked responsibility for the parents raising him or her. The parents have concerns of their own about issues of power, sexuality, changing physical status, the ability to let go or hold onto the youngster, as well as possible care of their own aged parents. The adult in mid-life is dealing with issues that may lead to a mid-life crisis. Compared to earlier years, many of the middle aged have lower lung capacity, narrower blood vessels, and more opacity of the lens. Their sexuality may be at a peak level or may be beginning to decline. Some of them may have arthritis, coronary artery disease, alcoholism, diabetes, hypertension, cancer, or sequelae of injuries or surgery that limit them further.

Some of the parents' questions about adolescent behavior have to be viewed through the prism of the parents' skewed views about themselves and their early stage of declining physical strength and sexual ability. Their bodies are becoming less powerful while the youngsters' bodies are quite lissome, nubile, virile, and powerful. These differences are a threat to the parents, who are declining in the areas of physical and sexual domination, and there is rivalry between the two generations. The middle-aged woman, who is menopausal, beginning to have wrinkles, or absent a uterus, has to contend with the burgeoning beauty of her fertile adolescent daughter. The father has to consider his son now as being more powerful, taller, or heavier than he and that the son may no longer be intimidated by parental threats as he was a few years ago. Thus, the adolescent is on the rise, and the adult is on the decline.

Parents usually have aspects of their residual oedipal conflicts rekindled when their offspring reenter the same arena in adolescence. The two generations then resonate to similar issues. Fathers often withdraw emotionally from their daughters at this crucial time; sons withdraw from their fathers; while both sons and daughters put more

399

distance between themselves and the mother. Parents in mid-life may have much unconscious envy and jealousy of their offspring, which is reflected in their concerns about power and control rather than in anxieties about the adolescents' sexuality. These conjectures stem from the percentage of questions about these topics by parents. We see these configurations clinically when parents have inordinate difficulties in allowing their youngsters appropriate autonomy and treat them as if they were grade-school children. Of course, this may be intertwined often with the parent's own difficulties in separation.

The adolescent and the parents alike have to adapt to shifts in social groups. The cohesiveness of their separate groups is loosening, which increases separation anxiety or the tendency toward it. The parents may have experienced the death, retirement, or relocation of their own parents, extended kin, and close friends. There may have been marked changes in interests—vocational and avocational—in the parents. The adolescent may have made a shift from the close ties to parents and grade-school friends to another set of friends or a rapidly changing grouping of new friends as part of his or her trying out new ideas and interests.

The parents' troubled reactions to their teenager's sexuality may stem from envy and jealousy as well as from displaced feelings about the youngster separating emotionally and beginning more autonomous functioning. This may also be a partial basis for the parental concerns with power, which would keep the youngster in a bind with them.

The two generations have some similar frightening, anxious issues to consider: physical and sexual changes, separation from love objects, and going in different directions regarding those issues. The parents question their success in their position and wonder what they are going to do with the rest of their lives. The mother worries about what to do now that the children have gone. With her reproductive days over, what is to be her future role? This is related to the crisis of generativity versus stagnation (Erikson 1950). Thus, there are questions about adult identity and future roles that are commingled with the questions they have about the youngster's identity and future. The parents may have some questions about their own abilities, marketability, or worth now, just as the youngsters are having questions about their value in relations with the opposite sex, their value in the marketplace, how they will be able to establish themselves vocationally, and what they will do with their lives.

The youngster has to develop and mature, drop off unnecessary baggage, and accommodate to feelings of potentially being able to achieve heretofore hidden or forbidden wishes. The ego has to mediate between these and the available sources for achieving such goals. The teen's superego has to reorganize in the face of inner and outer needs. What was formerly forbidden now becomes a subtle demand on the part of adults "to grow up," "get through school," "get a job," "get married," and so forth. Simultaneously, the youngster has peer pressure urging him or her, at times unflatteringly, to get his or her "act together."

Thus, there are many lines of coincident anxiety between the parents and the adolescents, which makes some of the clashes and difficulties in communication more understandable since the adult has two sources of anxiety to consider—the adolescent's and his or her own—while the adolescent has only one to consider—his or her own.

In contrast to Freud (1958), Masterson (1967) shows that turmoil in adolescence is not normative but is rather evidence of severe pathology. Of Offer's (1969) modal male adolescents, about 10 percent eventually were in psychiatric treatment. It is an axiom that it is routine in athletics to have the jitters prior to competing in an event, similar to stage fright in actors and exam anxiety in students. Considering the multiple tasks of adolescent development, it should not be a surprise to note that youngsters have moments or periods of anxiety. But this does not psychopathology make.

Perhaps we can consider that turmoil is going on in the unconscious, related to normal development; that the vast majority of adolescents cope, adapt, and function suitably despite the ongoing internal rearrangements; and that, when there is clinical turmoil, the dysfunction is evidence of psychopathology and not part of normal development (Masterson 1967).

Conclusions

From this material it appears that early and midadolescents' questions in rap sessions reflect their normative developmental anxieties about the various areas that are important to them. Sexuality makes up the majority of these, but there are also very significant concerns about physical changes, drug abuse, and relationships.

Parents' anxieties about their adolescents are reflected in their questions and represent two intertwining strands. One is a subtle or covert one having to do with the parents' anxieties about themselves, their status, and changes in physical, emotional, sexual, social, and vocational arenas. The other is overt and in part reflects concerns about the adolescent's changes in physical, emotional, hormonal, sexual, social, and vocational arenas. The generations are not usually aware of each other's developmental anxieties, which may compound the adolescents' difficulties in growth and development into mature adults.

From this standpoint, the concerns of the parents and other authorities about the further development of the youngster's ego, superego, and ego-ideal, as well as about helping with educational, social, and vocational preparation and pursuits, are appropriate. The confluence of parental problems or developmental anxieties that may impinge on and interfere with attending properly to the youngster needs clarification if parents are to respond more suitably to the adolescent, especially when the anxieties in the parents do not derive from the adolescent.

There is a need for more sex education for youngsters as well as support for both generations. Adolescent developmental anxieties need to be separated from psychopathology, just as they are for other developmental periods.

REFERENCES

Benson, M. D.; Perlman, C.; and Sciarra, J. J. 1986. Sex education in the innercity. *Journal of the American Medical Association* 255:43–47.

Block, J. 1971. *Lives through Time*. Berkeley, Calif.: Bancroft.

Blos, P. 1962. *On Adolescence*. New York: Free Press.

Erikson, E. 1950. *Childhood and Society*. New York: Norton.

Freud, A. 1958. Adolescence. *Psychoanalytic Study of the Child* 13:255–278.

Masterson, J. F. 1967. *The Psychiatric Dilemma of Adolescence*. Boston: Little, Brown.

Offer, D. 1969. *The Psychological World of the Teenager*. New York: Basic.

Offer, D., and Simon, W. 1975. Stages of sexual development. In H. Kaplan and A. Freedman, ed. *Comprehensive Textbook of Psychiatry*. 3d ed. Philadelphia: Williams & Wilkins.

Piaget, J., and Inhelder, B. 1958. *The Growth of Logical Thinking from Childhood to Adolescence*. New York: Basic.

Report of the President's Commission on Mental Health. 1978. Vol. 1. Washington, D.C.: U.S. Government Printing Office.

Scharff, D. E. 1980. Between two worlds: emotional needs of adolescents facing the transition from school to work. In M. Sugar, ed. *Responding to Adolescent Needs*. New York: Spectrum.

Sugar, M. 1968. Normal adolescent mourning. *American Journal of Psychotherapy* 22:258–269.

Tanner, J. M. 1978. *Foetus into Man: Physical Growth from Conception to Maturity*. Cambridge, Mass.: Harvard University Press.

Vaillant, G., and McArthur, C. 1972. Natural history of male psychologic health. I. the adult life cycle from 18–50. *Seminars in Psychiatry* 4:415–427.

22 CONSISTENCY AND CHANGE IN PERSONALITY CHARACTERISTICS AND AFFECT FROM MIDDLE TO LATE ADOLESCENCE

BERNARD A. STEIN, HARVEY GOLOMBEK,
PETER MARTON, AND MARSHALL KORENBLUM

This report is a continuation of a longitudinal study of personality development in a nonclinical sample of children followed from latency to young adulthood. We have previously reported that, although early adolescence is regarded as a difficult phase, functioning improves with time and passage into middle adolescence (Golombek, Marton, Stein, and Korenblum 1987). We have also indicated that, in the context of the response to developmental factors, a significant minority (20 percent) of early adolescents demonstrate marked personality dysfunction that may be related to the physiological, psychological, and social changes associated with pubescence (Golombek, Marton, Stein, and Korenblum 1986). This disturbed group demonstrated significantly more dysphoria, negative attitudes, more primitive defense mechanisms, and distant relationships with peers and parents than the majority (55 percent), who demonstrated competent personality functioning with minimal dysphoria, positive attitudes, higher-level defense mechanisms, and good involvement with peers and parental figures (Stein, Golombek, Marton, and Korenblum 1986).

Over the three-year period from early to middle adolescence, the proportion of teenagers with marked personality disturbance fell to 15 percent, and the proportion of those showing competent personality functioning rose to two-thirds (Golombek et al. 1987). Thus, our findings support the view of middle adolescence as a period of stabilization with less dysphoria and less disturbance, a greater sense of comfort with self and others, and a greater facility for coping and adaptation (Esman 1985). It was also found, however, that those early adolescents with significantly more observable depressed mood showed the least improvement over time (Stein, Golombek, Marton, and Korenblum 1987). Thus, we were able to trace developmental trends in the functioning of the whole group of adolescents as well as characteristics that identify individuals who function poorly compared to their age-mates.

Late adolescence is a period when important aspects of personality mature and become consolidated. This process involves a synthesis of experiences, relationships, conflicts, drives, and defenses, all of which are affected by inherent strengths and weaknesses (Blos 1972). Many of the internal and external struggles of earlier adolescence have been somewhat resolved, resulting in some stabilization of character structure (Blotkey and Looney 1980).

By late adolescence, the older teenager has usually confronted issues of independence, sexuality, vocation, and the nature of intimate relationships (Arnstein 1979; Bettelheim 1971). There often follows a period when there is a sense of urgency and when important life decisions must be made. It has been suggested that the element of choice is perhaps the key factor underlying the process of becoming an adult (Arnstein 1980). These changes must inevitably influence the emotional tone, attitudes, and the nature of significant relationships of the late adolescent. "The responsibility of independent choice and its consequences can bring about a period of perplexity, turmoil and sometimes profound despair" (Lidz 1976, p. 355). Clinicians and research investigators (Moriarity and Toussieng 1976) have suggested that it is at both the entry into and the exit from adolescence when there is the greatest stress and challenge to the stability and integrity of the personality.

It has not been clearly established how various affects and attitudes in older adolescents with healthy and adaptive personality functioning differ in their presentation from those characteristics in teenagers with more disturbed functioning. In particular, the increasing recognition of affective disorders in adolescence points to the need to determine whether dysphoria occurs randomly, in isolation from other aspects of personality, or is associated with certain personality problems and, therefore, occurs in a matrix of overall disturbed functioning.

This report presents findings of the clinical presentation and personality functioning of this same research sample as they reach late adolescence. The purpose is to determine whether a nonclinical sample of adolescents continues to improve in personality functioning in a continuous fashion as maturation occurs or whether the period of late adolescence, because of the stresses unique to that age, demonstrates increased personality problems. A further aim is to establish whether attitudes and affect change from middle to late adolescence and how these are related to personality functioning.

Method

SUBJECTS

The subjects in this study were participants in a longitudinal study of personality development. All grade 5 children in one region of an urban school board were screened using teacher (Arnold and Smeltzer 1974; Conners 1969) behavior rating scales. The children were stratified according to degree of behavior problems (high, middle, and low), and a study sample of seventy-two children was selected by sampling randomly from each of the three strata. The children included in the study sample did not differ in behavior ratings from the strata from which they were selected. The sample was judged to be representative of the whole range of behavioral presentation found in regular classrooms, from very quiet and nondisturbing to very boisterous and troublesome. The study sample was equally balanced for gender. The socioeconomic status of the sample was found to be predominantly middle and lower class, using the Blishen (1967) scale.

PROCEDURE

At ages thirteen, sixteen, and eighteen, each of the adolescents was interviewed by a psychiatrist, employing a semistructured interview based on a modified object relations scale (Giovacchini and Borowitz 1974). This interview was videotaped and subsequently rated by the interviewer and independently and blindly by a second psychiatrist on seven areas of personality functioning: maintenance of an internal sense of identity, reality testing, relatedness, verbal communication, self-esteem, identity, and role adequacy. Each area was rated as dysfunctional or clear of dysfunction. On the basis of these ratings, the adolescents themselves were classified into two groups: those who were clear of personality disturbance and those who demonstrated disturbance in more than one area. Following each psychiatric interview, ratings on a five-point scale were made on thirty-two items that assessed a broad range of affects and attitudes. Reliability of the two raters was determined for all ratings, and only items with adequate reliability were used. The average kappa statistic was .63. A more detailed report of this study can be found in Golombek et al. (1987).

DATA ANALYSIS

We present data on fifty-nine adolescents who were assessed at both age sixteen and age eighteen. In order to determine how the presentation of adolescents changed from age sixteen to age eighteen, we used a multivariate analysis of variance with repeated measures (group × sex × age). The individual items were clustered into two scales, one measuring affect and another measuring attitudes. Univariate analyses of variance with repeated measures (group × sex × age) were used to compare changes over time in individual scale items. These analyses also enabled us to examine the features that distinguished the presentation of adolescents who were clear of personality function disturbance in both middle and late adolescence, those who manifested disturbance at both phases, and those who manifested disturbance at only one phase. Pearson product-moment correlations were used to examine the predictability of affect and attitudes at age eighteen from their presentation at age sixteen.

Results

PERSONALITY FUNCTIONING

Comparison of the adolescents at ages sixteen and eighteen revealed that, of the total sample (N = 59), thirty were clear of disturbance at both ages and were classified as the "consistently clear" group; seventeen showed some disturbance at both ages and were classified as the "consistently disturbed" group. Twelve adolescents fluctuated between showing disturbance at one age and being clear at another age; these were classified as the "fluctuating" group.

We have previously reported that in middle adolescence the teenagers presented as being more competent in personality functioning when compared to their early adolescence (Stein et al. 1986). However, at age eighteen, they presented as being similar in personality functioning when compared to their middle adolescence. The proportion of adolescents with personality disturbance was approximately the same at both ages. As previously reported (Stein et al. 1986), in their early adolescence the late adolescent girls continued to be rated as demonstrating a similar level of competence in personality functioning to the boys.

CHANGES IN AFFECT AND ATTITUDES FROM MIDDLE TO LATE ADOLESCENCE

There were significant changes in affect from middle to late adolescence (table 1). At eighteen, the adolescents demonstrated more anxiety and more depression. There were a few differences found in attitudes (table 2). At eighteen, they were more curious, dominant, and pessimistic. They also demonstrated greater interest in significant persons in their lives.

PREDICTABILITY OF INDIVIDUALS FROM MIDDLE TO LATE ADOLESCENCE

Having established that there are developmental changes in affect and attitudes in our group of adolescents from age sixteen to age eighteen, we then wished to describe the predictability of functioning of eighteen-year-olds on the basis of observations at age sixteen. Examination of the correlation of the ratings obtained by individuals at

TABLE 1
CHANGE IN AFFECT FROM MIDDLE TO LATE ADOLESCENCE

Variable	Age 16[a]	Age 18[a]	Significance[b]
Depression	1.7	2.3	.00001
	(.9)	(.8)	
Anxiety	2.8	3.3	.00001
	(.9)	(.6)	

[a] Mean scale score (standard deviation).
[b] Analysis of variance.

TABLE 2
Change in Personality Traits from Middle to Late Adolescence

Variable	Age 16[a]	Age 18[a]	Significance[b]
Curiosity.......................	2.9	3.2	.005
	(.6)	(.6)	
Dominance.....................	2.4	2.7	.003
	(.7)	(.6)	
Pessimism......................	2.1	2.3	.02
	(.8)	(.8)	
Interest in others	3.0	3.2	.029
	(.5)	(.5)	

[a] Mean scale score (standard deviation).
[b] Analysis of variance.

the two ages on affect, attitudes, and personality functioning indicated that there was considerable predictability, with correlations of .69, .69, and .70, respectively. These correlations were highly significant at the .00001 level.

PERSONALITY FUNCTIONING AND AFFECT

We examined those characteristics that differentiated three groups of adolescents: those who were clear of disturbance in both middle and late adolescence ($N = 30$), those who were disturbed in both middle and late adolescence ($N = 17$), and those who were disturbed at only one period, either middle or late adolescence ($N = 12$). The consistently clear group presented as more adaptive than those who were consistently disturbed, and the fluctuating group usually fell in between. In affect (table 3), the consistently clear group demonstrated less anxiety, depression, and hate and more affection and pleasure. There were also differences in attitudes (table 4) among the three groups. The consistently clear group were found to be more cooperative, curious, approving, optimistic, and introspective and more interested in significant others.

Having established that there were differences in affect and attitudes associated with personality competence, we wished to identify those characteristics that would be associated with the development of more personality disturbance over time. We examined whether any affect or attitude of adolescents who were clear at age sixteen would differentiate those subjects who would continue to be clear at age eighteen ($N = 30$)

TABLE 3

AFFECT ASSOCIATED WITH STATUS OF PERSONALITY FUNCTIONING FROM MIDDLE
TO LATE ADOLESCENCE

Variable	Stable Clear $(N = 30)^a$	Stable Disturbed $(N = 17)^a$	Unstable Fluctuating $(N = 12)^a$	Significance[b]
Depression..............	1.6	2.7	2.0	.00001
	(.6)	(.6)	(.3)	
Pleasure	3.5	2.7	3.2	.00001
	(.4)	(.4)	(.2)	
Affection...............	3.4	2.7	3.2	.00001
	(.4)	(.5)	(.5)	
Anxiety................	2.9	3.5	2.8	.0015
	(.6)	(.5)	(.5)	
Hate...................	2.2	3.0	3.0	.00001
	(.4)	(.7)	(.7)	

[a] Mean scale score (standard deviation).

[b] Analysis of variance.

TABLE 4

PERSONALITY TRAITS ASSOCIATED WITH STATUS OF PERSONALITY FUNCTIONING FROM
MIDDLE TO LATE ADOLESCENCE

Variable	Stable Clear $(N = 30)^a$	Stable Disturbed $(N = 17)^a$	Unstable Fluctuating $(N = 12)^a$	Significance[b]
Cooperativeness	3.7	3.0	3.3	.0001
	(.4)	(.4)	(.3)	
Curiosity...............	3.3	2.6	3.1	.00001
	(.4)	(.5)	(.4)	
Approval...............	3.5	2.5	3.1	.00001
	(.5)	(.5)	(.5)	
Optimism	3.6	2.6	3.2	.00001
	(.4)	(.4)	(.3)	
Introspectiveness	2.8	2.1	2.7	.00001
	(.4)	(.5)	(.5)	
Overall relatedness.......	3.1	2.4	3.0	.00001
	(.4)	(.4)	(.4)	

[a] Mean scale score (standard deviation).

[b] Analysis of variance.

from those who would shift toward personality disturbance ($N = 9$). The comparison indicated that the one differentiating factor was that those who developed personality disturbance at age eighteen had shown significantly more feelings of hate at age sixteen. Those who remained clear of disturbance had a mean hate score of 2.1 (S.D. = .6), and those who became disturbed had a mean hate score of 2.8 (S.D. = .4). There was .003 level of significance to this difference.

Discussion

During the period from middle to late adolescence, overall competence of personality functioning tends to remain quite consistent. Older teenagers tend to be similar in personality functioning to the way they were in middle adolescence. Early adolescence appears to be a period of greater difficulty in the area of personality functioning, and there is improvement in the period from early to middle adolescence that is then maintained into late adolescence. Nevertheless, in terms of affect and attitudes, there are indications that late adolescence is a period of greater stress, whereas middle adolescence is more likely to be a period of relative stability and tranquility. In this respect, our findings confirm the observations of Lidz (1976) and Moriarity and Toussieng (1976).

Late adolescents demonstrate more dysphoria in the form of anxiety and depression than do middle adolescents. This increase in dysphoria parallels that seen in early adolescence but is qualitatively different and occurs in a different context. Very often, the older teenager is dealing with a number of stressful issues, such as educational or vocational decisions and commitment in personal relationships. Although identity formation with its internal and external tasks continues to be an important task, the conflicts in late adolescence are more clearly formed and crystalized. These may become outwardly manifest in the form of tension and sadness.

The attitudes observed in late adolescence have for the most part remained fairly consistent with those seen in middle adolescence. The changes in attitude that do occur point to an outward orientation, with an attempt at mastery rather than inner preoccupation. The finding that older teenagers have become more curious and dominant is consistant with the observation that they have become more emotionally involved with significant others and wish to take an active role in determining the nature of these relationships.

The increase in pessimism in late adolescence is consistent with the finding of more dysphoria. Previously, we had described an increase in optimism from early to middle adolescence, but two years later it appears that older teenagers are less hopeful in their perceptions of themselves and the world about them. It is likely that these feelings and attitudes are closely related to the "critical deidealization" (Blos

411

1977) of significant adults in their lives. The realistic appreciation of limitations in themselves and in significant others may have a sobering effect. It may be that the difficulties of identity resolution in late adolescence are a significant contributing factor in the development of depressive syndromes, which are seen much more frequently in this age group.

The continuity in personality functioning exhibited by these groups of adolescents is also apparent in the study of the individual teenager over the period from middle to late adolescence. An older adolescent is more likely to appear similar in a clinical interview and to have the same attitudes as two years earlier than to manifest dramatic changes.

An adolescent who does remain clear of personality function disturbance through the period from middle to late adolescence exhibits less dysphoria, more positive attitudes, and more adaptive coping skills. This finding is similar to the pattern seen in the period from early to middle adolescence and is further evidence that there is a relation and a continuity between personality functioning and affective regulation in adolescence. A well-functioning teenager does not tend suddenly to develop moodiness or different methods of dealing with situations or relationships during the adolescent years.

Those characteristics that are best able to distinguish personality competence from disturbed functioning in middle adolescence together constitute a pattern of involvement, identification, and approval of the surrounding world. In late adolescence, involvement and identification remain as powerful discriminators of personality functioning and are assisted by optimism and lack of dysphoria. At both ages, therefore, the ability of the adolescent to remain connected in a positive manner to the world around him is a very strong indication of personality competence.

The main differentiating characteristic of those middle adolescents who deteriorated in their personality functioning was increased hate. By comparison, the main differentiating characteristic of those early adolescents who improved in their personality functioning was decreased depression. In this nonclinical sample of teenagers, a relative increase in depressed mood in early adolescence and a relative increase in hatred in middle adolescence are both predictors of personality problems. This is an indication to take seriously those mood fluctuations that have in the past been relegated to the vicissitudes of normal adolescent development. These findings support other studies (Kashani, Carlson, Beck, et al. 1987) of community samples that have found clinically significant levels of dysphoria that are often undetected.

Blos has suggested that much of the rebellious behavior seen in late adolescents, especially angry activists, derives from the narcissistic rage provoked by the failure of society to live up to the fantasies of parental perfection (Blos 1972). The presence or absence of hate and depression, emotions that are related to and perhaps mirror images of one another, is a significant indicator of the nature of individual personality functioning and its changeability over time.

Conclusions

Both consistency and change are characteristic of personality functioning in teenagers as they grow from middle to late adolescence. The presence of prominent hatred in middle adolescence is an indicator that the individual is more likely to experience greater personality problems in late adolescence. More dysphoria in older teenagers without a concomitant increase in personality dysfunction points to the presence of greater stress associated with tasks at this stage of life: establishing intimacy with significant others and making important life decisions. Families, educators, and physicians should be aware that approximately one out of seven teenagers at both stages of life shows marked personality problems that might, therefore, come to the attention of a clinician to receive assessment and treatment.

REFERENCES

Arnold, L., and Smeltzer, D. 1974. Behavior checklist factor analysis for children and adolescents. *Archives of General Psychiatry* 30:799–804.

Arnstein, R. L. 1979. The adolescent identity crisis revisited. *Adolescent Psychiatry* 7:71–84.

Arnstein, R. L. 1980. The student, the family, the university and the transition to adulthood. *Adolescent Psychiatry* 8:160–172.

Bettelheim, B. 1971. Obsolete youth. *Adolescent Psychiatry* 1:14–39.

Blishen, B. 1967. A socioeconomic index for occupations in Canada. *Canadian Review of Social Anthropology* 4:41–53.

Blos, P. 1972. The function of the ego ideal in adolescence. *Psychoanalytic Study of the Child* 27:93–97.

Blos, P. 1977. When and how does adolescence end: structural criteria for adolescent closure. *Adolescent Psychiatry* 5:5–17.

Blotkey, M., and Looney, J. 1980. Normal female and male adolescent psychological development: an overview of theory and research. *Adolescent Psychiatry* 8:184–199.

Conners, C. 1969. A teacher rating scale for use in drug studies for children. *American Journal of Psychiatry* 126:152–156.

Esman, A. H. 1985. A developmental approach to the psychotherapy of adolescents. *Adolescent Psychiatry* 12:119–133.

Giovacchini, P. L., and Borowitz, G. H. 1974. An object relationship scale. *Adolescent Psychiatry* 3:186–195.

Golombek, H.; Marton, P.; Stein, B. A.; and Korenblum, M. 1986. A study of disturbed and nondisturbed adolescents: the Toronto Adolescent Longitudinal Study. *Canadian Journal of Psychiatry* 31:532–535.

Golombek, H.; Marton, P.; Stein, B. A.; and Korenblum, M. 1987. Personality functioning status during early and middle adolescence. *Adolescent Psychiatry* 14:365–377.

Kashani, J. H.; Carlson, G. B.; Beck, N. C.; et al. 1987. Depression, depressive symptoms and depressed mood among a community sample of adolescents. *American Journal of Psychiatry* 144(7): 931–934.

Lidz, T. 1976. *The Person: His and Her Development Throughout the Life Cycle*. New York: Basic.

Moriarity, A. E., and Toussieng, P. 1976. *Adolescent Coping*. New York: Grune & Stratten.

Stein, B. A.; Golombek, H.; Marton, P.; and Korenblum, M. 1986. Personality functioning and clinical presentation in early adolescence. *Canadian Journal of Psychiatry* 31:536–541.

Stein, B.; Golombek, H.; Marton, P.; and Korenblum, M. 1987. Personality functioning and change in clinical presentation from early to middle adolescence. *Adolescent Psychiatry* 14:378–393.

PART IV

PSYCHOPATHOLOGY AND PSYCHOTHERAPY OF ADOLESCENT EMOTIONAL DISORDERS

EDITORS' INTRODUCTION

This part includes a number of chapters concerned with various psychotherapies chosen to deal with adolescent psychopathology. Using a developmental approach, it is important to consider the pathological turn in growth as well as the conflict.

Richard C. Marohn reviews the determinants, consequences, and efficacy of violent delinquency in adolescents and compares the relation between adolescent and adult violence. He finds that adolescent violence presents unique formulations of psychopathology and treatment. Aggressive behavior appearing in the young can be predictive of adult disorder of a serious nature. Marohn discusses the determinants (socioeconomic factors, substance abuse, condoning groups and families, psychiatric disorders, and developmental traumas and delays), the consequences (juvenile violence leading to adult violence and a shifting of intervention to the correctional and juvenile justice systems), and treatment (psychotherapy, psychopharmacology, and milieu approaches). The author concludes that violent and unrestrained adolescents lead dangerous, risky lives. Difficult to handle, they are frequently shunted out of the mental health system; psychiatry should be able to provide the limits, contacts, and empathy they require.

Nancy H. Weil and Andrew M. Boxer describe a treatment program for impaired mothers: those who lack a remembered "good enough mother" who can function as a cohesive self- and selfobject introject. The women in their study were often overly dependent or hyperindependent in their relations. An interdependent relationship, characterized by maturity and reciprocity, was a task often difficult to achieve.

The structure of the treatment modality provides the opportunity for the development of a substitutive coparenting alliance between therapist and patient in the actual presence of the child. The authors relate the several dyadic relationships involved in this form of treatment: mother and child, mother and therapist, and child and therapist. While the therapist made considerable effort not to neglect either the mother or the child, both began to assert their needs and demand attention simultaneously. This eventually led to development in self-representation and finally transference and countertransference issues.

Susan J. Bradley studies panic disorder in children and adolescents, reviewing the biological basis, cognitive factors, and therapeutic response to both biological and psychological approaches. She confirms the existence of panic disorder in children and adolescents and notes that the disorder may coincide with other psychiatric disorders. She also supports early intervention to avoid development of avoidance or hypochondriacal behavioral patterns.

Demosthenes A. Lorandos reports that crime reports, incidence/prevalence data, and anecdotal evidence from social workers and psychologists describe children in community-based residential treatment programs as more pathological each year. This study proposes a null hypothesis: that boys in residential treatment do not differ significantly year to year or in five-year increments. Restrictive intake protocol and referral steering are discussed as possible reasons for resident homogeneity. It is concluded that boys in trouble are much the same as they have always been.

Kevin R. Ronan and Philip C. Kendall present a cognitive-behavioral approach to the therapy of impulsive, uncontrolled adolescents. This therapeutic regimen attempts to teach adolescents to control impulsive behavior through the use of problem-solving self-instructions aimed at reducing deficits in verbal mediation, social problem solving, and perspective taking. The procedures are designed to help the youngster cognitively mediate (stop and think about) problematic situations before embarking on a course of action.

23 VIOLENCE AND UNRESTRAINED BEHAVIOR IN ADOLESCENTS

RICHARD C. MAROHN

Most mental health professionals comprehend the sense and character of adolescent violence, but to understand and appreciate the extent of violent delinquency, its determinants, its consequences, and the efficacy of its treatment requires that the clinician be familiar with the work of others and reflect on the difficulties of working with this population.

The earliest and most significant therapeutic work with impulsive individuals was that of Aichhorn (1925, 1964), who had been impressed with Freud's ideas about the perversions and tried to apply them to the wayward youths of Vienna. Although we have moved beyond Aichhorn's ideas about transference gratification to achieve an internal dysphoria and now rely more on techniques of limit setting, we, nonetheless, continue to build on his discovery of narcissistic pathology and the idealizing transference in our appreciation of adolescent delinquency and behavioral disorders (Marohn 1977).

Our knowledge about these disabilities assists us in a general way to understand adolescent violence and unrestrained behavior, but there are differences, and one must recognize that adolescent violence presents unique formulations of psychopathology and treatment.

It is in the nature of the adolescent to act rather than to speak (Blos 1966), and, in this sense, adolescent violence is simply an exaggeration of this predilection for action and, even, impulsivity. Whether or not such a bent is manifested in "turmoil" (Freud 1958; Offer 1969), we can expect that a quiescence will descend with the closure of adolescence. Yet, in many, it does not, and I will examine in this chapter the relations between adolescent and adult violence, between violent behavior and death by violence, and between violent and suicidal behavior.

The relative tranquillity of young adulthood results from maturation and the development of self-regulating systems. Such healthy development emerges from complex biological, psychological, and social foundations, and there is much that can go awry. The assessment of adolescent health and psychopathology therefore becomes a matter of relative deviation rather than clear-cut syndromes. Our perspective, then, must be dynamic and systemic rather than classifying and sorting.

Finally, I will examine what happens to the violent delinquent when there is no intervention, which is rare, in the correctional system, and with various therapeutic approaches.

Extent

Approximately 25 percent of serious crimes, such as homicide, rape, robbery, aggravated assault, and arson, are committed by persons under eighteen years of age: 10 percent of all the murders, 19 percent of the rapes, 32 percent of the robberies, 17 percent of the aggravated assaults, and 32 percent of the arsons, even though this age group accounts for only about 15 percent of the population (Marohn 1979, 1982; Zimring 1978). About half the children brought to treatment are there because of aggressive behavior (O'Donnell 1985). Such behavior is often associated with attention-deficit disorders, with and without hyperactivity, schizophrenic and paranoid disorders, unipolar and bipolar affective disorders, seizure disorders, and "episodic dyscontrol" disorders. "Aggressivity is the most frequent and immediately distressing referral problem; and . . . nearly all reports of use and research into the pharmacology of conduct disorders focus on children with aggressive behaviors" (O'Donnell 1985, p. 253).

The earlier a child manifests a pattern of violent behavior, the longer and more extensive the career of violence will be (Loeber and Stouthamer-Loeber 1987; Monahan 1981; Ryan 1986; Temple and Ladouceur 1986). In fact, adult violence does not appear unless the child or adolescent was violent, except for very specific, newly developed disorders. "Early conduct problems—aggression, stealing, truancy, lying, drug use—are not only predictive many years later of

420

delinquency in general, but especially of serious delinquency, and in certain cases of recidivism" (Loeber and Stouthamer-Loeber 1987, p. 53).

Determinants

Although society and the government seem preoccupied with unemployment, racism, poor schools, and poverty as causing serious delinquency (Marohn 1979) and behavioral scientists and clinicians are routinely ignored when public policy is being formulated, other, more psychologically related factors need to be emphasized. Many violent adolescents use chemical substances to soothe and regulate themselves (Marohn 1983), and violent death, a serious problem for violent adolescents (Marohn, Locke, Rosenthal, and Curtiss 1982), is associated with alcohol use about 43 percent of the time in the fifteen to nineteen age group (Abel and Zeidenberg 1985).

Violent behavior is more likely to appear in those cultures and families that condone violence. Violence seems to gain greater approval as the child moves toward adolescence (Bush 1985). More violent boys think of themselves as healthy, whereas violent girls do not, and even treatment staff find something likable, or at least gratifying, in the violent patient (Offer, Marohn, and Ostrov 1975). While association with a delinquent peer group does not cause serious delinquency, it is predictive of it (Austin 1984).

Although adjudicated and institutionalized delinquents have higher than average rates of having been abused (i.e., 26–55 percent), there is no evidence that abuse leads to serious delinquency, for less than 20 percent of abused children become delinquent (Austin 1984). Family violence correlates closely with diagnosable psychiatric illness, particularly alcoholism with an antisocial personality disorder or recurrent depressions and suicide attempts (Bland and Orn 1986). Johnson and Szurek (1952) demonstrated that adolescents will enact the delinquent urges of their parents. Families that dismiss a child's temper tantrums, aggressive behavior, and noncompliance as "phases" will be confronted with further serious deviant behavior (O'Donnell 1985). When early separations from parents are more frequent, and when they occur at an earlier age, the child and adolescent are more likely to be behaviorally aggressive than self-destructive (Nielsen, Harrington, Sack, and Latham 1985). Fire setting often occurs at a time of family stress and disintegration (Bumpass, Brix, and Preston 1985; Bumpass,

421

Brix, and Reichland 1985; Bumpass, Fagelman, and Brix 1983; Bumpass, Via, Forgotson, and Fagelman 1974). Future delinquency in children was predicted by poor supervision at home, parental rejection of the child, lack of discipline and involvement by the parents, parental criminality and aggressiveness, and marital discord (Loeber and Stouthamer-Loeber 1987, p. 54).

Lewis and her colleagues (Lewis 1983; Lewis and Balla 1976; Lewis, Moy, Jackson, Aaronson, Restifo, Serra, and Simos 1985; Lewis, Pincus, Shanok, and Glaser 1982; Lewis and Shanok 1976; Lewis, Shanok, Pincus, and Glaser 1979; see also Lewis 1987 as cited in Adams 1987) have emphasized the neurological disorders and psychosis that underlie serious and violent delinquency. Their work is important because it serves to spotlight the serious needs of the violent and incarcerated delinquent. However, it is important to recognize that the history of head injury and other abuse that they describe also occurs in a family atmosphere that psychologically affects the developing child and adolescent. The prevalence of neurologic "soft signs" has not been replicated. Benedek, Cornell, and Staresina (1987) found a significantly lower incidence of psychosis in a population of adolescent murderers.

Other biological factors that have been associated with violence include an XYY chromosomal pattern, testosterone, seizure disorders with or without abnormal EEGs, and altered serotonin levels.

The effort to elucidate the individual psychodynamics of serious delinquent behavior has a long history. Winnicott (1958, 1973) described the "antisocial tendency" of the delinquent to test destructively and to seek out a stable, structured relationship. Redl (1966; Redl and Wineman 1957) wrote repeatedly about the possibility of understanding violent behavior and reversing the process by providing auxiliary psychological functions through caretakers.

Our own work at the Illinois State Psychiatric Institute concentrated on the understanding and management of adolescent violence. There is a close correlation between verbal threats of violence, damage to property, and assault on person, and threats, if unchecked, will escalate to physical assault (Marohn, Dalle-Molle, McCarter, and Linn 1980), whereas the verbal catharsis of angry feelings, without threat, does not correlate with further violent behavior (Curtiss, Rosenthal, Marohn, Ostrov, Offer, and Trujillo 1983; Ostrov, Marohn, Offer, Curtiss, and Feczko 1980).

Just as we must not assume that the more serious and socially unacceptable behavior is indicative of necessarily serious psychopathology, we should not equate violence with hostile or destructive motives. Many adolescents behave violently because they experience periods of traumatic overstimulation, often from strong wishes for affectionate contact that overwhelm them (Marohn 1974). Institutional riots result in part from such problems in tension regulation as well as from the tendency of property violence to intensify to personal violence (Marohn, Dalle-Molle, Offer, and Ostrov 1973; Zinn and Miller 1978).

Nonetheless, there are adolescents who express in their violence rage and destructiveness, the rage of a primitive narcissistic personality. They destroy an offending other, one who fails to mirror or sustain them, or one who fails to live up to their idealized expectations; or they try to reconstitute a crumbling self by actively turning an injury into an assault, utilizing a familiar behavior pattern, destructiveness, to do so (Kohut 1972; Marohn 1977; Newman 1974). Infant research has reemphasized the importance of the "self-regulating other" in the development of internal regulating systems (Stern 1985), and the regulation of primitive drive and narcissistic constituents is crucial to the growth of a nonviolent child and adolescent. Stechler (1987; Stechler and Halton 1987) has proposed another interesting model for the establishment of destructive aggression, that the parental responses to the child's assertiveness confuse or thwart such self-expression and that assertiveness, a motivation, becomes contaminated with aggression, a reaction like Kohut's narcissistic rage. In some, assertiveness is inhibited or stimulates guilt; in others, aggression may itself become an assertive mode of self-expression, and violence to others is the outcome.

Many clinicians and theorists have believed that depression and violence are diametrically opposed, that the violent individual is not suicidal, and that the depressed individual, having internalized his aggression, is not violent. Indeed, one treatment for depression involved helping the patient express his or her anger and aggression verbally or in an acceptable activity. We now know that such is not the case (Marohn et al. 1982; Shaffer, Garland, Gould, Fisher, and Trautman 1988). Violent adolescents are often suicidal, and the violent, delinquent adolescent is at great risk for suicidal behavior.

Violent behavior is multiply determined and complex, and there are many contributing factors to the final common pathway of violent delinquency. Fundamental is the realization that all behavior has psychological meaning and that the violent act can be understood psychodynamically (Marohn et al. 1980; Offer, Marohn, and Ostrov 1979).

Violent acts are occasional, and few delinquents are chronically violent, but these recidivists are responsible for the greatest proportion of juvenile violence and pose serious social and health problems. The violence of the older adolescent, of the minority, especially black, adolescent, and of the poor adolescent is more likely to be serious. Most violent adolescents are not psychotic, although they demonstrate poor impulse control; many, if not most, have learning problems (Strasburg 1978).

Consequences

The most reliable predictor of adult violence is juvenile violence (Wolfgang 1978). Yet for interventions in juvenile violence to be rational and effective some understanding of the natural history of the condition is required. Rarely is juvenile violence untreated. Any intervention—by the police, by the school, by the juvenile court—affects the outcome. Perhaps our focus can be only the consequences of juvenile violence altered by various and different interventions, some correctional, some psychiatric, some other.

Another problem that the student of outcome faces is that in many states juvenile delinquency data do not follow the person into his or her adulthood (Maltz 1984). There are many adult criminals who when arrested for their first adult crime are characterized as "first offenders" whether or not they had previous juvenile offenses, even violent. Thus, we may not find valid juvenile follow-up data in the adult records.

A third difficulty is the many layers in the juvenile justice system—police discretion on the street, the caseworker's discretion in preparing the presentence investigation report, the biases of the juvenile officer who investigates, or the options and preferences of the juvenile court judge—which cannot be controlled and which increase the variability of the data. Solid comparisons between diverse intervention systems become difficult, if not impossible (Maltz 1984). Girls are often excused for their behavior; therefore, when a girl's acting out finally comes to the attention of authorities, it may have become quite serious. Boys' behavior is taken more seriously because it is more of a threat. Black male adolescent violence is often considered normative by both black and white professionals, whereas white violence is often considered a manifestation of an underlying psychopathology.

Apparently, children who had been treated in the mental health system shift to the correctional and juvenile justice systems as they become adolescents, probably because their behavior becomes more violent and their size makes them more difficult to manage. Many disturbed adolescents in correctional facilities were transferred there from therapeutic settings because their behavior had become threatening to staff, and such correctional settings are now expected to function as psychiatric treatment units for disturbed and violent adolescents (Lewis and Shanok 1976).

A study of over 1,400 eleven- to seventeen-year-olds by Elliott, Huizinga, and Morse (1986) produced a subsample of about 120 seriously violent offenders and demonstrated that the involvement in violent activity lasted less than one year, that individual offense rates increased over time, and that the variety of crimes became more diversified over time. They conclude that incarcerated violent delinquents do not represent the population at large committing such offenses.

Although in a general sense adolescent violence does predict adult violence, the pattern of violence must have evolved by a critical period. It seems that an aggression pattern at age thirteen or grades five or six is more predictive of later adult violence than it is at age eight or grades three or four: "Early adolescence probably is a time when aggressiveness has crystallized and becomes highly predictive of aggression and delinquency. . . . Children who have not outgrown their aggressiveness by early adolescence appear at high risk for delinquency and aggressiveness later. . . . Although juvenile arrest or conviction is a predictor of arrest or conviction in adulthood, the seriousness of the juvenile offense appears a better predictor of the continued, serious delinquency in adulthood" (Loeber and Stouthamer-Loeber 1987, pp. 41, 54).

Treatment

Violent adolescents are difficult to treat; their adjustment is fragile, and, when threatened, they may become violent. Their hostility, negativism, and violence are inevitably repeated in their treatment, and, as a result, many therapists avoid this kind of patient (Marohn 1981). Yet to avoid these patients' violence or to try simply to support them is to fail them (Kernberg 1975). Whether their rage is the result of a destructive inner drive (Kernberg 1974, 1979) or the rage attendant on an inevitable narcissistic injury, it must be met by a confident and secure therapist (Marohn 1985).

Often, violent adolescents lack the personal resources or the psychological support of peers or family to confront their pathology and violence in office therapy, and then they need the selfobject relationships of a hospital or residential treatment staff (Easson 1969). Here, the staff perform extremely important sustaining functions for violent patients, who are invariably structurally deficient; they help to complete the adolescents' self. The psychotherapist focuses on the associative material brought to him or her, not just verbally in the office session, but also by the patient's behavior on the treatment unit (Marohn et al. 1980).

Many violent adolescents are alexithymic and simply experience affect but cannot use affect as a communication. They have little awareness of an inner psychological world, cannot name affects or differentiate one from another, and often confuse thought, feeling, and deed. This kind of adolescent does not "act out" because "inside" and "outside" are one and to think is to feel is to do something. When these adolescents say that they did something because they "felt like it," they are often accurately describing their psychological state. Our task is to help them accomplish an important adolescent transformation, experiencing affect as part of themselves and developing the capacity to manage affect and use it effectively as a self-communication (Krystal 1974, 1975, 1978; Marohn 1983). When we try to engage these adolescents in a verbal treatment, not only do we try to help them begin to experience and learn about an inner psychological world, but we try to facilitate certain maturational steps, converting motor behavior to verbal behavior.

Medication can be readily integrated into such a milieu and psychotherapy approach, not only for the physiological indications in certain situations, but also to facilitate pacifying and organizing the patient's inner psychological world. Physical restraints, patient holding, and seclusion rooms can also be part of the therapeutic armamentarium in working with the hospitalized violent adolescent, even though in some situations they may be subject to abuse and misuse or used too hastily

426

or frequently instead of more difficult assessment and intervention (Bornstein 1985; Tomkiewicz 1984).

A careful diagnostic assessment is essential to successful treatment of the violent adolescent. The prevalent psychiatric condition, for example, a bipolar affective disorder or a narcissistic behavior disorder, becomes the focus of the treatment, not the violence as such, and an integrated treatment approach of psychotherapy, psychopharmacology, and milieu is formulated. Careful supervision of the treatment staff and of the psychotherapist provides the sustenance needed to work with these difficult and demanding patients.

There are no research or clinical data that justify the use of psychopharmacologic agents alone in treating the violent adolescent, without appropriate psychosocial and behavioral interventions (O'Donnell 1985). Neuroleptics, such as thioridazine, perphenazine, haloperidol, and the benzodiazepines; lithium, which is especially useful because it is not sedating; anticonvulsants, such as diphenylhydantoin, primidone, or carbamazepine; central nervous system stimulants, such as dextroamphetamine, pemoline, or methylphenidate; antidepressants, such as the tricyclics; and the beta blockers, such as propranolol or metoprolol, have all been recommended for treating violent behavior, depending on the underlying neurophysiological pathology.

Conclusions

Violent and unrestrained adolescents lead risky lives and face violent death more frequently than average teenagers. When we confront them in treatment, they are usually difficult to work with; they are resistant, they frustrate us; they, and we, do not understand their motives or their behavior; and, because they are often psychologically damaged and severely deficient, they are not "attractive" patients. When they show up in the public sector, they are usually shunted out of the mental health system (which can attend only to psychotic or suicidal patients) and into the correctional system, where they are faced with no or uncertain diagnosis, little or no psychotherapy, poorly monitored psychopharmacology, and an attitude that behavior is consciously determined and under one's voluntary and moral control. If psychotherapy is attempted, the therapist is often confronted with a negativistic, hostile, sometimes violent patient, who is thought to be incapable of establishing a treatment alliance and is accordingly untreatable.

The challenge is extensive and serious, but not hopeless. Violent and delinquent youths continue to search for the lost contact, the self-regulating other. Their behavior often expresses that search, their efforts to recapture the selfobject. Because they continue to search for those missing parts of themselves, we must respond by offering the limits, contact, and empathy that they require.

They may include the therapist in their search.

REFERENCES

Abel, E. L., and Zeidenberg, P. 1985. Age, alcohol and violent death: a postmortem study. *Journal of Studies of Alcohol* 46:228–231.

Adams, J. 1987. Risk of violence in teens can be identified early. *Clinical Psychiatric News* (December), pp. 1, 16.

Aichhorn, A. 1925. *Wayward Youth*. New York: Viking.

Aichhorn, A. 1964. *Delinquency and Child Guidance—Selected Papers*. New York: International Universities Press.

Austin, J. 1984. Statement before the Select Committee on Children, Youth, and Families, House of Representatives, May 18, 1984. In *Youth and the Justice System: Can We Intervene Earlier?* Washington, D.C.: U.S. Government Printing Office.

Benedek, E. P.; Cornell, D. G.; and Staresina, L. 1987. Violence and adolescence. *Psychiatric Times* (October), pp. 2, 4.

Bland, R., and Orn, H. 1986. Family violence and psychiatric disorder. *Canadian Journal of Psychiatry* 31:129–137.

Blos, P. 1966. The concept of acting out in relation to the adolescent process. In E. N. Rexford, ed. *A Developmental Approach to the Problems of Acting Out*. New York: International Universities Press.

Bornstein, P. E. 1985. The use of restraints on a general psychiatric unit. *Journal of Clinical Psychiatry* 46:175–178.

Bumpass, E.; Brix, R. J.; and Preston, D. 1985. A community based program for juvenile firesetters. *Hospital and Community Psychiatry* 36:529–533.

Bumpass, E.; Brix, R. J.; and Reichland, R. E. 1985. Triggering events, sequential feelings and firesetting behavior in children:

proceedings for papers and new research posters. *Journal of the American Academy of Child Psychiatry* 10:18.

Bumpass, E.; Fagelman, F. D.; and Brix, R. J. 1983. Intervention with children who set fires. *American Journal of Psychotherapy* 37:328–345.

Bumpass, E.; Via, B. M.; Forgotson, J. H.; and Fagelman, F. D. 1974. Graphs to facilitate the formation of a therapeutic alliance. *American Journal of Psychotherapy* 28:500–516.

Bush, D. M. 1985. Victimization at school and attitudes toward violence among early adolescents. *Sociological Spectrum* 5:173–190.

Curtiss, G.; Rostenthal, R. H.; Marohn, R. C.; Ostrov, E.; Offer, D.; and Trujillo, J. 1983. Measuring delinquent behavior in inpatient treatment settings: revision and validation of the adolescent antisocial behavior checklist. *Journal of the American Academy of Child Psychiatry* 22:459–466.

Easson, W. M. 1969. *The Severely Disturbed Adolescent*. New York: International Universities Press.

Elliott, D. S.; Huizinga, D.; and Morse, B. 1986. Self-reported violent offending: a descriptive analysis of juvenile violent offenders and their offending careers. *Journal of Interpersonal Violence* 1:472–514.

Freud, A. 1958. Adolescence. *Psychoanalytic Study of the Child* 13:255–278.

Johnson, A. M., and Szurek, S. A. 1952. The genesis of antisocial acting out in children and adults. *Psychoanalytic Quarterly* 21:323–343.

Kernberg, O. 1974. Further contributions to the treatment of narcissistic personalities. *International Journal of Psycho-Analysis* 55:215–240.

Kernberg, O. 1975. *Borderline Conditions and Pathological Narcissism*. New York: Aronson.

Kernberg, O. 1979. Psychoanalytic psychotherapy with borderline adolescents. *Adolescent Psychiatry* 7:294–321.

Kohut, H. 1972. Thoughts on narcissism and narcissistic rage. *Psychoanalytic Study of the Child* 27:360–400.

Krystal, H. 1974. The genetic development of affects and affect regression. *Annual of Psychoanalysis* 2:98–126.

Krystal, H. 1975. Affect tolerance. *Annual of Psychoanalysis* 3:179–219.

Krystal, H. 1978. Self-representation and the capacity for self-care. *Annual of Psychoanalysis* 6:209–246.

Lewis, D. O. 1983. Neuropsychiatric vulnerabilities and violence, juvenile delinquency. *Psychiatric Clinics of North America* 4:707–714.

Lewis, D. O., and Balla, D. 1976. *Delinquency and Psychopathology*. New York: Grune & Stratton.

Lewis, D. O.; Moy, E.; Jackson, L. D.; Aaronson, R.; Restifo, N.; Serra, S.; and Simos, A. 1985. Biopsychosocial characteristics of children who later murder: a prospective study. *American Journal of Psychiatry* 142:1161–1167.

Lewis, D. O.; Pincus, J. H.; Shanok, S. S.; and Glaser, G. H. 1982. Psychomotor epilepsy and violence in a group of incarcerated adolescent boys. *American Journal of Psychiatry* 139:882–887.

Lewis, D. O., and Shanok, S. S. 1976. Medical histories of delinquent and nondelinquent children. *American Journal of Psychiatry* 134:1020–1025.

Lewis, D. O.; Shanok, S. S.; Pincus, J. H.; and Glaser, G. G. 1979. Violent juvenile delinquents: psychiatric neurological, psychological and abuse factors. *Journal of the American Academy of Child Psychiatry* 18:307–319.

Loeber, R., and Stouthamer-Loeber, M. 1987. The prediction of delinquency. In H. C. Quay, ed. *Handbook of Juvenile Delinquency*. New York: Wiley.

Maltz, M. D. 1984. *Recidivism*. New York: Academic.

Marohn, R. C. 1974. Trauma and the delinquent. *Adolescent Psychiatry* 3:354–361.

Marohn, R. C. 1977. The "juvenile imposter": some thoughts on narcissism and the delinquent. *Adolescent Psychiatry* 5:186–212.

Marohn, R. C. 1979. A psychiatric overview of juvenile delinquency. *Adolescent Psychiatry* 7:425–432.

Marohn, R. C. 1981. The negative transference in the treatment of juvenile delinquents. *Annual of Psychoanalysis* 9:21–42.

Marohn, R. C. 1983. Adolescent substance abuse: a problem of self soothing. In *Clinical Update in Adolescent Psychiatry,* vol. 1, no. 10. Princeton, N.J.: Nassau.

Marohn, R. C. 1985. Assertiveness in the treatment of juvenile delinquents. *Psychiatric Annals* 15:606–613.

Marohn, R. C.; Dalle-Molle, D.; McCarter, E.; and Linn, D. 1980. *Juvenile Delinquents: Psychodynamic Assessment and Hospital Assessment*. New York: Brunner/Mazel.

Marohn, R. C.; Dalle-Molle, D.; Offer, D.; and Ostrov, E. 1973. A hospital riot: its determinants and implications for treatment. *American Journal of Psychiatry* 130:631–636.

Marohn, R. C.; Locke, E. M.; Rosenthal, R.; and Curtiss, G. 1982. Juvenile delinquents and violent death. *Adolescent Psychiatry* 10:147–170.

Monahan, J. 1981. *The Clinical Prediction of Violent Behavior.* Rockville, Md.: National Institute of Mental Health.

Newman, K. 1974. Some applications of concepts of the self to management of adolescents in the hospital. Paper presented to the Chicago Society for Adolescent Psychiatry, February 23, 1974.

Nielsen, G.; Harrington, L.; Sack, W.; and Latham S. 1985. A developmental study of aggression and self-destruction in adolescents who received residential treatment. *International Journal of Offender Therapy and Comparative Criminology* 29:211–226.

O'Donnell, D. J. 1985. Conduct disorders. In J. M. Weiner, ed. *Diagnosis and Psychopharmacology of Childhood and Adolescent Disorders.* New York: Wiley.

Offer, D. 1969. *The Psychological World of the Teenager.* New York: Basic.

Offer, D.; Marohn, R. C.; and Ostrov, E. 1975. Violence among hospitalized delinquents. *Archives of General Psychiatry* 32:1180–1186.

Offer, D.; Marohn, R. C.; and Ostrov, E. 1979. *The Psychological World of the Juvenile Delinquent.* New York: Basic.

Ostrov, E.; Marohn, R. C.; Offer, D.; Curtiss, G.; and Feczko, M. 1980. The adolescent antisocial behavior check list. *Journal of Clinical Psychology* 36:594–601.

Redl, F. 1966. *When We Deal with Children.* New York: Free Press.

Redl, F., and Wineman, D. 1957. *The Aggressive Child.* Glencoe, Ill.: Free Press.

Ryan, G. 1986. Annotated bibliography: adolescent perpetrators of sexual molestation of children. *Child Abuse and Neglect* 10:125–131.

Shaffer, D.; Garland, A.; Gould, M.; Fisher, P.; and Trautman, P. 1988. Preventing teenage suicide: a critical review. *Journal of the American Academy of Child and Adolescent Psychiatry* 27:675–687.

Stechler, G. 1987. Clinical applications of a psychoanalytic systems model of assertion and aggression. *Psychoanalytic Inquiry* 7:348–363.

Stechler, G., and Halton, A. 1987. The emergence of assertion and aggression during infancy: a psychoanalytic systems approach. *Journal of the American Psychoanalytic Association* 35:821–838.

Stern, D. N. 1985. *The Interpersonal World of the Infant.* New York: Basic.

Strasburg, P. A. 1978. *Violent Delinquents.* New York: Sovereign.

Temple, M., and Ladouceur, P. 1986. The alcohol-crime relationship as an age-specific phenomenon: a longitudinal study. *Contemporary Drug Problems* 13:89–115.

Tomkiewicz, S. 1984. Violences et negligences envers les enfants et les adolescents dans les institutions (Violence and negligence to children and adolescents in institutions). *Child Abuse and Neglect* 8:319–335.

Winnicott, D. W. 1958. The antisocial tendency. In *Collected Papers.* New York: Basic.

Winnicott, D. W. 1973. Delinquency as a sign of hope. *Adolescent Psychiatry* 2:364–371.

Wolfgang, M. E. 1978. An overview of research and violent behavior. Testimony before the U.S. House of Representatives, Committee on Science and Technology.

Zimring, F. 1978. Background paper. In *Confronting Youth Crime: Report of the Twentieth Century Fund Task Force on Sentencing Policy toward Young Offenders.* New York: Holmes & Meier.

Zinn, L. D., and Miller, D. H. 1978. Riots on adolescent inpatient units. *Journal of the National Association of Private Psychiatric Hospitals* 9:42–51.

SUSAN J. BRADLEY

The study of panic disorder today is an examination involving all the currently salient areas in psychiatry. Family studies, infusion techniques, inhalation studies, and drug response all suggest a biological basis for this disorder. Cognitive factors, however, also appear to be important. The co-occurrence of panic disorder with most other major psychiatric disorders raises issues as to whether panic anxiety is simply severe anxiety or, as Klein (1981) has argued, a unique biological entity, central to the development of other psychopathology. Finally, the fact that panic disorder responds to both biological and psychotherapeutic interventions has added to the interest in this disorder. Despite an immense amount of study in adults, relatively little attention has been directed to this entity in children and adolescents.

Background Literature—General

Panic disorder (PD) is defined in DSM-III-R (American Psychiatric Association 1987, p. 235) as recurrent discrete "periods of intense fear or discomfort with at least four characteristic associated symptoms." Most commonly reported symptoms are heart pounding, trembling and shaking, sweating, hot or cold flashes, fear of dying, dizziness, and breathing difficulty. Age of onset peaks around age sixteen; this holds true for individuals with simple attacks, for those with severe and recurrent attacks, and for those with full-blown PD. The male to female ratio is roughly 1:2.5. In adults, the past-six-months prevalence is 3 percent for any type of panic attack, 1.5 percent for severe and recurrent attacks, and 0.6–1 percent for PD (Von Korff, Eaton, and Keyl 1985).

Panic disorder has been associated for many years with mitral valve prolapse. Although this relation has been most logically explained as being due to a common autonomic dysregulation, some doubt now exists as to whether the connection is real (Margraf, Ehlers, and Roth 1988; Sevin 1987) or meaningful (Gorman, Goetz, Fyer, King, Fyer, Liebowitz, and Klein 1988; Margraf et al. 1988; Weissman, Kramer-Fox, Devereaux, and Shear 1987). Panic disorder patients may, however, be at increased risk for death due to cardiovascular causes (Coryell, Noyes, and House 1986), and patients with idiopathic cardiomyopathy (undergoing cardiac transplant) appear to have an increased frequency of PD compared to transplant patients with other types of heart disease (Kahn, Drusin, and Klein 1987).

Many symptoms of PD overlap with symptoms of hyperventilation. This fact has led to a number of studies attempting to explore whether PD causes hyperventilation or hyperventilation causes PD or whether both have a common etiology (Cowley and Roy-Byrne 1987). It is clear that hyperventilation of room air can induce panic attacks in some individuals (Gorman, Fyer, Goetz, Askanazi, Liebowitz, Fyer, Kinney, and Klein 1988). However, not all PD patients experience panic attacks with hyperventilation. This has led Gorman, Fyer, et al. (1988) to suggest that a subgroup of PD patients may be primarily hyperventilators and that breathing retraining may be specifically useful with this subgroup. Others suggest that PD and hyperventilation are both part of a hypersensitive alarm response, which may be mutually reinforcing (Cowley and Roy-Byrne 1987).

Panic disorder occurs much more frequently in patients with other psychiatric disorders than it does in the normal population. The odds of having PD are increased 4.3 times with alcohol abuse or dependency, eighteen times with agoraphobia, nineteen times with depression, twenty-one times with obsessive/compulsive disorder, twenty-four times with mania, thirty-eight times with schizophrenia, and ninety-six times with somatization disorder (Boyd, Burke, Gruenberg, Holzer, Rae, George, Karno, Stoltzman, McEvoy, and Nestadt 1984). Other psychiatric symptomatology and disorders are also found frequently in patients with PD. These include anticipatory anxiety and generalized anxiety disorder, depression, alcoholism, obsessive/compulsive disorder, and hypochondriasis (Breier, Charney, and Heninger 1984; Katon, Vitaliano, Russo, Jones, and Anderson 1987; Mellman and Uhde 1987). Family studies support these connections as well (Crowe, Pauls, Slymen, and Noyes 1980; Leckman, Weissman, Merikangas, Pauls, and Prusoff 1983; Munjack and Moss 1981; Noyes, Clancy, Crowe, Hoenk, and Slymen 1978). The fact that PD responds to tricyclic antidepressants, to monoamine oxidase inhibitors (Pohl, Berchou, and Rainey 1982), and, more recently, to both alprazolam (Ballenger, Burrows, DuPont, Lesser, Noyes, Pecknold, Rifkin, and Swinson 1988) and clonazepam (Fontaine and Chouinard 1984) adds further interest to the debate about whether PD is a unique disorder (Aronson 1987). Finally, a linkage between separation anxiety/school phobia and PD (especially PD with agoraphobia) has been suggested by the apparently high frequency of these disorders in the childhood histories of patients with PD (Casat 1988; Klein 1964; Perugi, Deltito, Soriani, Musetti, Petracca, Nisita, Maremmani, and Cassano 1988).

Panic attacks frequently become associated with phobically avoided situations or triggers. Individuals may learn to suppress or avoid further attacks by avoiding these situations. Fears of being alone, of being in a crowded place, and of heights are common examples. Panic attacks can also be induced in vulnerable individuals through lactate infusion, carbon dioxide inhalation, and yohimbine and isoproterenol administration as well as by such self-administered agents as caffeine, alcohol, nicotine, over-the-counter cold preparations, cannabis, and cocaine. Sleep deprivation, dieting, exercise, relaxation, hyperventilation, fluorescent lighting, and life stressors have also been found to induce panic attacks. (For a review of exogenous factors, see Roy-Byrne and Uhde 1988.) Temporal lobe seizures have been suggested as an etiologic factor by others (Edlund, Swann, and Clothier 1987; Signer 1988; Weilburg, Bear, and Sachs 1987). Pregnancy, on the contrary, may have an ameliorating effect on PD (George, Ladenheim, and Nutt 1987). Cognitive factors may also be important in exacerbating or ameliorating the experience of panic attacks (Rachman, Levitt, and Lopatka 1987; Vitaliano, Katon, Russo, Maiuro, Anderson, and Jones 1987). Vitaliano et al. (1987) found that patients with PD tended to use less problem-focused strategies and more wishful thinking than patients with simple panic attacks and non-PD controls. As well, within the PD group, the presence of anxiety and depression correlated negatively with problem-focused coping and positively with wishful thinking.

Studies of Children and Adolescents with Panic Attacks or PD

As mentioned previously, the child and adolescent literature is scant. Anecdotal reports covering a total of nine children and adolescents with PD have focused on such issues as connections with neurological disorders (Herskowitz 1986), mitral valve prolapse (Vitiello, Behar, Wolfson, and Delaney 1987), and response to treatment (Biederman 1987). In the only published empirical study in this area, Alessi, Robbins, and Dilsaver (1987) conducted interviews with sixty-one adolescent psychiatric inpatients using DSM-III diagnostic criteria. They found ten cases (15 percent) who met criteria for definite PD and fifteen cases (24 percent) with definite or possible PD. Of the ten cases with definite PD, nine also met criteria for a depressive disorder. When they compared their depressed with their nondepressed patients, nine out of twenty-eight depressed patients had definite PD, whereas only one out of twenty-eight nondepressed patients did. Borderline personality disorder was the most frequent DSM-III, Axis II, diagnosis, occurring in 50 percent of the PD cases.

In an unpublished study, Bradley, Wachsmuth, Swinson, and Hnatko (1986) examined the prevalence of panic attacks and PD in an outpatient sample of 295 child and adolescent psychiatric patients. In this questionnaire survey of child psychiatrists, the overall prevalence rate for panic attacks was 26 percent in patients between four and nineteen years of age. The male to female ratio was 1:1.8. Panic disorder was reported in 10 percent of the total patient sample (5 percent of males, 17 percent of females). The percentage of patients with panic attacks, according to sex, age, and diagnostic category, is shown in table 1. This study was limited by a low response rate among the psychiatrists surveyed and by an inability to validate diagnoses.

Nelles and Barlow (1988) have questioned whether children can experience panic attacks. Although they acknowledge that children may experience the somatic manifestations of panic attacks, they suggest that children's cognitive development may limit their capacity

TABLE 1

PERCENTAGE OF PATIENTS WITH PANIC ATTACKS
ACCORDING TO SEX, AGE, DIAGNOSTIC GROUP

		Panic Attacks	
	Sample (N)	(N)	(%)
Sex:			
Males	171	33	19
Females	124	44	35**
Total	295	77	26
Age:			
11 years or under	83	12	14
12–15 years	115	22	19
16–19 years	97	43	44***
Total	295	77	26
Diagnostic group:			
Conduct disorder	51	7	14*
Anxiety disorder	45	22	49***
Adjustment disorder	43	9	21
Affective disorder	40	13	33
Oppositional disorder	13	0	0*
Attention deficit disorder	13	1	8
Psychotic disorder	12	6	50
Developmental disorder	11	2	18
Eating disorder	13	3	23
Personality disorder	13	7	54*
Total	254	70	28

Source.—Bradley, Wachsmuth, Swinson, and Hnatko (1986).
* $p < .05$.
** $p < .01$.
*** $p < .001$.

to conceptualize their experience as "panic." While it may be important to clarify how children experience panic attacks, the conclusion that they do not experience panic attacks because of cognitive immaturity does not seem justified. Nonfearful panic attacks have been described in adults (Beitman, Basha, Flaker, DeRosear, Mukerji, and Lamberti 1986) and do not appear to differ in other respects from panic attacks with true "panic." Also, reduction in hypochondriasis in the treatment of PD in adults suggests that many individuals do not label their experience as "panic" (Aronson and Logue 1988; Noyes, Reich, Clancy, and O'Gorman 1986).

More intensive study of individual cases and empirical investigations are needed to address the obvious questions of relevance of PD to the practice of adolescent psychiatry. Careful case study may help define the intricate interplay between PD and other psychopathology. The following cases provide some examples of this intricacy as well as demonstrating some of the ways in which this interesting disorder may be manifest.

CASE EXAMPLE 1

A sixteen-year-old female was referred because of somatic complaints and a fear of going into class and taking tests. She was contemplating leaving school because of her inability to control these feelings. The patient reported her first attack at age ten during a test situation. She recalled a sudden onset at that point of her heart beating fast, a sense of burning pain in her stomach, a feeling of her head pounding, and her hands sweating. She acknowledged worry about failing her test but was shocked and puzzled by the intensity of her feelings. This attack lasted for the duration of the test, which she estimated to be about thirty minutes. She reported several of these attacks in grades 5–8, largely related to tests or times when she had to give an oral presentation. In addition to the spontaneously reported symptoms, on direct questioning she reported a sense of difficulty breathing, chest pain, dizziness, and tingling feelings in her hands as well as feeling shaky. She denied a fear of dying or of going crazy but instead reported shock at the intensity of these experiences, which she felt were an intensification of her worry about herself. The most obvious precipitating factor related to the onset of her first attack appeared to be the death of her maternal grandmother. In addition, she identified loss of her paternal grandmother and maternal grandfather as precipitants for bouts of further attacks two to three years prior to the assessment. At the time of the loss of her grandparents, she reported feeling "down," with trouble sleeping, a reluctance to go out, and a sense that people were looking at her. These feelings lasted for approximately a month at the time of the deaths of her grandparents.

In the year prior to the assessment, the patient had been investigated thoroughly for somatic complaints involving pain in her knees and stomach. Because of this, she had missed a lot of school. Coincident with this, her panic attacks increased to the almost daily basis that she reported at the time of the assessment. She also indicated further increases to several times a day if she was having tests. She related that she would normally get up in the morning with a slight feeling of stomach discomfort. When she went to school she would experience a full-blown panic attack that would gradually alleviate with her sitting down and telling herself that it would go away. She reported that she experienced the same feelings if she had to go on an elevator alone. She was aware of worries about being trapped and, in such a circumstance, normally would avoid having to go on an elevator alone. She indicated, however, that, if she had to do this, she would simply have to force herself. The patient was unaware of any precipitants related to her panic attacks. There was no use of coffee, tea, or street drugs or any relation to exercise. Avoidance behavior centered around the beginning sense that she might have to leave school in order to control these feelings. There were no particular socially phobic behaviors, and she appeared to be performing adequately in school given a low average IQ.

Psychiatric assessment did not reveal any other significant psychopathology. Exploration of family history revealed psychiatric illness in a paternal uncle; her father was judged to be depressed at the time of the initial assessment. There was no other family history of panic attacks or PD. Early history of separation anxiety in the patient was absent. Although there was no formal testing done of her coping strategies, it was the examiner's impression that one of the protective factors, despite the long history of panic attacks, was that this girl and her parents had an expectation that one had to do one's best in a difficult situation. There was little reinforcement of an avoidance response. The patient was placed on imipramine, 100 milligrams at bedtime. This produced a complete remission of her panic attacks. She also reported that, since that time, she had been going to school regularly with no further difficulties and she was no longer experiencing the somatic concerns for which she had been investigated. Although she acknowledged occasional recurrence of panic anxiety, it was of such diminished intensity that she was quite able to cope. The patient was comfortable with the information given to her about her disorder and seemed willing to accept medication as a necessary way of dealing with her illness.

CASE EXAMPLE 2

A sixteen-year-old Caucasian male admitted to the medical ward because of longstanding headaches and obesity was referred for psychiatric assessment. During the assessment, he described having "attacks." These occurred on looking up at tall buildings or down from a height. He described a feeling of the building swaying around him and a fear that it would fall down on him. He experienced a sensation of being dizzy, weak, and faint. He described feeling his heart beating faster and sweating all over, with chest pain and shivers going up and down his spine. He also sensed that everyone was looking at him. These panic attacks began at age four, when he first came to a large city with skyscrapers. In addition, he reported a similar type of feeling, although not as intense, when he was fishing with his father, looked over the side of the boat, and thought how deep the water was. These attacks were infrequent at the time of assessment as he was living in a small town.

The patient described himself as an anxious youngster who was never able to climb on monkey bars or go on swings as he was always falling and worrying about being hurt. He avoided fights but stated that, if he were forced into fighting, he could be very vicious. He had always had a quick temper and reported feeling very irritated at times of physical discomfort, for example, with a headache. He saw himself as a person who was awkward in social situations and very fidgety in such circumstances. He was aware of some separation anxiety at the time of kindergarten, with several days of intense crying when his mother left him at school. Subsequent to this, however, he did not have any school phobia or other behavior that interfered with his going to school. He did report, however, that the idea of people leaving him caused him to feel scared. He was aware of these feelings when his sister left for university and became very worried about something happening to her. He also worried about his mother going off from the ward at the hospital back to the hostel and stated that he could not entirely relax until he saw her coming back again. He stated that he had other global worries around things like nuclear war. He saw himself as a sensitive individual experiencing guilt about some of his behaviors and easily hurt by many things. The patient had had ongoing difficulties with enuresis, which he related, in part, to his anxiety. He saw his difficulty losing weight as being driven in a similar way. He perceived himself as having no willpower and as being clumsy. His headaches appeared to be migrainous in nature and had been present since age four or five. He had been advised to avoid caffeine and chocolate, to which he was allergic, and felt that this helped in part.

The patient expressed much frustration with his parents but had great difficulty talking openly about his anger even in the interview during which he was seen alone. He felt that his parents did not allow much freedom and that he could not talk to them about this. He was concerned that his mother was overburdened, and he did not want to aggravate her situation. He was very frustrated with his father's inflexibility and felt unable to talk to him. The patient experienced suicidal feelings in grade 8 that he resolved when he realized that doing something to himself would contradict his religious beliefs. He believed that his father had cancer and struggled with ambivalent feelings about this. Recommendations were made for supportive therapy in his local town. He was advised that his attacks were panic attacks and could be treated if they were of concern to him, if he were to return to an aggravating situation such as a larger city.

CASE EXAMPLE 3

A thirteen-year-old reported the onset of panic attacks around the age of eleven. She described these episodes as "so awful she wished she could die." She described "sensations of feeling not real, sweating, her heart beating hard, her face going pale, and fluttering in her stomach." Her interpretation of these attacks was that she was unable to handle normal upsets, and she had become worried about her difficulty in this regard. She had developed a pattern of having regular attacks most evenings, when she would become extremely distressed and look to her parents to comfort her and to resolve her upset. She was angry that her brother saw her behavior as attention seeking. At the time of referral, the patient acknowledged that she was having difficulty sleeping and trouble concentrating and was experiencing frequent headaches. She had a psychiatric assessment at age nine because her parents felt that she was not happy. The patient, in that circumstance, denied that she was unhappy, and the psychiatrist corroborated this, indicating that he felt that she was normal. At age eleven, she was seen by her father's psychiatrist. The father also suffered from PD. That psychiatrist, who was apparently unaware of her father's PD, saw her in individual psychotheraphy for eighteen months, but the contact was deemed ineffective by the family.

The initial diagnosis of the patient was PD with agoraphobic behaviors. Depression and personality traits of dependency, histrionic features, and oppositional behaviors were noted. The patient was placed on imipramine, with doses gradually increased to 175 milligrams per day. She was seen supportively, as were her parents, and the panic attacks decreased significantly on the medication. As the panic attacks alleviated, other difficulties began to emerge. A longstanding pattern of avoidance of difficult tasks began to lead to skipping classes in subjects that she disliked. This produced a decline in her marks, which escalated her anxiety and depression. Panic attacks recurred as this self-defeating pattern of behavior worsened. As the father's panic attacks alleviated and his wife's hopes for a return to normal functioning did not materialize, the patient's mother became progressively more disillusioned with the marriage and eventually decided to request a separation. Her own sense of distress and need to try to resolve the marital separation, being strongly resisted by her husband, led to preoccupation and some withdrawal on mother's part. This worsened the relationship with her daughter, the patient, as she resented her mother's apparent rejection and irritability. The parental separation coincided with an increase in demands at school, which the patient tried to avoid. Her mother initially tried to support her by providing excuses and notes for her, but, ultimately, she became very frustrated with her daughter, who appeared not to be working. This led to an increase in frustration and anxiety in the patient, who only narrowly missed failing her year. Summer provided a break from school demands, some smoothing out in the mother-daughter relationship, and a renewed interest in preventing a similar occurrence in the next school year. At the time of writing, panic attacks were experienced infrequently with very diminished intensity and were well tolerated by the patient. She remains on 125 milligrams of imipramine daily. Treatment has focused on the pattern of avoidance that includes avoidance of negative affect seen as relevant to her periods of depression.

CASE EXAMPLE 4

The patient, a sixteen-year-old white female, was referred by her family doctor for "attacks," described as periods of feeling hot, her heart beating hard, and feeling sweaty all over. These episodes lasted from a few seconds up to several minutes and were experienced most typically while at school or in crowded areas. Attacks ceased quickly when the patient could remove herself from such a situation. She was tired and rather depressed when the panic stopped. The attacks, which began when the patient was fifteen, led to worry about having other attacks and a sense of depression about her inability to control these bouts. She felt that other people avoided her because of her nervousness. The patient denied any concerns about what she might do during an attack or fears of going crazy or dying. This adolescent was the third youngest in a traditional European family. Despite minor conflict between the father and his daughters with respect to the amount of freedom that was acceptable, the family was described by the patient and her mother as reasonably comfortable and happy. The mother had been trying to encourage her daughter to go out more to dances and shopping, but the patient was resistant to going to crowded places. Relevant developmental factors were clinginess and early separation anxiety, which improved by the time the patient was school aged. Her mother felt, however, that the patient had always been an anxious girl and the patient described herself as quite shy. There were no other difficulties with respect to school functioning, but she was beginning to have difficulties maintaining friendships, partly because of her phobic avoidant behaviors. The patient reported stress-related difficulties with sleep. The patient's father had a history of headaches and an ulcer. A maternal aunt had committed suicide, and a maternal cousin had a history of depression and phobic avoidant behavior.

The patient was placed on imipramine, with gradually increased doses up to 250 milligrams a day, and seen supportively by the school counselor. On this regimen, the panic attacks alleviated somewhat, but she continued to be quite anxious. Alprazolam was added, with the final dosage reaching 3 milligrams per day, and the imipramine was reduced. With this, the patient noticed an almost complete disappearance of her panic attacks and seemed to be functioning reasonably well, although with some phobic avoidance. Because of the complete disappearance of her attacks, the patient decided not to renew her medication and experienced a grand mal convulsion several days after sudden withdrawal. She was placed back on medication and appeared to return to a good level of functioning once more. The mother had ongoing concerns about the high level of medication, but both she and her daughter realized that medication was helpful to her and that any future attempts at discontinuation had to be done very gradually. At last contact, the patient was not entirely free of panic attacks, but they had diminished in intensity, and she was, therefore, not limited in her

443

daily function. She reported, however, that, under situations of anger or marked discomfort, she continued to feel very anxious and worried that she would experience a recurrence of panic attacks. Dealing with negative affect was a persisting difficulty for her. She was also extremely sensitive and easily personally slighted. Aware of some of these problems, she was making efforts to deal with them in supportive therapy.

Discussion

Although some authors (Nelles and Barlow 1988; Werry 1986) have questioned whether panic attacks occur in childhood or adolescence, there should no longer be any doubt about their existence. In fact, the need for routine inquiry of children and adolescents for panic attacks is supported both by studies of adults that examined age of onset and by the few studies of children cited. As is clear from these case examples, panic attacks are experienced by children and adolescents but are frequently not recognized as such at their first appearance. In my experience, children and adolescents are less likely than adults initially to label this experience as panic. They appear, however, to be distressed by their experience, particularly by the sense that these attacks, although sometimes predictable, are out of their control.

The fact that PD co-occurs with other psychiatric disorders is important particularly in a young population, in which prevention of subsequent morbidity is always a goal. It is clear that panic attacks do induce avoidant behaviors and that these avoidant behaviors can become particularly crippling. It is also clear that panic attacks, which are primarily interpreted as somatic distress, can lead to what might be labeled as a hypochondriacal pattern. Noyes et al.'s (1986) report of the alleviation of hypochondriacal symptomatology with the treatment of panic attacks, as shown in case example 1, would support the contention that early intervention, particularly with an adolescent population, would be well worth the effort in preventing the development of a pattern of behavior that may be difficult to change later on.

There are many ways of understanding the relation between PD and affective disorder. In some patients, the stress of repeated attacks that are embarrassing and uncontrollable appears to overwhelm a vulnerable individual, producing a depressive picture similar to the depressive posture that can be produced in overly stressed animals (Suomi 1984).

In other situations, patients will report onset of an affective disorder prior to, or separate from, bouts of PD. This would suggest the possibility of a shared vulnerability to both disorders, possibly triggered by different stressors. The fact that panic attacks occur in such a wide variety of disorders (exclusive of behavior disorders) would suggest that panic attacks are symptomatic of intense distress. Finally, on a more specific note, recent interest in comorbidity of panic attacks and eating disorders suggests that a careful inquiry in adolescents with anorexia nervosa for panic attacks may be clinically important in treatment of these disorders. I have seen three adolescent females referred because of reluctance to eat, with weight loss. All three had panic disorder that, when treated, led to the alleviation of intense nausea, the part of the panic attack that produced the avoidance of eating.

Although the patients in case examples 1, 3, and 4 were all treated and improved on tricyclic antidepressants, it is my clinical experience that other forms of intervention may be equally effective in specific cases. Cognitive behavioral strategies for identification of the stressors and methods of countering the anticipatory anxiety can be useful. Exposure to avoided situations may be necessary both with medication and in less severe forms of the disorder to prevent or deal with the avoidance that regularly accompanies PD. Reduction of anticipatory anxiety through such exposure may lead to significant reduction of panic attacks. Panic attacks that are the result of physiological disruption, for example, withdrawal from medication, and other disorders may remit with treatment of the primary disorder, for example, schizophrenia.

Despite anecdotal reports and clinical experience that suggest that children and adolescents appear to respond similarly to adults to the tricyclic antidepressants for panic attacks, there have been no systematic studies exploring the use of tricyclic antidepressants, MAO inhibitors, alprazolam, or clonazepam in children. Case example 4 highlights the problems inherent in using medications such as alprazolam with adolescents who may not be fully oriented to consultation with a physician with respect to stopping or monitoring medication.

Because of the potentially disabling nature of PD, it seems incumbent to study further the factors that cause an individual to progress from simple panic attacks to PD as well as the interconnections between PD and other psychiatric disorders. Long-term follow-up of children and adolescents vulnerable to panic attacks might yield important information in this regard. Presently, assessment of coping strategies appears to be an important factor to examine as it may also lead to nonchemical ways of dealing with panic attacks. This assessment of cognitive strategies may also clarify the relation between panic attacks and avoidant behavior. It is clear that many individuals experience panic attacks and do not become avoidant. Whether this has to do with coping strategies, as was suggested in case example 1, or whether it has a more biological basis is not clear. It is important, however, to understand whether there are strategies that can be promoted to prevent the development of avoidant behaviors. Clinicians who have tried to deal with avoidant patients will appreciate the difficulty in eradicating these behaviors once they are established. One of the most complex problems is to get avoidant patients to participate in treatment.

Conclusions

An overview of panic disorder has been presented, including issues of diagnosis, comorbidity, exacerbating factors, and treatment. The scant literature on this disorder in children and adolescents is reviewed. Case histories are reported to illustrate typical and atypical features in young people, cautions to be heeded with respect to medical treatment of PD in adolescents, and specific issues that require further investigation. I conclude that inquiry for panic attacks should be part of the routine assessment of all child and adolescent patients.

REFERENCES

Alessi, N. E.; Robbins, D. R.; and Dilsaver, S. C. 1987. Panic and depressive disorders among psychiatrically hospitalized adolescents. *Psychiatry Research* 20:275–283.

American Psychiatric Association. 1987. *Diagnostic and Statistical Manual of Mental Disorders*. 3d ed., rev. Washington, D.C.: American Psychiatric Press.

Aronson, T. A. 1987. Is panic disorder a distinct diagnostic entity? a critical review of the borders of a syndrome. *Journal of Nervous and Mental Disease* 175:584–594.

Aronson, T. A., and Logue, C. M. 1988. Phenomenology of panic attacks: a descriptive study of panic disorder patients' self-reports. *Journal of Clinical Psychiatry* 49:8–13.

Ballenger, J. C.; Burrows, G. D.; DuPont, R. L.; Lesser, I. M.; Noyes, R.; Pecknold, J. C.; Rifkin, A.; and Swinson, R. P. 1988. Alprazolam in panic disorder and agoraphobia: results from a multicenter trial. I. efficacy in short-term treatment. *Archives of General Psychiatry* 45:413–422.

Beitman, B. D.; Basha, I.; Flaker, G.; DeRosear, L.; Mukerji, V.; and Lamberti, J. 1986. Nonfearful panic disorder: panic attacks without fear. *Behavior Research and Therapy* 25(6): 487–492.

Biederman, J. 1987. Clonazepam in the treatment of prepubertal children with panic-like symptoms. *Journal of Clinical Psychiatry* 48:38–41.

Boyd, J. H.; Burke, J. D.; Gruenberg, E.; Holzer, C. E.; Rae, D. S.; George, L. K.; Karno, M.; Stoltzman, B.; McEvoy, L.; and Nestadt, G. 1984. Exclusion criteria of DSM-III: a study of co-occurrence of hierarchy-free syndromes. *Archives of General Psychiatry* 41:983–989.

Bradley, S. J.; Wachsmuth, R. J.; Swinson, R.; and Hnatko, G. 1986. A pilot study of panic attacks in a child and adolescent psychiatric population. Paper presented at the annual meeting of the Canadian Academy of Child Psychiatry, Vancouver, B.C., September.

Breier, A.; Charney, D. S.; and Heninger, G. R. 1984. Major depression in patients with agoraphobia and panic disorder. *Archives of General Psychiatry* 41:1129–1135.

Casat, C. D. 1988. Childhood anxiety disorders: a review of the possible relationship to adult panic disorder and agoraphobia. *Journal of Anxiety Disorders* 2(1): 51–60.

Coryell, W.; Noyes, R.; and House, J. D. 1986. Mortality among outpatients with anxiety disorders. *American Journal of Psychiatry* 143:503–510.

Cowley, D. S., and Roy-Byrne, P. P. 1987. Hyperventilation and panic disorder. *American Journal of Medicine* 83:929–937.

Crowe, R. R.; Pauls, D. L.; Slymen, D. J.; and Noyes, R. 1980. A family study of anxiety neurosis: morbidity risk in families of patients with and without mitral valve prolapse. *Archives of General Psychiatry* 37:77–79.

Edlund, M. J.; Swann, A. C.; and Clothier, J. 1987. Patients with panic attacks and abnormal EEG results. *American Journal of Psychiatry* 144:508–509.

Fontaine, R., and Chouinard, G. 1984. Anti-panic effect of clonazepam. *American Journal of Psychiatry* 141(1): 149.

447

George, D. T.; Ladenheim, J. A.; and Nutt, D. J. 1987. Effect of pregnancy on panic attacks. *American Journal of Psychiatry* 144:1073–1079.

Gorman, J. M.; Fyer, M. R.; Goetz, R.; Askanazi, J.; Liebowitz, M. R.; Fyer, A. J.; Kinney, J.; and Klein, D. F. 1988. Ventilatory physiology of patients with panic disorder. *Archives of General Psychiatry* 45:31–39.

Gorman, J. M.; Goetz, R. R.; Fyer, M.; King, D. L.; Fyer, A. J.; Liebowitz, M. R.; and Klein, D. F. 1988. The mitral valve prolapse—panic disorder connection. *Psychosomatic Medicine* 50:114–122.

Herskowitz, J. 1986. Neurologic presentations of panic disorder in childhood and adolescence. *Developmental Medicine and Child Neurology* 28:617–623.

Kahn, J. P.; Drusin, R. E.; and Klein, D. F. 1987. Idiopathic cardiomyopathy and panic disorder: clinical association in cardiac transplant candidates. *American Journal of Psychiatry* 14:1327–1330.

Katon, W.; Vitaliano, P. P.; Russo, J.; Jones, M.; and Anderson, K. 1987. Panic disorders: spectrum of severity and somatization. *Journal of Nervous and Mental Diseases* 175:12–19.

Klein, D. F. 1964. Delineation of two drug-responsive anxiety syndromes. *Psychopharmacologia* 5:397–408.

Klein, D. F. 1981. Anxiety reconceptualized. In D. F. Klein and J. G. Rabkin, eds. *Anxiety: New Research and Changing Concepts*. New York: Raven.

Leckman, J. F.; Weissman, M. M. ; Merikangas, K. R.; Pauls, D. L.; and Prusoff, B. A. 1983. Panic disorder and major depression: increased risk of depression, alcoholism, panic, and phobic disorders in families of depressed probands with panic disorders. *Archives of General Psychiatry* 40:1055–1060.

Margraf, J.; Ehlers, A.; and Roth, W. T. 1988. Mitral valve prolapse and panic disorder: a review of their relationship. *Psychosomatic Medicine* 50:93–113.

Mellman, T. A., and Uhde, T. W. 1987. Obsessive-compulsive symptoms in panic disorder. *American Journal of Psychiatry* 144:1573–1576.

Munjack, D. J., and Moss, H. B. 1981. Affective disorder and alcoholism in families of agoraphobics. *Archives of General Psychiatry* 38:869–871.

Nelles, W. B., and Barlow, D. H. 1988. Do children panic? *Clinical Psychology Review* 8:359–372.

Noyes, R.; Clancy, J.; Crowe, R.; Hoenk, P. R.; and Slymen, D. J. 1978. The familial prevalence of anxiety neurosis. *Archives of General Psychiatry* 37:77–79.

Noyes, R.; Reich, J.; Clancy, J.; and O'Gorman, T. W. 1986. Reduction in hypochondriasis with treatment of panic disorder. *British Journal of Psychiatry* 149:631–635.

Perugi, G.; Deltito, J.; Soriani, A.; Musetti, L.; Petracca, A.; Nisita, C.; Maremmani, I.; and Cassano, G. B. 1988. Relationship between panic disorder and separation anxiety with school phobia. *Comprehensive Psychiatry* 29(2): 98–107.

Pohl, R.; Berchou, R.; and Rainey, J. M. 1982. Tricyclic antidepressants and monoamine oxidase inhibitors in the treatment of agoraphobia. *Journal of Clinical Psychopharmacology* 2:399–407.

Rachman, S.; Levitt, K.; and Lopatka, C. 1987. Panic: the links between cognitions and bodily symptoms. I. *Behavior Research and Therapy* 25:411–423.

Roy-Byrne, P. P., and Uhde, T. W. 1988. Exogenous factors in panic disorder: clinical and research implications. *Journal of Clinical Psychiatry* 49(2): 56–61.

Sevin, B. H. 1987. Mitral valve prolapse, panic states, and anxiety: a dilemma in perspective. *Psychiatric Clinics of North America* 10:141–150.

Signer, S. F. 1988. Seizure disorder or panic disorder? *American Journal of Psychiatry* 144:508–509.

Suomi, S. J. 1984. The development of affect in rhesus monkeys. In N. A. Fox and R. J. Davidson, eds. *The Psychobiology of Affective Development*. Hillsdale, N.J.: Erlbaum.

Vitaliano, P. P.; Katon, W.; Russo, J.; Maiuro, R.; Anderson, K.; and Jones, M. 1987. Coping as an index of illness behavior in panic disorder. *Journal of Nervous and Mental Disease* 175:78–84.

Vitiello, B.; Behar, D.; Wolfson, S.; and Delaney, M. A. 1987. Letter to editor: panic disorder in prepubertal children. *American Journal of Psychiatry* 144(4): 525–526.

Von Korff, M. R.; Eaton, W. W.; and Keyl, P. M. 1985. The epidemiology of panic attacks and panic disorder: results of three community surveys. *Amerian Journal of Epidemiology* 122(6): 970–981.

Weilburg, J. B.; Bear, D. M.; and Sachs, G. 1987. Three patients with concomitant panic attacks and seizure disorder: possible clues to the neurology of anxiety. *American Journal of Psychiatry* 144:1053–1056.

Weissman, N. J.; Kramer-Fox, R.; Devereaux, R. B.; and Shear, M. K. 1987. Contrasting patterns of autonomic dysfunction in patients with mitral valve prolapse and panic attacks. *American Journal of Medicine* 82:880–888.

Werry, J. S. 1986. Diagnosis and assessment. In R. Gittelman, ed. *Anxiety Disorders of Childhood*. New York: Guilford.

25 WHO MOTHERS YOUNG MOTHERS? TREATMENT OF ADOLESCENT MOTHERS AND THEIR CHILDREN WITH IMPAIRED ATTACHMENTS

NANCY H. WEIL AND ANDREW M. BOXER

"I can't imagine becoming a mother," a patient spontaneously remarked; "I don't even have a mother of my own." Another patient arrived in treatment for her first consultation carrying her eight-month-old child. As she walked in the door, she said, "Here, take him. I can't take care of myself." Another patient continued this theme of young mothers and infants when she began her treatment session by saying, "I have a new baby. I'd like to throw him down the stairs." Finally, a young woman whose own mother had been emotionally unavailable throughout her life watched her ongoing pregnancy with increasing fear, as she said, "I'm afraid I will be the kind of mother my mother was. I want so much to be different, but I just don't know how." It has proved useful to bring these mothers together with their children into the treatment room over a prolonged period of time. This may provide a "holding environment," in the broadest sense (Winnicott 1960b), in which these mothers, who typically experience a sense of psychological deprivation, can themselves feel mothered.

Benedek (1959) pointed out that unresolved, unconscious preoedipal conflicts are revived in every individual who parents a child (see also Anthony and Benedek 1970; Benedek 1970). Others (Fraiberg, Adelson, and Shapiro 1980) explain this by describing the infant as a "transference object" for its parents, an identity fostered by the special meaning that the baby serves, one based on the parents' own experiences. This may account for parents' fantasied (in contrast to the "real") baby leading to largely unconscious conflicts of unresolved preoedipal issues, specifically issues of dependency and separation.

In this chapter, we offer some examples of a therapeutic intervention of conjoint psychoanalytic psychotherapy with mothers and infants, which we conducted through a major medical center outpatient psychiatric clinic and in a private practice. The young mothers and their children, all under four years of age, were from both lower-class, black, urban and middle-class, white, suburban populations.

What these women seemed to have in common was the absence of a remembered "good enough mother" who could function as a cohesive self- and selfobject representation throughout the vulnerable early stages of motherhood. These young women came into treatment without an explicit complaint about their mothering capacities, although they frequently evinced difficulties providing care and nurturance to their children. The feeling of exquisite vulnerability in the mothering role emerged only after treatment was underway.

The women in our study came to adolescence with many preoedipal vulnerabilities. Adolescence and the transition to adulthood have been frequently conceptualized in terms of the developmental task of separation from the family (i.e., parents) and the successful assumption of new autonomous social roles (Bettelheim 1965; Blos 1962; Freud 1914). Erikson (1956), for example, describes this process as the "selective repudiation and mutual assimilation of childhood identifications, and their absorption in a new configuration" (p. 65). Following the tradition of Mahler (1972a, 1972b; Mahler, Pine, and Bergman 1975), Blos (1962, 1967) characterizes adolescence as a second individuation process, recapitulating many of the conflicts of earlier parental ties and attachments. As he states, it is "the shedding of family dependencies, the loosening of infantile object ties in order to become a member of society, or simply of the adult world" (Blos 1967, p. 163).

As attachments to parental figures decrease during this transition, attachments to others increase (Freud 1914). However, newer conceptualizations of adolescence have criticized the earlier dichotomized views of adolescence in that the successful transition to adulthood is presumed to entail a disruption of, if not an end to, attachments between generations (Greene and Boxer 1986). Alternative views of adolescence suggest that one of the tasks associated with the transition to adulthood is the achievement of not familial autonomy but rather familial interdependence (Cohler and Geyer 1982; Weissman, Cohen, Boxer, and Cohler 1987), a state of differentiation rather than separation, in which the maintenance of parental bonds and the maintenance of independent functioning are dual achievements. The important question is thus one not of separation or its timeliness but of the processes by which the individual's interdependence is renegotiated over successive mutual transitions (Greene and Boxer 1986; Lerner and Ryff 1978). The women in our study were often overly dependent or hyperindependent in their relations with the therapist, their parents, significant others, and their own children. An interdependent relationship, characterized by mutuality and reciprocity, was a task that they often had been unable to achieve.

The women that we discuss in this report had typically entered adolescence with a number of unresolved conflicts relating to earlier preoedipal development, particularly at the phallic narcissistic stage. Their self-representations were often vulnerable, and they were unable, without difficulty, to bear the stresses and strains associated with motherhood. These women's motivations for mothering were, therefore, confounded with many other narcissistic needs. They typically looked to their children for sources of confirmation, soothing, and repair to injured aspects of the self, characteristics that were beyond what is normally expected between mothers and small children. Their early difficulties could be characterized by deficits in self-structure, which did not resolve during the oedipal and latency periods and resulted in further deficits in their peer relations during early adolescence.

These young women were typically without a husband or partner with whom to share the psychological tasks of parenting; there was a marked absence of a parenting alliance (Cohen and Weissman 1984) with any partner, which added to these women's vulnerability and sense of isolation. While many of these mothers' own mothers took an active role in parenting their grandchildren, this was usually not in the form of a parenting alliance; rather, the grandmother became a surrogate mother for her grandchild.

Enhancing the mother's self-esteem regulation through therapeutic interaction between therapist, mother, and child facilitated the formation of a co-parenting alliance (Cohen and Weissman 1984; Weissman and Cohen 1985) as well as of a more reliable self-representation in the mother. Cohen and Weissman (1984) have defined the parenting alliance as "a paradig-matic self-self object relationship vital to the evolving parenthood experience and other adult tasks. It encompasses interactions . . . which pertain to childbearing, with the provision that these behaviors are appropriate to the developmental needs of children. It is a contributing process for the continuous mastery of developmental issues for the adults and children involved in it. . . . it clearly involves the issue of self-esteem and its vicissitudes which can endanger the adult's feeling of competence, effectiveness, and well-being" (pp. 33, 35).

The structure of the treatment modality that we delineate provides the opportunity for the development of a substitutive co-parenting alliance between therapist and patient in the actual presence of the child. Such an alliance, we believe, is the outcome of the therapeutic process, not the basis of it. In this conceptualization, a treatment alliance is, of course, a necessary but insufficient condition for the development of a parenting alliance.

Patients engaged in this treatment modality with their infants eventually made the choice to give up their children's presence in the treatment room. The therapist had, in effect, assisted in the regulation of tension and in the control of aggressive and destructive behavior directed to the children. Through this conjoint therapy, the therapist provided basic confirmation that the mother was "good enough" (Winnicott 1960a, 1960b, 1967), which had the effect of enhancing the mother's experience of herself being able to provide "good enough mothering." A co-parenting alliance was possible after the patients themselves had experienced a holding environment in a therapeutic setting. This alliance then had the advantage of assisting the mothers to feel that they were able and worthy as mothers. In the safety of the treatment room, the patients were able to experience decreased deprivations of the mothering functions themselves and, thereby, were able to learn to provide these experiences for their own children. Evidence suggests (Galenson and Swibel 1984) that treatment outcome depends on the extent to which the mother-child reciprocal relationship has been supported and improved. Treatment failures were found to correlate in great part with the degree to which the therapist had substituted for the mother in her therapeutic relationship with the child and therapeutic failure to engage the mother as a "co-parent." The question then arises as to whether this is due to parental psychopathology or poor treatment design.

Several key issues that this treatment modality raises are examined and described. First, we briefly review psychoanalytic perspectives on the treatment of parents and children. We then consider the several dyadic relationships on which this modality is based and their complications because of the need to follow each dyad (i.e., mother and child, mother and therapist, and child and therapist, at any given moment) to determine the points at which appropriate interventions need to be made. The experience for the mother of having her child present during psychotherapy holds many intrapsychic meanings that must be examined as well, particularly in the realm of her self-representation. Finally, transference and countertransference issues, in the broadest sense, are a significant part of this form of treatment and will be discussed as they pertain to mother and child.

Brief Review of Existing Paradigms

The psychoanalytic theory that forms the basis for this method of treatment, or paradigm, has been explored from a slightly different perspective by Bergman (1982), Brinich (1984), Loewald (1982, 1985), and Weil (1970). For Bergman, Brinich, and Weil, treatment of the children was the primary aim of therapy. The mothers were there only to provide a continuity for the therapeutic alliance. In Loewald's (1982) example, the mother was the primary patient, and the baby appeared occasionally. However, the mother's conflicts around mothering remained the focus of treatment regardless of whether the baby was present during sessions.

Our treatment strategy is in some respects similar to the concept of simultaneous analysis, which has been examined extensively by clinicians at the Hampstead Child Therapy Clinic (see, e.g., Burlingham, Goldberger, and Lussier 1955). Some of these treatment outcomes and strategies have been published in reports that focus either on the perspective of the child (e.g., Hellman, Friedmann, and Shepheard 1960) or on that of the mother (Levy 1960). Others (e.g., Johnson and Szurek 1942) have described collaborative psychiatric treatment for disturbed children and their parents in which the therapeutic interventions were made by two therapists, one dealing with the child and the other with the parent, in psychotherapy rather than psychoanalysis. In nearly all these reports, the patient is identified most frequently as the child, although often the mother was providing the unconscious background to which the child was responding. It should be noted, however, that recent research has examined the effect of disturbed offspring on parents' psychosocial development (Cook and Cohler 1986). In our cases, the mother is identified as the patient, and the child is brought in to support the mother's treatment.

Multiple Dyads in the Treatment

As stated previously, this form of treatment, which has as its premise several dyadic relationships, has complications that arise from the need to follow each dyad, that is, mother and child, mother and therapist, and child and therapist, at any given moment. The mother-infant dyad is to be supported because of the mother's experience of having felt that she was poorly mothered herself and her fearful clinging to or outright rejection of the child. The alliance between mother and therapist is therefore critical at all times. This is the stable primary dyadic relationship in the treatment room. It is the ease and comfort with which the therapist can deal with the mother that makes the other work move forward. The therapist-child dyad is the hardest one to monitor because of the deprived condition in which one frequently finds the infant and the therapist's eagerness to step in and do the mothering better. The therapist must avoid setting too good an example for the patient so as to avoid making her feel that she cannot achieve this level of comfort in her own mothering (see also Brinich 1984).

Case Example 1

The treatment of a young, black, unemployed, separated mother, who had consistently brought her two-and-a-half-year-old daughter with her to treatment, illustrates the delicate balance that the therapist must attend to at all times when treating a mother-child dyad. A limited number of play materials had been provided in the room: a dollhouse with a few pieces of furniture, some miniature dolls, and some modeling clay.

When she first entered treatment with her mother, the child had been reluctant to engage in play and had clung closely to her mother. The therapist extended many efforts to engage the child in play. The mother assisted in this effort, feeling that her daughter needed to be out of the way. Gradually, the little girl came to approach these materials herself, as she entered the treatment room for each session. A rhythmic cycle developed whereby the girl would play alone and alternatively engage the therapist and her mother in her play, showing each what she had created or asking one of the adults for help. Slowly, over time, the child began to engage in triadic play with both mother and therapist, as the therapist supported the child's efforts.

The therapist was careful to neglect neither mother nor child; however, both began to assert their needs and demand the attention of the therapist simultaneously. It was this type of mother-daughter competition that required careful intervention from the therapist. At these times, the mother's use of the child as a bad selfobject would emerge and disrupt the cyclic interaction and play. When the patient perceived that Rachel, her child, was getting too much attention, she would break into aggressive language and threaten the child, admonishing her to sit down, shut up, and be good, or she would get a "whoping."

During one session, the little girl had made some figures out of clay and asked the therapist for help. The therapist drew the mother into this interaction by saying, "Let's all work on this together and help Rachel." The mother felt affirmed and eagerly began to assist the little girl and the therapist in their joint creative venture. At the end of the session, the little girl asked if she could make some more "people" out of clay. The therapist told her that it was time to stop for today but that she could make more figures next time. The mother, sensing the therapist's pleasure in working with the child as well as the child's wish to return, felt injured and neglected by the therapist's comment. She quickly interjected, "Well, I don't know if Rachel will be able to come here next week. She may have to be at home." Rachel, hearing her mother's words, became silent and withdrawn, looking very sad.

DISCUSSION

The narcissistically vulnerable mother may easily feel wounded in the sector of the grandiose self when attention is directed to the child. Tremendous efforts of attention and planning are necessary to keep the mother feeling intact while simultaneously attending to the child. It appears that careful attention to the needs of the patient, the mother, during this entire psychotherapeutic process (which has, at times, gone on for four or five years) is key. Many extraordinary efforts may be necessary to ensure that the patient feels well cared for. The "parameters" of psychoanalysis (Eissler 1958) are useful. Such things as providing milk and other beverages to a nursing mother, for example, help establish for the patient that her sense of being calmed is assured.

The Meaning of the Child to the Mother in the Treatment

For each of the young mothers with whom we were engaged in treatment, the meaning of having a child seems to recreate the early frustrated mother-daughter relationship. That is, one sees the regressive pull in the transference at the same time that there is a flow of material about current or past relations with the young mother's own mother. Benedek (1959) has written on the recapitulation of the mother-daughter dyad with the birth of a child of either sex. This no doubt continues beyond the birth of a child, and there is evidence that it recurs with the birth of grandchildren. Thus, the concept of mothering may be defined in this context as a "holding environment" (Winnicott 1960b) that intends to sooth the memories that recur of the frustrated attachment to the patient's own mother.

Modell (1976) summarizes the experience of the holding environment and the therapeutic action of psychoanalysis. Winnicott introduced the term "holding environment" as a metaphor for certain aspects of the analytic situation and the analytic process. The term derives from the maternal function of holding the infant, but, taken as a metaphor, it has a much broader application and extends beyond the infantile period, during which holding is literal, not metaphoric, "to the broader caretaking functions of the parent in relation to the older child" (Khan 1974, p. 290). We suggest that the mother or, more accurately, the caretaking adults stand between the child and the actual environment and that the child and its caretaking are an open system joined by means of communication of affects. "The analyst is holding the patient and this often takes the form of conveying in words at the appropriate moment something that shows that the analyst knows and understands the deepest anxiety that is being experienced, that is waiting to be experienced" (Winnicott 1960b, p. 240). The holding environment provides, in Sandler's (1960) terms, "a background of safety" because to have a child requires the presence of a holding environment.

This treatment modality that we are describing, using the child to enhance the mother's self-esteem and self-cohesion, seems necessary until the patient has a more reliable self-representation. When that occurs, the patient frequently makes the choice to give up the child's ongoing presence in the treatment room. That is, there is a move forward from the early narcissistic phase to more advanced levels of separation-individuation, which the mother then attempts to master in the dyadic relationship with the therapist.

Patients' whose aggression and hostility toward their infants became modified through treatment can then safely take the child out of the treatment room. The therapist has, in fact, acted both to regulate tension and to modify the aggressive and destructive fantasies of the mother.

Case Example 2

Mrs. D., a nineteen-year-old white female, came into treatment prior to her pregnancy. She was a highly intelligent but nonverbal patient whose history included running away from home at the age of sixteen and whose own mother had been orphaned when she was five. The first two years of treatment were generally nonverbal, but very meaningful communication nevertheless ensued. The patient would arrive late and sit down with a kind of bravado, daring the therapist to get her to talk. The therapist sensed an enormous sadness under this power struggle, concentrated primarily in the feeling that Mrs. D. could not trust her. Gradually, over the first two years of treatment, the patient began to talk, and one could see her reluctance to tell the therapist anything that might be criticized as being less than perfect. Her earliest memories were of an experience of constant retreat into a world of fantasy without active speech.

It was with some trepidation that the therapist heard the news of the patient's pregnancy, which she and her husband had planned. The treatment shifted as the therapist began to wonder about the patient's relationship to her own mother, who had not spoken to her in several years. The patient claimed little interest in this relationship and none in actually seeing her mother. She anticipated the baby with pleasure but said very little about it for the first three months. There was no increase in memories of early childhood, no change in feelings about her mother, and no effort to communicate with her mother, who lived nearby. Treatment went on as if the pregnancy had nothing to do with her own past experience of childhood. At this point, the therapist realized that the patient was denying experiencing ordinary fears about her new role.

The therapist anticipated the baby's arrival with great pleasure, planning to go to the hospital, where she taught, to see the patient and the newly born infant. When the baby arrived, the patient chose not to see the therapist in the hospital, although she now claims to have watched and waited for her. The patient, Mrs. D., began to bring the baby to treatment one week after his birth. She clung fiercely to the baby, as she explained it, twenty-four hours a day. He was alert and responsive, and the mother quickly tuned into his various cries of hunger or discomfort. The therapist carefully abstained from holding or touching the baby until she was asked to do so; this occurred two weeks after joint treatment had begun. The patient appeared less angry at the therapist for not having been to visit her at the hospital. She handed her the baby and with enormous pleasure watched the therapist hold, touch, and interact with her son. The meaning of this was clear when the patient said, "We've been through so much together; we've gone so far. These moments are golden to watch with you and the baby and then to watch the three of us."

The beginning termination problems came eight months later when the patient abruptly chose to come to sessions alone. Within a few weeks, the mother reported that the child had begun a disturbing habit; he was banging his head against the bedroom door repeatedly during the day. The therapist suggested that she observe the timing of his head banging and its relation to her. It occurred to the therapist that the bond that she had established with the baby had been abruptly broken and that the baby was experiencing an anaclitic depression.

It was suggested to the patient that she bring the baby back to treatment. The rapprochement meeting had been significant. The first time the baby returned to a session, he exhibited relative stranger anxiety on seeing the therapist, crying when she attempted to pick him up and playing around his mother's feet. When he arrived for the next session a week later, he had a wonderful smile, greeted the therapist openly, and, when held, melded into her arms. The mother reported after these rapprochement sessions that she was having trouble leaving the baby to go off to school. At first she anticipated that the separation would be bad for the baby and then understood that the separation was bad for her. She was afraid that the baby would become too attached to the baby-sitter. Further, she admitted shyly that she was even afraid that the baby would become too attached to the therapist. She could later recall that the fear of the baby liking the therapist more than her had gone on throughout the treatment relationship, although she felt that she needed the therapist in the treatment room to correct her own fears that she could not mother alone.

In the following session, Mrs. D. arrived alone and reported a dream in which she met the therapist on the stairway leading to the office. In her dream, the therapist was on her way downstairs, having forgotten her appointment date with the patient. The therapist looked surprised as the patient approached but agreed to return with her to the office, where the patient sat in her regular chair. The therapist then turned off all the lights and left her alone in the office for several hours.

The dream had distressed the patient, and she displayed an angry residue. It occurred to the therapist that the dream had something to do with the patient's fear that the therapist was becoming too attached to her son and that perhaps the therapist's forgetting her appointment and turning the lights off were indications that the therapist had been perceived as not "seeing" her during the period of eight months that she and her son had been in treatment together.

DISCUSSION

It is common for the mother to recommence bringing the child with her to treatment when her own aggressive impulses feel out of control. It is then the therapist's task to reconfirm the mother's capacity to "hold" by again forming an alliance with her to co-parent the child.

The parenting alliance, as a paradigmatic self-selfobject relationship, affords each parent the opportunity to make use of the other in coping with the stresses and strains of parenting. It is in a different framework that one talks of "mothering young mothers"; that is, there is only the therapist-patient dyad, and the infant is outside this concept except as it is represented as part of the self system.

The question, Who mothers young mothers? requires understanding of early mother-infant interaction. In attempting to establish self-constancy (cohesive self), the therapist may provide a "gleam in the mother's eye" (Kohut 1968) that over a period of time is internalized by the mother and can be replicated, at least in partial function, with her own child. Mutual gazing is a dimension of the nonverbal aspects of the so-called holding environment (Modell 1976; Winnicott 1960b) that seems similar to preverbal mother-child interaction (see also Weil 1984). Kohut (1968) has extensively described the creation of the gleam

461

in the mother's eye, and Winnicott (1967) elaborated on the "mirror role" of the mother, which has been further investigated by Brazelton (1981), Cohler (1982), Mahler, Pine, and Bergman (1975), and Pollock and Breuer (1968). Freud (1919) considered eye contact an important sign, communicating a feeling that "betrays itself by a look even though it is not put into words" (p. 240). While the idea of the mirror role of the mother probably began with Freud's (1911) discussion of the mother and infant as a physical system, it was further considered in his later work (1931) on the mother-daughter relationship. Winnicott's (1967) use of the mother's face as a mirror suggests a dialogue of gaze between patient and therapist. He suggested that the baby sees himself relative to what he finds in the face of the mother. There seems reason to assume that the patient in a therapeutic setting may experience similar phenomena in relation to the therapist.

Our report will not examine the degree of difficulty in providing a gleam in the mother's eye, that is, the gleam in the therapist's eye, except to mention that this experience is thwarted by the structural weakness and developmental deficits that these mothers exhibit. This gleam is often missing in the mother, but it can be provided by the therapist's experience with the baby, and the pleasure is then reflected back in the experience of the mother.

To the mother, the meaning of the child appears to be in the realm of the mother's self-representation (Fraiberg et al. 1980). Often, the baby represents the part of the self that is healthy, functioning, and conflict free. The baby may also, at times, represent a part of the mother's more hated self-representation, which is defective, conflictual, and depreciated—the "bad" mother. These splits in self- and object representations may occur regularly. In Kohut's (1968) terms, the baby contains the part of the self that has grandiose and exhibitionistic qualities that other people can admire and enjoy, even though the mother cannot reflect pleasure through the child alone. It becomes the therapist's task to provide many of these missing functions for the mother.

Transference and Countertransference to Mother and to Child

Transference and countertransference, in the broadest sense, are the significant parts of this form of treatment. These transferences represent the range of diversity found in any one-to-one therapeutic relationship. However, we believe that there are three dimensions to the transference and countertransference issues in the treatment of mother-infant dyads. These include the transferences from and countertransferences to each of the individuals, mother and child. However, there is an added dimension, which is the transference from the mother and child as a dyad and the consequent response to them. While, of course, within each individual such dimensions are blurred together, conceptually they appear quite distinct. That is, mother and child may, together, come to hold some shared fantasies and wishes about the therapist based on their relationship with each other. In consequence, countertransference to the dyad may be expected.

There is a general sequence of emergence of these transferences. Initial transference is at the narcissistic level until the mother-infant dyad has reached a symbiotic level. In the early phases of treatment, when mother-infant bonding is not clearly established, there is an early maternal transference to the treatment on the part of the mother, which is a transference different from the dyadic level of her relationship with her infant. Individualized transferences emerge outside the mother-infant dyad. This is expected since the typical reason that these mothers have sought treatment is, in part, the failed symbiosis with their infants.

As stated previously, the mother's transference precedes the shared dyadic level with the child, until a symbiotic merger is achieved with the child, which may take considerable time. In case example 2, there was an emergent wish on the part of the mother for a merger with the therapist. This was viewed as a primitive state that existed and required treatment before a completed symbiosis between the mother and the infant could proceed.

A typical countertransference response to the situation of an aggressive mother, we have found, is the therapist's feelings of a need to remove one of the individuals from the treatment room, an impulse that, if acted on, would, we believe, actually serve to further erode the healthy basis of the mother-infant symbiosis that does exist.

Winnicott's (1949) discussion of hate in the countertransference is highly relevant to our treatment of mothers and infants. As a consequence of treating such pairs, mothers have come to some understanding of their feelings of rage and hate toward their own infants. The process of treating the dyad has enabled these women to experience their hate without "having to pay the child out" (Winnicott 1949). Hate in the countertransference, in response to the mothers' aggression directed toward their children, has served a liberating function for the mothers. Such feelings can serve as the basis for understanding and interpreting the mothers' aggressive feelings toward their children, enabling normal symbiosis to be restored and developed toward individuation of mother and child.

The issue of aggression is a salient one when treating mothers and infants. With regard to treating mothers and children together, Brinich (1984) has stated, "A child's difficulties in dealing with aggressive impulses come into focus very quickly (sometimes too quickly) when the therapist sees the child and mother together in joint sessions. . . . Of course once the aggressive impulses and angry feelings emerge in actions or words, the therapeutic work has just begun. It is common for the mothers of these children to find themselves profoundly upset by their children's aggression" (p. 501).

In one of the mother-infant pairs that we treated, the mother became very upset when her four-year-old daughter played aggressively with dolls and blocks. Her response to the daughter's behavior, in the presence of the therapist, was to become counteraggressive in an attempt to stop the aggression in her daughter, possibly due to the therapist's presence. The mother did not wish to be evaluated as a bad mother on the basis of her daughter's behavior. Her wish to be valued as a good mother by the therapist may have led to her aggressive attempts to thwart her daughter's own aggression. The mother's transference to the therapist at this early phase of treatment was at the early maternal level and was viewed as a negative maternal transference. In this case, the therapist's countertransference response was to the dyad and was focused around the wish to stop the mother's aggression from being leveled at the child. The therapist's response in this example is to the mother-infant relationship.

Many therapists believe that bringing a child into the treatment room when the mother is the identified patient may serve as defense and resistance and thus act as an impediment to the normal psychoanalytic therapeutic process. However, allowing the mother to bring her child (whom she views as either a selfobject or a part object; Tolpin 1974) with her enables her to feel some new mastery in that sector of her development, even in the face of seemingly disruptive aspects of her interaction with the small child.

Case Example 3

Mrs. B., a thirty-six-year-old black, unemployed, mother of three who had been separated from her husband for several months, came to an outpatient psychiatric clinic because of increasing anxiety and depression. Mrs. B. was finding it more and more difficult to leave her home, to go to the store, or to go out for a walk. She felt that the external world beyond her apartment was full of danger, and she described feeling like she was in a shell. When the therapist met her for their first appointment in the waiting room, he was surprised to see that she had brought with her a little two-and-a-half-year-old girl named Shelly. Mrs. B. spoke in a thick Southern dialect and, as became apparent later, was also suffering from a developmental speech deficit. The shyness that she said she felt made it even more difficult for the therapist and patient to communicate with one another.

After Mrs. B. and her Shelly came into the treatment room, Shelly began to explore the office, and Mrs. B. admonished her, lightly striking her on the hand and bottom for attempting to open the drawers to the desk or climb on the furniture. Shelly soon told her mother, "Pooh, Mommy," indicating that she wanted to go to the bathroom. Mrs. B. became infuriated with the child and told her, "Shhs, not now Shelly," until the therapist indicated that she could take her to the bathroom, which was right down the hall.

The many interruptions, the difficulty in communication, and the high level of aggression expressed by Mrs. B. to her daughter made the therapist feel that psychotherapy could not ensue unless the baby was taken out of the room. Mrs. B. had told the therapist at the beginning of her first session that there was no one who could watch Shelly and that she had to bring her to the clinic. While trying to be a "dedicated" therapist (Searles 1967), he could not help but engage with Shelly, who was warm, friendly, and eager for a response to her smiles and explorations. The therapist had complimented Shelly on the pretty red dress she was wearing, to which Mrs. B. broke into a large smile and said, "Say thank you, Shelly."

The therapist's immediate reaction following this first session was frustration and dismay. He wondered how he could do his job as a psychotherapist with the disorganizing interactions and disruptions that were constantly occurring between mother and child. He decided that he would have to keep the child out of the treatment room in order for psychotherapy to begin. It was hard for him to imagine, at that time, that he would be seeing Mrs. B. and Shelly together for the next three years. The therapist's initial reaction was one of anger at having to deal with the child, whom he found disruptive and who left him feeling like a baby-sitter for the mother; he felt out of his normal role as therapist.

DISCUSSION

The attention that the therapist pays to the child complicates treatment in many ways. Countertransference issues, in the broadest sense, are also a critical part of this treatment modality. The pleasure that the therapist may feel in working with a healthy infant or child, as contrasted to the work with the "disturbed" mother, at times makes it difficult to turn from the infant back to the angry, frightened, sometimes psychotic mother. Further, the later bonding between mother and infant can leave the therapist feeling left out.

It seems clear that the baby's attachment to the therapist is as much a therapeutic alliance as the mother's attachment to the therapist. It must be handled separately and with the appropriate emphasis on the frequency of sessions and termination procedures, as if it were an individual psychotherapy. This is borne out by the intensity of the countertransference responses experienced toward these babies. Although the attachments have in the main been very positive, occasionally they have been negative, with equally negative responses from the child. It might be added that, when the therapist has negative feelings about the baby (we recall one child in particular whose destructiveness in the office was fairly uncontrollable), the baby has done poorly outside the office as well.

Conclusions

We have been describing the results of an intervention utilizing a psychoanalytic psychotherapeutic approach to the treatment of a group of adolescent mothers and their children with impaired attachments. These women manifested many difficulties providing care and nurturance to their children and often displaced hostile and aggressive impulses onto them. Enhancing the mother's self-esteem regulation through therapeutic interaction between therapist, mother, and child eventuated in the development of a co-parenting alliance as well as a more reliable self-representation in the mother. Through this conjoint treatment, the therapist provided basic confirmation that the mother was good enough, which had the effect of enhancing the mother's experience of herself receiving good enough mothering. Eventually the mothers were able to take their children out of the treatment room, and therapy continued with the mothers alone.

We have underscored three key and complex aspects of this therapeutic modality: the several dyadic relationships and their complications in the treatment room (i.e., mother and child, mother and therapist, and child and therapist), which must all be monitored closely to determine the points at which appropriate interventions need to be made; the experience for the mother of having her child present during psychotherapy and the many intrapsychic meanings that this holds for her, which must be examined, particularly in the realm of her self-representation; and, finally, transference and countertransference issues, which are a significant part of this form of treatment. This treatment modality appears to assist the mothers in the regulation of tension, the modification of destructive impulses directed at the children, and the formation of a more reliable self-representation.

In our treatment cases, it is the mother who is identified as the patient, and the child has been brought in to support the mother's treatment and her working through self-esteem issues made more acute by the mothering role. We would like to emphasize the difficulty in returning to the dyadic relationship of mother and therapist alone, without child. It has been anticipated that this would be relatively easy since these patients had reached a stage of their own development as mothers that would permit them to feel that the mothering aspect of their self-representation was now good enough. It had been hypothesized early in these treatment cases that the therapist would have a feeling of satisfaction with a new piece of development that had occurred. What was not taken into account was the absence of the child as the healthiest part of the treatment relationship, that is, the part that was least inhibited, least impaired, and, therefore, most pleasurable in terms of moment-to-moment interaction. These infants became developmentally age appropriate quickly, with all the attendant pleasures that the therapist may experience.

For example, a three-year-old returned after several months of absence to the treatment room with her mother. She had been in regular attendance for the first year of her life, starting at the age of four days. This child demonstrated age-appropriate behavior and had traversed through major developmental milestones with resilience. At the end of this session, she said that she wanted to come back, "before it starts snowing." This was in September, so she herself had set the pace and timing of her presence in the treatment—about every three months. The child herself was able to demonstrate her own internal regulation as she interacted with the therapist.

Modell (1978) has stated that a patient "who is forced into premature self-sufficiency does so by means of an illusion for which the ego pays a price" (p. 495). Adolescent mothers, in particular, may frequently choose to have a baby to repair or restore a defect in themselves. What is missing is the capacity of self-structure to achieve an object relationship inherent in a more mature parenting relationship. The self-defect of a young woman who becomes a mother is built on a fantasy (see Galenson and Swibel 1984) that the baby will be healthy and a conflict-free area of self-representation. What these mothers often fail to take into account is the hated or bad-mother aspect of their self-representation, which under stress becomes split off. So, instead of a fantasied good mother in symbiotic merger with a good baby, one finds instead bad-mother aspects fused with bad-baby representations because of splits in self-representations.

We have found more shame tension (Piers and Singer 1953) related to self-representations than guilt tensions related to the object. We hypothesized that, in lower-functioning women, shame tension would be a more frequent outcome than guilt, which is less related to narcissistic vulnerabilities. This seems to have been borne out in the outcomes of our treatment cases, in which a heightened sense of exposure produced narcissistic rage out of shame tension (see also Kohut 1968).

It appears that, under stress, the first function to go is the newly developed mothering capacity. Because it was the most difficult to achieve and the most tenuous, it is not surprising that it is the first function in the mother that shows impairment. It then becomes appropriate to bring the child back to the treatment room again to allow the mother to experience that holding environment, which assists in reintegration at the very earliest level of a cohesive self.

468

NOTE

During the preparation of this manuscript, Andrew M. Boxer was supported by a predoctoral fellowship from the Clinical Research Training Program in Adolescence, National Institute of Mental Health training grant 5T32-MH14668-10, sponsored by the Center for the Study of Adolescence at Michael Reese Hospital and the Committee on Human Development at the University of Chicago.

REFERENCES

Anthony, E. J., and Benedek, T. 1970. *Parenthood: Its Psychology and Psychopathology.* Boston: Little, Brown.

Benedek, T. 1959. Parenthood as a developmental phase: a contribution to the libido theory. *Journal of the American Psychoanalytic Association* 7:389–417.

Benedek, T. 1970. Parenthood during the life cycle. In E. J. Anthony and T. Benedek, eds. *Parenthood: Its Psychology and Psychopathology.* Boston: Little, Brown.

Bergman, A. 1982. Beyond autism: the study of a psychotic child treatment and follow-up. Paper presented at the World Congress on Infant Psychiatry, Glasgow.

Bettelheim, B. 1965. The problem of generations. In E. Erikson, ed. *The Challenge of Youth.* New York: Anchor.

Blos, P. 1962. *On Adolescence: A Psychoanalytic Interpretation.* New York: Free Press.

Blos, P. 1967. The second individuation process of adolescence. *Psychoanalytic Study of the Child* 22:162–186.

Brazelton, T. B. 1981. Early infant social interaction with parents and strangers. *Journal of the American Academy of Child Psychiatry* 20:132–152.

Brinich, P. 1984. Aggression in early childhood: joint treatment of children and parents. *Psychoanalytic Study of the Child* 39:493–508.

Burlingham, D.; Goldberger, A.; and Lussier, A. 1955. Simultaneous analysis of mother and child. *Psychoanalytic Study of the Child* 10:165–186.

Cohen, R., and Weissman, S. 1984. The parenting alliance. In R. S. Cohen, B. J. Cohler, and S. Weissman, eds. *Parenthood: A Psychodynamic Perspective.* New York: Guilford.

469

Cohler, B. J. 1982. On being therapeutic: issues of person and setting in the psychotherapy of developmental arrests. University of Chicago, Committee on Human Development. Typescript.

Cohler, B. J., and Geyer, E. S. 1982. Psychological autonomy and interdependence within the family. In F. Walsh, ed. *Normal Family Process*. New York: Guilford.

Cook, J. A., and Cohler, B. J. 1986. Reciprocal socialization and the care of offspring with cancer and with schizophrenia. In N. Datan, A. L. Greene, and H. W. Reese, eds. *Life-Span Developmental Psychology: Intergenerational Relations*. Hillsdale, N.J.: Erlbaum.

Eissler, K. R. 1958. Symposium: remarks on some variations of psychoanalytic technique. *International Journal of Psycho-Analysis* 39:222–229.

Erikson, E. 1956. The concept of ego identity. *Journal of the American Psychoanalytic Association* 4:56–121.

Fraiberg, S.; Adelson, E.; and Shapiro, V. 1980. Ghosts in the nursery. In S. Fraiberg, ed. *Clinical Studies in Infant Mental Health*. New York: Basic.

Freud, S. 1911. Formulation on the two principals of mental functioning. *Standard Edition* 12:213–227. London: Hogarth, 1958.

Freud, S. 1914. On narcissism: an introduction. *Standard Edition* 14:69–102. London: Hogarth, 1955.

Freud, S. 1919. The uncanny. *Standard Edition* 17:219–256. London: Hogarth, 1957.

Freud, S. 1931. Female sexuality. *Standard Edition* 21:223–247. London: Hogarth, 1961.

Galenson, E., and Swibel, T. 1984. In J. Hall, E. Galenson, and R. Tyson, eds. *Frontiers of Infant Psychiatry*. New York: Basic.

Greene, A. L., and Boxer, A. M. 1986. Daughters and sons as young adults: restructuring the ties that bind. In N. Datan, A. L. Greene, and H. W. Reese, eds. *Life-Span Developmental Psychology: Intergenerational Relations*. Hillsdale, N.J.: Erlbaum.

Hellman, I.; Friedmann, O.; and Shepheard, E. 1960. Simultaneous analysis of mother and child. *Psychoanalytic Study of the Child* 15:359–377.

Johnson, A., and Szurek, S. 1942. Collaborative psychiatric therapy of parent-child problems. *American Journal of Orthopsychiatry* 12:231–236.

Khan, M. 1974. Ego-distortion, cumulative trauma, and the role of reconstruction in the analytic situation. In M. Khan, ed. *The Privacy of the Self*. New York: International Universities Press.

Kohut, H. 1968. The psychoanalytic treatment of narcissistic personality disorders. *Psychoanalytic Study of the Child* 23:80–113.

Lerner, R. M., and Ryff, C. D. 1978. Implementation of the life-span view of human development: the sample case of attachment. In P. B. Baltes, ed. *Life-Span Development and Behavior,* vol. 1. New York: Academic.

Levy, K. 1960. Simultaneous analysis of mother and child. *Psychoanalytic Study of the Child* 15:378–389.

Loewald, E. 1982. The baby in the mother's treatment. *Psychoanalytic Study of the Child* 23:80–113.

Loewald, E. 1985. Psychotherapy with parent and child in failure-to-thrive: analogies to the treatment of severely disturbed adults. *Psychoanalytic Study of the Child* 40:345–364.

Mahler, M. 1972a. On the first three phases of the separation-individuation process. *International Journal of Psycho-Analysis* 53:333–338.

Mahler, M. 1972b. Rapprochement subphase of the separation individuation. *Psychoanalytic Quarterly* 41:487–506.

Mahler, M.; Pine, F.; and Bergman, A. 1975. *The Psychological Birth of the Human Infant*. New York: Basic.

Modell, A. 1976. The "holding environment" and the therapeutic action of psychoanalysis. *Journal of the American Psychoanalytic Association* 24:285–307.

Modell, A. 1978. The conceptualization of the therapeutic action of psychoanalysis: the action of holding environment. *Bulletin of the Menninger Clinic* 42:493–504.

Piers, G., and Singer, M. 1953. *Shame and Guilt: A Psychoanalytic and a Cultural Study*. Springfield, Ill.: Thomas.

Pollock, G., and Breuer, J. 1968. The possible significance of childhood object loss in the Joseph Breuer–Bertha Poppenheim "Anna O" Sigmund Freud relationship. In J. Gedo and G. Pollock, eds. *Freud: Fusion of Science and Humanism: The Intellectual History of Psychoanalysis*. New York: International Universities Press.

Sandler, J. 1960. The background of safety. *International Journal of Psycho-Analysis* 41:61–72.

Searles, H. 1967. The "dedicated physician" in the field of psychotherapy and psychoanalysis. In R. W. Gibson, ed. *Psychiatry and Psychoanalysis*. Philadelphia: Lippincott.

Toplin, M. 1974. The spotter: the role of the mirroring object in the beginning of the cohesive self. Paper presented at the fifth regional conference of the Chicago Psychoanalytic Society, Chicago.

Weil, A. 1970. The basic core. *Psychoanalytic Study of the Child* 25:442–460.

Weil, N. 1984. The role of facial expressions in the holding environment. *International Journal of Psychoanalytic Psychotherapy* 10:75–89.

Weissman, S. H., and Cohen, R. S. 1985. The parenting alliance and the adolescent. *Adolescent Psychiatry* 12:24–45.

Weissman, S. H.; Cohen, R. S.; Boxer, A. M.; and Cohler, B. J. 1987. The parenthood experience and the child's transition to young adulthood: intergenerational perspectives from a self-psychology framework. Paper presented at the annual meeting of the American Society of Adolescent Psychiatry, Chicago, May.

Winnicott, D. W. 1949. Hate in the counter-transference. In *Through Paediatrics to Psycho-Analysis*. New York: Basic, 1975.

Winnicott, D. W. 1960a. Ego distortion in terms of the true and false self. In *The Maturational Processes and the Facilitating Environment*. New York: International Universities Press, 1965.

Winnicott, D. W. 1960b. The theory of the parent-infant relationship. In *The Maturational Processes and the Facilitating Environment*. New York: International Universities Press, 1965.

Winnicott, D. W. 1967. Mirror-role of the mother and family in child development. In *Playing and Reality*. London: Tavistock, 1971.

26 ADOLESCENTS IN RESIDENTIAL TREATMENT: A SIX-YEAR COMPARISON

DEMOSTHENES A. LORANDOS

Anecdotal evidence from social workers and psychologists involved in the residential treatment of adolescents informs us that kids are getting "sicker" all the time. In the past, orphans, runaways, shoplifters, and kids with special needs were referred to residential programs (Barker 1978), but now, say the workers in these homes, kids who have exhausted outpatient counseling, community day treatment, and foster care and ended up in the residential treatment programs are involved in criminal sexual conduct, felonious assaults, and murder. With the movement to deinstitutionalize the mentally ill, more and more kids from state mental hospitals are being referred to community-based residential treatment programs, and the counselors point to sexual and assaultive incidents in their homes that did not occur a mere ten years ago.

This view is sustained in part by the *Uniform Crime Reports,* printed annually by the Federal Bureau of Investigation (1987), where violent aggravated assaults by juveniles have increased by 8 percent since 1978. Rape by juveniles has increased 20 percent since the late 1970s. Familial pathology is seen as an indication of an overall malaise in the health of the American family, and, if one were to listen to the fundamentalists on the air waves, the number of broken homes creating "sick kids" is at an all-time high. Indeed, single-parent, female-headed homes are said to be at epidemic proportions.

Are these kids "sicker" than they were ten years ago? A review of the computerized data bases such as Medline and Psych-info with key words like "pathology" and "adolescent pathology" lends little to answer this question. In her review of the literature, Johnson (1982) stops short of describing a basal pathology level in adolescents in residential treatment. In discussing adolescents at the Anneewakee residential program, Stewart and Poetter (1976) describe remediation in reactive characterological disorders but fail to provide data to utilize in a 1976–1986 comparison.

In an attempt to describe adolescents in residential settings, Wurtele, Wilson, and Prentice (1983) discuss parental pathology, incidence of broken homes, below-average IQ scores, and academic difficulties. While a comprehensive attempt to describe children in residency was made, little in the way of data useful for replication and later comparison was offered.

With just over twenty years' experience in residential treatment of adolescents and adults, I have been of the opinion that times change, behaviors change, but kids making an attempt to better themselves in residential treatment remain very much the same. This view is seen as heretical among the younger therapists and social workers within these programs. Reviewing national incidence and prevalence reports of adolescent crime and punishment, the casual observer could easily be drawn into a sense of kids as "sicker and sicker."

The purpose of this study was to test a null hypothesis that there is no real difference in cognitive, intellectual, academic, and pathology-indicating variables in adolescents within residential treatment in the last six years. The study was conducted at Teen Ranch, a seventy-bed residential treatment program in three Michigan counties. Teen Ranch uses the teaching-parent model and has been providing high-quality residential and outreach treatment to adolescents and their families for a generation.

Method

SUBJECTS

The subjects in this study were 534 boys referred to the Teen Ranch residential treatment program from January 1983 through June 1988. They ranged in age from eleven to seventeen years, with a mean age of fourteen years six months at onset of treatment. Assessments revealed a mean Wechsler Intelligence Scale for Children–Revised (WISC-R) full-scale IQ of ninety-eight, and the subjects' average length of stay was fifteen months.

Typically, most boys were removed from their parents' care prior to placement at the ranch. Most came from single-parent and dysfunctional families and had spent time in a variety of foster homes and treatment and detention centers before placement at Teen Ranch. Unlike teenagers in other studies (Barker 1978; Wurtele et al. 1983), a history of substance abuse and violent crime was common among Teen Ranch residents. Typically, mental health and community day treatment alternatives had been exhausted prior to placement. Teen Ranch accepted all referrals, and any boy willing to try to change his life was accepted into the program.

PROCEDURE

Within thirty days of the onset of treatment, each boy was given a full battery of psychological tests, including a Mental Status Examination, Bender-Gestalt Test, Slosson Drawing Coordination Test, WISC-R, Wide Range Achievement Test–Revised (WRAT-R), H-R Stress Test, Projective Drawings, Self-Description Inventory, Sentence Completion Test, and a Minnesota Multiphasic Personality Inventory (in Overall's abbreviated "168" version; MMPI-168). The most clearly objective of these measures, the WISC-R, WRAT-R, and MMPI-168, were utilized for this study as their standard and T-scores could be easily codified.

The 534 test batteries were divided into groups by year 1983–1988 inclusive, and each boy's chronological age and his score on the WISC-R, WRAT-R, and MMPI-168 entered into N. H. Analytical Software's Stastix II program in an IBM AT. Each boy's onset of treatment assessment was reduced to twenty-nine variables, including chronological age in years and months, eleven WISC-R scores, three WRAT-R standard scores, and thirteen MMPI-168 individual scale T-scores. A brief descriptive statistics package analyzed this data and produced means and standard deviations for these variables for each year.

Results

Twenty-nine mean variable values from age in years through intelligence scores and mean response levels to the personality tests for my

475

sample of 534 cases were placed in a matrix for each year 1983–1988. This matrix of 174 values was fed into the N. H. Analytical Software's Stastix II program as described.

Pearson r product-moment correlations were run intercorrelating a year-by-year matrix to examine the variables in linear association. The results (table 1) indicate that the variables bear essentially the same relation to one another year after year. That is, the typical resident in 1983 presents almost identically to the typical resident in 1984, 1985, and so on through 1988.

As some could argue, it may be possible for the linear association between the variables to maintain the same relation while residents are becoming slightly worse. A chi-square matrix was run on all twenty-nine mean/year variables times each of six years.

The chi-square process was utilized to generate an expectation probability and compare that to the cell values. These values, when compared to the chi-square table at degrees of freedom, offer a number that informs us of the probability of getting a value by chance. As my null hypothesis held that there is no difference between the mean values for the 1983 resident, 1984 resident, and so on, the chi-square process was utilized to provide an indication of the sum of the variance between what we could expect if the residents presented as essentially the same over time and the reported mean variable values. The lower the chi-square score, the less variance between the null hypothesis and the obtained values.

The overall chi-square value was 11.38, with 140 degrees of freedom. This is clearly not significant and informs us that the residents are not changing appreciably over time. In 174 individual chi-square cells, there was not one significant difference.

TABLE 1
PEARSONr CORRELATIONS OF MEAN/YEAR VARIABLES COMPARED YEAR TO YEAR

	Year 1	Year 2	Year 3	Year 4	Year 5	Year 6
Year 1	1.0000					
Year 2	.9988	1.0000				
Year 3	.9975	.9985	1.0000			
Year 4	.9950	.9941	.9973	1.0000		
Year 5	.9964	.9968	.9981	.9982	1.0000	
Year 6	.9869	.9868	.9916	.9957	.9948	1.0000

Discussion

Certainly, the argument could be made that Teen Ranch has accepted the same sort of boy month after month, year after year, into its residential treatment program. This is not supported by the intake data. Every boy who is ambulatory, has an IQ above fifty, and is willing to make some attempt, any attempt, to better himself (often just getting out of detention is seen by the prospective resident as motivation enough to say that he will change) is accepted into the ranch program. The family-style treatment milieu and strong undercurrent of basic values often has a surprisingly positive effect on the residents. No, it is not that the ranch is taking only a clone of each resident before him; it is trying to help just about all the boys who are referred. The homogeneity among adolescents referred is not due to an intake policy at the ranch.

Perhaps the social workers and juvenile court personnel who make referrals to Teen Ranch all see the ranch the same way and refer only a specific type of boy. This idea is also unsupported by the data. Sitting in public relations and informative luncheons put on by the ranch over the last few years, I have heard widely diverging ideas about who does best in the ranch program from foster care, delinquency, and adoption workers throughout Michigan. It is not a particular form of steering a certain type of adolescent to Teen Ranch that accounts for this homogeneity.

Interestingly, it is the old hands, the therapists, program directors, and directors emeriti, who understand this homogeneity best. "Sure, times change and the trouble they're in changes, but the boys are the same, down in their hearts they're the same," say the old-timers. This research supports their understanding.

REFERENCES

Barker, P. 1978. The impossible child: some approaches to treatment. *Canadian Psychiatric Association Journal* 23:1–21.

Federal Bureau of Investigation. *Uniform Crime Reports*. Washington, D.C.: U.S. Department of Justice, 1987.

Johnson, S. 1982. Residential treatment for emotionally disturbed children and adolescents: a review of the literature. *Canada's Mental Health* 5:8–19.

Stewart, H., and Poetter, L. 1976. Therapeutic process with adolescents at Anneewakee. *Adolescence* 11:213–216.

Wurtele, S. K.; Wilson, D. R.; and Prentice, D. S. 1983. Characteristics of children in residential treatment programs: findings and clinical implications. *Journal of Clinical Child Psychology* 12:137–144.

27 NON-SELF-CONTROLLED ADOLESCENTS: APPLICATIONS OF COGNITIVE-BEHAVIORAL THERAPY

KEVIN R. RONAN AND PHILIP C. KENDALL

How best to interact therapeutically with adolescents? Adolescence is itself a period of dramatic personal, physical, and cognitive change (e.g., Sprinthall and Collins 1984; Steinberg and Silverberg 1986). Psychologically, adolescent clients are neither children, who may need external adult controls, nor full adults, whose independence would be assured. Medications may be helpful in certain instances, though there are cases in which medications effective with adults are not potent with adolescents. Adolescents are a special sample.

We do not propose to have a singular answer to our opening question. We do, however, have a proposal that is based on both the theory of adolescent development and evidence of related clinical outcome. The cognitive-behavioral approach outlined herein was developed for use with non-self-controlled, impulsive children and adolescents. Young people of this type have been classified as attention disordered, overactive, disobedient to authorities, externalizing (Achenbach 1966), undercontrolled, and/or aggressive toward others. They may carry formal DSM-III-R diagnoses of attention-deficit hyperactivity disorder (ADHD), undifferentiated attention-deficit disorder, or conduct disorder.

This therapeutic regimen attempts to teach adolescents to control impulsive behavior by training them in the use of problem-solving self-instructions aimed at reducing deficits in verbal mediation, social

479

problem solving, and perspective taking. As will be discussed, the intervention utilizes cognitive and behavioral methods, including formal and informal coping modeling, affective education, practice and role playing, and reinforcement via tangible and social reward contingencies to help the adolescent learn the self-guided problem-solving skills. Put simply, the purpose of the cognitive-behavioral training program is to help the adolescent stop and think before acting. We believe that the adolescent's acquisition, implementation, and generalization of stop-and-think skills is achieved most efficiently via the repetitious modeling and practice of reflecting thinking skills in a setting providing clear incentives and strong social support.

Owing to space considerations and the importance of spelling out in some detail the particulars of the intervention itself, discussion of related issues necessarily must be curtailed. Therefore, we briefly discuss theoretical formulations focusing specifically on the cognitive-developmental features implicated as targets for treatment and research assessing the efficacy of the intervention itself, including its utility with clinical populations and as adjunctive to pharmacologic intervention. Salient issues, including assessment, desirable therapist attributes, coping with impulsive behavior, therapeutic applications of directed discovery principles, and other issues related to the intervention, are discussed.[1]

Cognitive Features

A cognitive-behavioral model of child/adolescent psychopathology places a major emphasis on the youth's learning environment, along with the attendant influences of external contingencies and models, and the prominence of information-processing and mediation factors in the development, maintenance, and treatment of childhood/adolescent disorders such as ADHD and conduct disorder (Kendall 1985; Kendall and Ronan 1990). While the model does not place primary emphasis on biological, neurological, and genetic factors, they are nevertheless acknowledged as being of potential etiological importance in the development of some disorders of childhood and adolescence. Affective processes, family and social contexts, and developmental considerations are assigned meaningful places alongside cognitive and behavioral processes in understanding and treating childhood and adolescent disorders. A cognitive-behavioral representation of child/adolescent disorders does indeed consider numerous aspects of the youngster's world.[2] We will focus here specifically on one of the areas that has received recent theoretical interest and renewed therapeutic attention—the cognitive/developmental features implicated in the non-self-controlled disorders of childhood and adolescence.

A number of recent theorists have focused on cognitions as an information-processing system (e.g., Ingram and Kendall 1986; Kendall and Ingram 1987; Marzillier 1980; Turk and Speers 1983). One such model (Ingram and Kendall 1986; Kendall and Ingram 1987) based on an information-processing system distinguishes between the conceptual heuristics of cognitive structures, cognitive contents (events), cognitive processes (operations), and cognitive products. *Cognitive structures* may be viewed as the means by which incoming information is internally represented. One way to look at cognitive structures is by the metaphor of the hardware of a system—its indexing and filing functions. *Cognitive contents* refers not to the hardware of representation but to the actual information or propositions that are stored within the cognitive structures. *Cognitive processes* are the methods or means by which the information-processing system carries out its various functions or operations (e.g., input, processing, and output). Finally, the interface between incoming information and cognitive structures, content, and operations results in *cognitive products*. The thoughts or internal dialogue that one experiences in everyday life (e.g., current concerns, attributions, problem solving) are content and product, depending on their relation to the target event.

A recent formulation implicates the interface between cognitive processing and cognitive products in the development, maintenance, and remediation of childhood disorders such as ADHD and conduct disorder. The potentially significant delineation has been referred to as *cognitive distortions* versus *cognitive deficiencies* (Kendall 1985). As the term suggests, cognitive distortions point to inaccurate thinking processes manifested as dysfunctional and often negative self-talk. Cognitive distortions tend to invite overcontrolled behavior patterns based on misperceptions of environmental demands, excessive self-criticism, and an undervaluation of abilities. Disorders associated with distorted cognitive processing and overcontrolled behavior include those that are associated more with anxious, depressed (Kendall, Stark, and Adam in press), withdrawn, and/or isolated patterns of behavior (e.g., anxiety, depression, eating disorders).

481

Cognitive deficiencies, the primary focus of the present treatment, are not erroneous processing but rather a generalized lack of mental activity in which engagement in careful and planned cognitive processing (e.g., forethought) would be quite beneficial (e.g., perspective taking, interpersonal problem solving). Cognitive deficiencies, then, point to a lack of cognitive planning and execution; consequently, the manifest problems are associated with a correlated lack of verbal mediation and a resultant lack of self-control. Disorders of this type point to the undercontrolled, acting-out nature characteristic of impulsive, hyperactive, and aggressive behavioral patterns often seen in non-self-controlled children (e.g., ADHD, conduct disorder).

Another cognitive feature holding promise is the concept of the *schema*. Representing the interdependence between cognitive structures and content, the schema works as an organizing principle, or template, from which each adolescent constructs his or her own view of himself or herself, others, the environment, and the past, present, and future. While much needs to be learned about the role of schemata in non-self-controlled disorders, the clinical assessment of each adolescent's unique cognitive template by various means (e.g., as reported by the youngster and significant others [see Kendall and Braswell 1985]) may allow the therapist access into the young client's private world. This "therapeutic perspective" allows for the structure of the therapy to be geared according to each client's individual needs (see Kendall, Ronan, and Epps, in press; Kendall and Siqueland, in press) and may further serve to promote the alliance between adolescent and therapist.

It is our belief that the therapeutic efforts aimed at ameliorating cognitive deficits and promoting positive structural change (e.g., increased self-perceptions of competence) are enhanced by the adolescent actively and thoughtfully inculcating the cognitive aspects of the training program rather than passively memorizing rote material. The cognitive process utilized in the present intervention to promote active involvement and optimal change is known as *directed discovery* (see also Brown, Bransford, Ferrara, and Campione 1983). As will be emphasized a number of times, it is crucial to gear the therapy program initially to match the adolescent's level of cognitive or schematic understanding. The adolescent must initially be able to assimilate new material within ongoing schemes before any change is possible (Piaget 1954). As Overton (1972) points out, any problem beyond the realm of structural assimilation is a "nonexperience" (Dewey 1938) having limited meaning for the child. For change and improvement to occur, the therapeutic environment must be such that the child is able to incorporate the material at his or her level of understanding (i.e., assimilation) and modify this level of understanding in accordance with the environmental material (i.e., accommodation). This delicate interplay between assimilative and accommodative activity requires that both therapist and therapy be concerned with providing, or "arranging," experiences that set problems for youngsters that invite their active involvement according to their level of understanding of the task involved and that result in structural schematic change that is linked to clinical improvement. In our case, of course, this arrangement of experiences targets the cognitive deficits and related behavioral and emotional problems of the non-self-controlled adolescent. We will discuss how to apply these principles more specifically when we detail the application of the therapy program.

An adolescent who learns to execute planned cognitive strategies may accrue several observable benefits. First, he or she becomes a more cautious self-monitor and more active cognitive processor who may make better sense of various situations (e.g., home, school) potentially resulting in more adaptive behavioral outcomes. Second, an adolescent who becomes proficient at utilizing self-paced self-instructions will have successfully coped with numerous personal and interpersonal difficulties. These success experiences may become inculcated within the adolescent's schema and thereby help shift his or her self-view from one of limited ability to one of a person who is capable within his or her environment. Increased self-esteem and self-perceptions of competence may then lead to further improvements. For example, the youngster might begin to view difficult situations as problems capable of being solved rather than as having an inevitable outcome based on the adolescent's view that he or she is a "bad" person who has seemingly no control over his or her behavior (e.g., "I can't help it, I'm hyper"). Accordingly, the ability to utilize cognitive strategies may also diffuse tension in the home and at school if various situations are framed as problems to be solved rather than as a function of a hopelessly difficult youngster. In a later section, we will look at empirical efforts that actually address the ameliorative potential of the treatment program. However, let us first turn our attention to detailing the components and structure of the cognitive-behavior therapy designed to help non-self-controlled adolescents discover how to stop and think.

Cognitive-Behavioral Treatment Program Components

The cognitive-behavioral training program for teaching self-control consists of six major components: a problem-solving approach, self-instructional training, coping modeling, affective education, role-play exercises, and behavioral contingencies. Although these strategies are implemented as an integrated treatment package, they are first described separately to clarify the role of each (see also Braswell and Kendall 1987). The following section describes the interplay between each when applied with the non-self-controlled adolescent.

PROBLEM-SOLVING APPROACH WITH ADOLESCENTS

A problem-solving approach toward difficult interpersonal-social situations is central to this therapeutic program. Arising directly from cognitive, behavioral, and developmental theorizing, it is a strategy to teach youngsters with cognitive deficits to engage and utilize adaptive planning strategies when encountering a vast array of problematic situations. The client acquiring the ability to apply this cognitive "attitude" across situations is the desired therapeutic outcome. It is desirable for the therapist to emphasize continually that difficult situations are merely problems that may often be solved by stopping and thinking rather than being outside the young client's control (see also D'Zurilla 1986; Spivack, Platt, and Shure 1976).

We should here make a few points regarding the role of the therapist. Use of directed discovery principles may help elucidate the nature of the problem-solving environment that we emphasize with adolescent clients. We find it desirable for the therapist to fulfill diverse but related roles—diagnostician, educator, consultant. As educator, the therapist is concerned with teaching the adolescent how to apply problem-solving self-instructions to a diverse array of problematic situations. The teaching of self-guided instructions to adolescents emphasizes the therapist—as consultant—actively pursuing a collaborative relationship and problem-solving alliance with the client. We find that reaching this goal requires an acknowledgment of the emerging issues of the adolescent client (e.g., cognitive development, identity formation, autonomy issues, physical development). Consistent with directed discovery principles, it is crucial for the therapist—as diagnostician—to assess and be sensitive to the unique developmental characteristics of the adolescent client. For example, Piaget points out that it is during adolescence that formal operational thinking is acquired. Adolescents begin to be able to reflect on their thinking (Flavell 1977); hypothetical rather than concrete reality becomes a primary issue (Overton 1972). It is important for the therapist to be sensitive to the fact that chronological age and physical development are not necessarily synchronous with cognitive development when considering the level of the adolescent's reasoning abilities. A fourteen-year old may appear physically to be adult-like; however, close scrutiny of his or her cognitive style may reveal a tendency to reason through problems in a more concrete than abstract fashion. A clinical assessment of the adolescent's problem-solving style may provide the therapist with the initial "data base" from which to pursue his or her role as educator and consultant during the teaching of individualized, self-guided, problem-solving instructions (to be discussed in the next section).

The growth in cognitive skills during adolescence is often accompanied by concurrent cognitive/emotional limitations that also have implications for the therapist as self-instructional educator and problem-solving consultant (Kendall and Williams 1986). As Elkind (1967, 1978) points out, the new-found ability to think about one's own thought may lead the adolescent to become somewhat obsessed with this discovery. At the same time, the adolescent is often not yet able to separate his or her thoughts fully from those of others. These limitations, in concert with an adolescent's increased concern about his or her social behavior, may lead the youngster to believe that others are also overly scrutinizing his or her actions. This "imaginary audience" phenomenon often contributes to another cognitive/developmental limitation—the personal fable. Elkind (1967, 1978) states that the personal fable is the adolescent's belief that his or her emotional experiences are most original and unlike those of any other. The personal fable is based on the adolescent's belief that, because so many others seem to be so scrutinizing and concerned with the adolescent's behavior (i.e., imaginary audience), he or she must be genuinely different and truly unique.

The therapist may find it very helpful to recognize and adjust to these cognitive features when problem solving with the adolescent client. For example, trying too hard to convey an understanding of the adolescent's thoughts and feelings may be counterproductive. The therapist may instead allow the adolescent more autonomy by acknowledging that the therapist may not fully understand or have the answers to the adolescent's problems; rather, it may be stressed that the adolescent is the only one who can decide what is right. The following brief interchange may be illustrative.

> *Client*. You have no idea what my problems really are. You can't tell me what to do.
> *Therapist*. You're right; I don't know what's right for you or even what you would like to have happen here. I'm here instead to help you try some different ways to think about problems like the ones we talked about a little earlier. You, and only you, can decide on what truly works best for you.
> *Client*. I don't believe you; you're going to tell me what to do, just like they do at school.
> *Therapist*. Well, you're an emerging adult, and you're going to have to make up your own mind what to do—I can't tell you what to do, and I won't. What I can do is maybe help you think things through so you can anticipate what might happen and make some good choices. You'll be more sure of what you want and how you might go about getting there.
> *Client*. Well, we'll see.

This introduction to therapy will have to be supplemented with a consistent follow-through as impulsive adolescents often can be quite persistent in testing their therapists. Consistently promoting adolescent autonomy may also serve to enhance therapist likability—a variable that has been implicated as a potentially important predictor of therapy outcome (Tramontana 1980).

SELF-INSTRUCTIONAL TRAINING

Self-instructional training is a step-by-step thinking strategy taught to guide the adolescent through the problem-solving process. Self-instructions are discrete steps that the youngster may apply to diverse problematic situations. As illustrated in table 1, the self-instructions move from the generation of a problem definition (identifying a

486

TABLE 1

CONTENT OF SELF-INSTRUCTIONAL PROCEDURES

Problem definition	"What's the problem? What do I have to figure out?"
Problem approach	"I need to think about different choices to this problem."
Focusing of attention	"Okay, now I have to concentrate and think how each choice will affect myself and others. What are the consequences?"
Choosing an answer	"Okay, I've thought about it, and I think this one is best."
Self-reinforcement or Coping statement	"I made a good choice—good job"
	"Okay, that choice wasn't the best for me to make. I just have to concentrate and stop and think through the problem. I can do it—I can make good choices for myself—I just need to stop and think. Let's try that one again."

Adopted from Braswell and Kendall (1987).

problem to be solved), to approaching the problem in a systematic fashion, focusing of attention and generating alternatives, and choosing an answer, followed by either self-reinforcement for correct responses or a coping response following a wrong answer.

This sequence is designed to encourage adolescents to reflect critically—to stop and think—about the following: the problem that needs to be analyzed, how to initiate a cognitive strategy, how to consider alternatives and the behavioral and emotional consequences of each, and how to make a choice of a possible solution and follow through on the thoughtful plan. Self-reinforcement is designed to strengthen the use of the stop-and-think process by reminding the adolescent that appropriate choices may often have positive, self-rewarding consequences. Coping statements are included to help reduce the possibility of "blowups" resulting from becoming overly frustrated following a mistake. The therapist can be helpful by demonstrating that everyone occasionally makes mistakes and that utilizing an appropriate coping self-statement can help get the problem solver "back on track" to more effective problem solving.

A crucial aspect of the self-instructional training includes individualizing the self-statements for the specific client. It is important for the therapist to collaborate with the adolescent to come up with suitable individualized self-directed statements rather than allowing the self-instructions to be taught and learned in a mechanical, rote fashion. The purpose of the individualizing of the self-instructional sequence is to make the self-statements the "personal property" of the adolescent potentially allowing him or her to carry and utilize these self-statements outside the therapy setting. In more technical terms, this process is designed to promote the acquisition, maintenance, and generalization of self-instructions.

Collaborating with the adolescent in choosing suitable self-instructions evolves out of the notions of directed discovery. The child, with the help of the therapist, is led to discover suitable self-instructional statements. Some research has supported the view that directed discovery training can be generalized to alternate cognitive tasks. In a study examining the interaction of Piagetian stage of the child (preoperational vs. concrete operations) with type of training, only concrete operational children who received a directed-discovery type of training demonstrated significant generalization to nontraining tasks (Schleser, Cohen, Meyers, and Rodick 1984). Another benefit of having the child choose suitable self-statements lies in the collaboration process itself. Encouraging the young client's involvement serves to enpower him or her with an active role in the therapeutic process. Indeed, research supports the notion that youngsters who are the most actively involved in therapy sessions also tend to display the most behavioral improvement following treatment (Braswell, Kendall, Braith, Carey, and Vye 1985).

Consistent with the foregoing, the cognitive/developmental level of each client must be taken into account when teaching self-instructions. When treating adolescents, the cognitive advance into formal operational, adult-like reasoning capacity may provide the clinician with the opportunity to gear the program toward a more conceptual and abstract level, taking into account nascent adolescent issues (e.g., physical development, identity formation, autonomy issues). In fact, research has indicated that a more abstract, conceptual approach to teaching self-instructions produced greater benefits with non-self-controlled children than a more concrete, task-focused approach (Kendall and Wilcox 1980).

A brief digression on therapy tasks may be helpful at this point. When teaching self-instructions, various tasks may be utilized. The actual tasks used may be of less importance than the understanding that they are therapeutic tools designed to help the adolescent learn and utilize the self-instructions in an interpersonally adaptive fashion. Nevertheless, a set of training materials, the *Stop and Think Workbook,* is available (Kendall 1989). During the first phases of therapy, tasks are generally psychoeducational, with little or no emotional arousing capacity. Later, the emphasis shifts to tasks involving interpersonal play situations (e.g., checkers, card games requiring forethought). The next sessions involve affective education. These sessions utilize tasks requiring the client to generate affective labels and behavioral alternatives and consequences to problematic interpersonal situations (see the section on affective education for examples). Finally, as will be discussed shortly, actual role plays are utilized as a forum for addressing both hypothetical and real-life problems. This task sequence is designed to ensure that the adolescent learns the application of thoughtful problem solving in relatively nonstressful situations before having to utilize the process in emotionally charged interpersonal situations.

COPING MODELING

Therapist modeling of cognitive and behavioral problem solving is designed to facilitate the adolescent's acquisition of these strategies. The therapist alternates performing tasks with the client and in so doing models the self-instructional problem-solving sequence. The therapist does not tell the youngster what to do or how to do it but rather solves problems himself or herself using the strategies that are being taught to the adolescent. The therapist as a problem-solving model actually demonstrates to the adolescent that stopping and thinking about problematic situations—seeking alternative solutions, evaluating these possibilities, and anticipating likely consequences—can be a valuable means by which both to resolve difficult situations and to reach desired goals.

Modeling serves a vital function by, in less structured contexts, calling for innovation, skill, and timing on the part of the therapist. He or she serves as an informal model to solve real-life problem situations that arise during the course of therapy. For example, the therapist may appear disorganized and initially frustrated at not being organized. Through overt modeling of a planned sequence, he or she may demonstrate how to cope with difficulties and how to reach a desired goal by stopping and thinking. The therapist presenting as a coping model—occasionally making a mistake but nevertheless demonstrating a strategy for preventing or correcting that misbehavior—is emphasized. Failure and frustration resulting from a pattern of poorly planned, impulsive acts are not uncommon in the history of many of these children/adolescents. The coping model allows the adolescent to observe that mistakes and frustration may be dealt with adaptively rather than being a catalyst for more frustration. Therapist modeling of patient and careful use of stop-and-think skills (including coping statements when necessary) demonstrates the capacity to cope with difficult situations even in the face of initial frustration or failure. This is in contrast to a mastery model in which problem situations are successfully dealt with in a facile, unconcerned manner. "Real-life" situations utilized to demonstrate self-corrective strategies may be planned prior to the therapy sessions.

AFFECTIVE EDUCATION

The therapy program is designed to help the adolescent accurately label his or her emotional states as well as those of others. The rationale for this component lies in the belief that the ability to identify feeling states will improve personal and interpersonal problem-solving effectiveness. The tasks for affective education may be pictures showing persons with various expressions and postures in problematic situations. We use and recommend cartoons with empty thought bubbles and contemporary magazine pictures. The crucial aspect is to generate a discussion of emotions, how emotions are related to thoughts and behaviors, and the role of self-talk in appropriately mediating emotional arousal. The affective educational component is usually introduced in the latter stages of therapy after the self-instructional problem-solving sequence has been learned. In a sixteen-session therapy, sessions 12 and 13 are usually devoted to this training. Of course, modifications in the timing of these sessions should be made where needed. Role plays, discussed next, may facilitate the integration of an adolescent's cognitive problem solving and feeling states in interpersonal problem-solving situations.

490

ROLE-PLAY EXERCISES

The performance-based component of the therapy—role playing—is introduced following affective education. The purpose here is to promote the generalization of self-instructions to emotionally charged real-life situations.

Role-play sessions can begin with common interpersonal problems listed on a set of index cards. These situations can reflect both typical adolescent concerns and those relevant to the problematic themes in the adolescent's life. Initially, it may be desirable to handle hypothetical situations before moving on to "real" problems: this may ease the client into a more active involvement in the role playing. Some of these "hypothetical" situations may in fact be real problem situations for the youngster but may be general enough so that he or she does not feel specifically singled out.

The therapist and adolescent begin role plays by alternating in the random selection of cards. After reading the card together, both then generate alternative solutions. After a number of alternatives have been suggested, the emotional and behavioral consequences are chained to each alternative from both the client's and the other's perspectives. The client and therapist then perform each alternative and its outcome, after which a discussion of their thoughts and feelings about each situation follows. The client then picks the response that he or she views as best. These role plays are brief (two to four minutes), with more extended discussion following the role play.

A few additional points must be mentioned to supplement the structure described. As in all phases of therapy, and particularly important here, the client's active involvement should be encouraged (let the client make suggestions, choose props, etc.). Additionally, it is advantageous to create an environment in which the client feels safe enough to act out potentially embarrassing thoughts, feelings, behaviors, and so forth. For adolescents resistant to role plays, the therapist may actually demonstrate that he or she is thinking and feeling awkward and reluctant but nonetheless copes with these thoughts and feelings (e.g., "I'll look stupid. . . . Well, maybe I can just try one. . . . Even if I don't do it right the first time, I can keep trying. . . . Besides, what's the worst thing that will happen anyway?"). It should also be conveyed to adolescent clients that some real-life situations have more than one desirable alternative and that others may not have a truly "best" choice—it will be up to them to decide on which alternative works best for them.

BEHAVIORAL CONTINGENCIES

Behavioral contingencies are specifically designed to motivate non-self-controlled, externalizing children and adolescents to learn and apply problem-solving self-instructions. The specific contingencies used in the treatment program include social reward, response cost, and self-reward. Additionally, concrete rewards are given for demonstrating self-evaluating behavior and problem-solving skills within the therapeutic setting and completing assignments between sessions. With adolescents, specific behavioral programs may be perceived as overly intrusive and/or punitive, possibly resulting in a heightened resistance to active participation in therapy. We first describe the contingencies as originally designed for younger children, where necessary, we then describe appropriate modifications for the adolescent client.

As with the other reward contingencies, social approval is designed to create an environment in which the young client feels secure and motivated to learn and use the strategies being taught. Smiles and comments such as "good job," "excellent," and other appropriate social messages are used liberally. Additionally, research suggests that remarks such as "keep it up" and "way to keep trying" may be particularly valuable (Braswell et al. 1985). Adolescent clients—by virtue of their cognitive/developmental characteristics—may overly scrutinize therapist comments as to their sincerity. A well-timed approval in some cases may be more advantageous than showering them with continual praise.

A response-cost contingency is included owing to the general nature of the externalizing youngster. Non-self-controlled children and adolescents tend to be quite impulsive when resolving a problematic situation, often failing to evaluate alternative solutions. If an impulsive child is rewarded only for correct answers, which may be due to luck or other factors, his or her target problem (i.e., failing to utilize a cognitive strategy) becomes spuriously rewarded. A response-cost procedure thus attempts to circumvent this potential problem. The client is given a specified number of chips at the beginning of each session, which may be saved for some agreed-on prizes. He or she is then told that chips may be lost for specific behaviors. For example, reward tokens might be lost for failing to use the self-instructions, going too quickly, or getting an incorrect answer to a therapy task. These are to be construed not as punishments but rather as cues to the child (logical consequences) that he or she needs to slow down and be cautious.

To promote the autonomy of the adolescent client, the response-cost contingency might be modified to downplay the possibility that the adolescent perceives the contingency as both externally controlled and overly punitive. For example, the adolescent may be told that he or she is responsible for monitoring his or her own behaviors in each session. After each therapy task—with the help of the therapist/consultant—the adolescent self-evaluates whether he or she utilized the self-guided problem-solving steps appropriately and then, if necessary, is responsible for enacting a response cost. Of course, the therapist might want to "drop hints" in cases in which the adolescent fails to see that his or her behavior warrants a response-cost enactment. As with other procedures, the therapist models the self-monitoring behavior necessary to self-direct this contingency. Of course, this includes modeling the self-corrective coping behaviors necessary for successful resolution of a problem following the enactment of the response-cost "consequence."

A brief word on concrete reinforcers used with adolescents—the tangible rewards utilized for "purchase" with adolescent clients may vary as long as they are agreed on by client and therapist. A "reward menu" is collaboratively drawn up by the therapist and adolescent in initial sessions that lists prizes, varying in "price," that may be purchased. Encouraging more social rewards (e.g., time spent playing computer games with the therapist) and using abstract purchasing "points" (e.g., stop-and-think points) may be more palatable to an adolescent than employing the more concrete rewards and bonus chips generally utilized with younger children.

Self-reward is encouraged. The exact wording may be flexible; the important point is that the adolescent acknowledge and self-reinforce after successful use of problem-solving strategies. To promote self-awareness skills necessary for both self-monitoring and intrinsic reward capacity, self-evaluation is included at the end of each session. The adolescent rates his or her behavior on a five-point scale. Verbal labels accompanying the numbers indicate behavior ranging from 1 ("not so hot") to 5 ("super"). The therapist also rates the client's behavior and provides stop-and-think points when the two ratings agree within one point. This procedure is typically explained early on, and a rationale for the therapist's choice of a particular rating (including referring to specific behaviors) is provided.

Therapeutic activity outside the therapy setting is desirable. Show That I Can (STIC) tasks (Kendall, Kane, Howard, and Siqueland 1989) are included to help the adolescent begin to use stop-and-think skills between sessions. We have found that framing assignments between sessions as STIC tasks rather than as specific homework assignments tends to enhance compliance. Typically, these assignments progress from the adolescent describing a situation between sessions in which self-instructions may have been appropriate to actually employing these skills in problematic situations. At the beginning of each session, the adolescent describes when and how he or she identified a problem and thought it through. Social and tangible rewards (stop-and-think points) are given for completed STIC assignments. The story that the adolescent offers does not have to be checked for validity; it is the appropriate use and elaboration of problem solving that should be rewarded since thinking about a social problem and the problem-solving sequence "at that moment" is by itself beneficial to the assimilation of these skills within the adolescent's cognitive repertoire.

Integration of Treatment Components

The cognitive, behavioral, and affective components described are not implemented separately but are interwoven within the entire treatment program (Braswell and Kendall 1987). We first describe the structure of individual sessions and then give an overview of the progressive phases of the intervention.

INDIVIDUAL SESSIONS

There is a fairly consistent order of events within each individual session. All sessions (other than the first, to be discussed shortly) begin with a brief period of pleasant conversation, followed by having the adolescent describe performance on the prior STIC task. Next, the task for the session is introduced. The therapist and adolescent collaborate to arrange the task, set any rules, and use appropriate self-instructions applicable to that task. Working together involves the therapist consulting with the adolescent to help the young client think through each problem. While encouraging the stop-and-think process is emphasized, the specific answer chosen is up to the adolescent. It may be desirable earlier in the therapy sequence for the therapist to begin the task focus by modeling the use of the problem-solving steps applicable to that task. Next, the therapist consults/collaborates with the client to solve the task (e.g., giving the adolescent well-timed hints). Finally, the adolescent can "solo" on that task while individually self-instructing. Therapist and client may then perform alternate tasks in this collaborative fashion, with the adolescent doing more as the session progresses. The adolescent is encouraged to be responsible for enacting response cost—with appropriate hints from the therapist/consultant. When response cost is warranted, a review of the problem-solving steps may be helpful, the therapist taking the lead in overtly talking through the problem-solving sequence for the next few tasks, encouraging the adolescent to do the same. The end of each session involves the therapist and client filling out the self-evaluation rating scale. Stop-and-think points earned during the session may be used to purchase a reward or "banked" for future use. Each session tends to have this same basic sequence of events; typically, earlier sessions are more structured than later sessions.

PHASES OF TREATMENT

As the child begins to assimilate new material, the therapy program is designed to "shift gears" to maintain pace with the changing client. The progressive nature of the treatment program may be broken down into the following four phases: introduction, skill building, skill expansion, and skill consolidation and termination. These stages derive from research experience with implementation of twelve- to twenty-session protocols (e.g., Kendall and Braswell 1982; Kendall, Reber, McCleer, Epps, and Ronan 1988).

INTRODUCTION

The introductory phase encompasses an average of 25 percent of total sessions. However, the number of sessions may be modified in either direction, depending on the adolescent's facility for acquiring

495

new information. The purposes of this phase are twofold: establishing a good therapeutic relationship and introducing the structure of the program. Early sessions allow for a presentation of all the treatment components. The time allowed for this collaborative effort may be modified depending on how quickly the client is able to understand the wealth of new material being presented.

Encouraging a positive affective tone to the therapeutic relationship during these discussions is essential. Therapist acknowledgment of the adolescent's unique characteristics can further the therapeutic alliance during this and later phases. Encouraging his or her participation in therapy as a young adult is desirable (taking responsibility for individualizing self-statements, enacting response costs, deciding on rewards, etc.). The therapist is also encouraged to frame the program as a collaborative effort wherein both participants are problem solvers working together. These points may be illustrated in the following exchange:

> *Therapist*. Okay, let's talk for a minute about how you and I can work together to help you decide how you can deal with some of these tough situations that we talked about.
> *Client*. Yeah, okay, but you can't really help me decide what to do—you don't know who I am or what my problems are.
> *Therapist*. I accept that—we'll both take turns solving problems. We'll use the stop-and-think method together. This method might help us look at different ways of handling problems. When it's your turn to solve a problem, we'll look at different ways to handle it and how these different solutions might affect you and others. Then you choose the plan that works best for you.
> *Client*. So you mean we both think about different answers but, when it's my turn, only I get to choose what to do?
> *Therapist*. You got it—we team up as we use the stop-and-think skills; then you pick the answer that works best for you.

At this point, it is also helpful to discuss the presenting problem by having the adolescents discuss their perceptions of why they are in treatment. Emphasis on addressing problematic situations should be encouraged rather than talking in a more general manner about life, school, or the reasons for therapy. These actual problematic situations are then framed as problems whose solutions, with the use of some thinking, are within reach of the adolescent.

496

SKILL BUILDING

The skill-building phase is initiated following the establishment of rapport and the forming of a trusting relationship and after the adolescent has become comfortable with session structure. At this point, the therapist fades self-instructions from overt to covert and introduces more social STIC assignments. It is important in this stage to emphasize the problem-solving strategy over the actual content of the problems being solved. Behavioral contingencies and verbal hints are both helpful in motivating the client to continue utilizing self-instructions. To facilitate compliance, the therapist can use any of several strategies (see Meichenbaum and Turk 1988). For example, two strategies involve paradox and solicitation of multiple public statements of commitment:

> *Therapist* [in the presence of another person]. You mean to tell me that you believe you can think a problem through from beginning to end?
> *Client*. Yeah, I can.
> *Therapist*. Come on, can you really?
> *Client*. Yeah, no kidding, I can do that.
> *Therapist*. You're pulling my leg.
> *Client*. Why, you think I can't?
> *Therapist*. Well, I guess I could be wrong, let's try some problems and see how you do.

It is encouraged during this phase that the therapist allow the adolescent's sharing of his or her views about home, school, and social life. Information abut how the youngster views his or her role in problematic situations can document any cognitive deficiencies, or possible distortions, that interfere with adjustment. The adolescent's coping style will also become apparent, and the therapist can later use appropriate coping modeling to coach the client in alternate and more adaptive coping strategies.

SKILL EXPANSION

This phase emphasizes interpersonal problems. In a sixteen-session protocol, this stage generally begins at approximately the twelfth

497

session, with a shift from impersonal problems to ones that more directly involve affective education and role playing regarding the solutions to interpersonal problems. Soliciting from the client examples of situations that he or she would like to problem solve individualizes the approach. Elaboration of behavioral alternatives and likely emotional consequences to each problematic interpersonal situation is emphasized. There are no right or wrong answers here; the therapist works to demonstrate how to think things through but does not require specific solutions—these are up to the adolescent. Praise is given for active cognitive problem solving—not for picking the socially appropriate solution.

SKILL CONSOLIDATION AND TERMINATION

The final phase of treatment involves having the adolescent apply problem-solving strategies to real problems that he or she may be experiencing outside therapy. The therapist and client can switch roles at points during this phase by having the youngster teach the self-instructions to the therapist (role playing another adolescent or child). Behavioral contingencies are more relaxed than in earlier sessions. Discussions are generally geared more toward how the adolescent might use the skills in present and future situations. Of course, termination issues should also be addressed at this point (e.g., planning a special activity for the final session, expression of feelings, discussion with the adolescent and parents about booster sessions of extending therapy).

Treatment Efficacy

Research efforts have assessed the efficacy of this type of treatment program with various populations of non-self-controlled children and adolescents (Hinshaw, Henker, and Whalen 1984; Hughes 1988; Kendall 1985; Kendall and Braswell 1982, 1985; Meyers and Craighead 1984). Recent reports regarding the status of cognitive-behavioral training as adjunctive to psychoactive medication have reached mixed, but generally favorable, conclusions. For example, Hinshaw et al. (1984) found that the combination of cognitive behavioral training (using procedures similar to those described here) and methylphenidate produced a significant increase in prosocial behaviors and a reduction

498

in negative social interactions in a sample of hyperactive boys. Further, this combination of treatments proved superior to the effects of all treatment conditions (including extrinsic reinforcement and placebo conditions) either alone or in combination in producing desired treatment benefits. In fact, subjects treated with the combination of cognitive-behavioral training and medication showed a reduction in levels of negative social behaviors below those of a sample of comparison boys. Thus, the frequency of negative social behaviors enacted by subjects were within normative limits following the combination of medication and cognitive-behavioral intervention.

A more recent report reached a more negative conclusion. Abikoff and Gittelman (1985) have reported that their version of cognitive training did not add meaningfully to the clinical efficacy of medications in treating hyperactive children. However, it has been pointed out (Kendall and Reber 1987) that the training program utilized by Abikoff and Gittelman was substantively different than the cognitive-behavioral package described. For example, behavioral contingencies were applied for participating only, not as a function of learning and applying the cognitive skills. Possible sources of inconsistency across studies include the nature of the target sample treated, the sensitivity of dependent variables, the experience and expertise of the therapist, and the length and quality of therapy provided.

The specific treatment detailed in this chapter has been empirically assessed to determine efficacy with various populations of non-self-controlled children and adolescents. The initial series of studies using samples of teacher-referred impulsive children produced favorable and encouraging results (e.g., Kendall and Finch 1976; Kendall and Braswell 1982; Kendall and Finch 1978; Kendall and Wilcox 1980; Kendall and Zupan 1981). Although the initial demonstrated effectiveness was with nonclinical samples of impulsive problem children, the studies nevertheless provided the impetus to assess further the treatment program's efficacy with psychiatric populations of disruptive children. For example, Kazdin, Esveldt-Dawson, French, and Unis (1987) reported positive findings with a psychiatric clinic sample of antisocial children. The treatment program was cognitive behavioral—combining, as here described, behavioral procedures with cognitive problem-solving training—and was found to be superior to a relationship-enhancement therapy and attention placebo across several parent and teacher reports.

A more recent study evaluated the cognitive-behavioral program with a population of day-hospitalized, conduct-disordered children and adolescents (Kendall, Reber, et al. in press). A twenty-session version of the cognitive-behavioral treatment was compared with current therapeutic modalities in treating twenty-nine youngsters diagnosed as conduct disordered (with or without concurrent ADHD). Results indicated the superiority of cognitive-behavioral therapy in producing significant gains across various domains, including teacher's blind ratings of prosocial behavior (e.g., self-control, adaptive functioning, appropriate behavior) and self-reports of perceived competence (e.g., social acceptance, scholastic competence). Further, the cognitive-behavioral therapy improved teacher-reported levels of self-control to within one standard deviation of those of a normative sample of nonreferred children.

The research findings summarized here support the ameliorative effect of properly focused cognitive-behavioral procedures with clinical samples of non-self-controlled children and adolescents. For those non-self-controlled youngsters diagnosed as in need of medication (e.g., ADHD), the evidence is not totally consistent, but some data do suggest that the combination of pharmacologic plus behavioral and cognitive-behavioral intervention is superior to either intervention alone in providing benefit for these young clients (see the review in Pelham and Murphy 1986).[3]

Conclusions

We have described a cognitive-behavioral program for use with clinical populations of impulsive, non-self-controlled adolescents (e.g., ADHD, conduct disorder). The procedures are designed to help the youngster cognitively mediate (stop and think about) problematic situations before embarking on a course of action. Future empirical efforts may want to address issues related to our opening question, How best to interact with the adolescent? We have a strategy, but, for example, given the often strong influence of peer groups on decision making within adolescence (Howard and Kendall 1988), might peer-run groups help in the assimilation of the cognitive skills outlined here? Adolescents are striving for autonomy, but family influences require attention. Would a cognitive-behavioral program for the family be more or less effective when compared with individual therapy (Masten

1979)? Additional program development and evaluation will address these and related questions regarding the efficacy of cognitive-behavioral procedures with adolescents.

NOTES

1. For a more extensive discussion of the methods, training tasks, and issues related to the cognitive-behavioral treatment, see Braswell and Kendall (1987), Kendall (1989), Kendall and Braswell (1985), and Kendall, Padawer, Zupan, and Braswell (1985).

2. For an elaborated discussion of all these facets of cognitive-behavioral theory, see Kendall 1985; Kendall, Howard, and Epps 1988; Kendall and Ronan 1990).

3. For more detail concerning the efficacy of cognitive-behavioral procedures with children and adolescents, see Hobbs, Moguin, Tyroler, and Lahey (1980), Hughes (1988), Kendall and Braswell (1985), and Urbain and Kendall (1980).

REFERENCES

Abikoff, H., and Gittelman, R. 1985. Hyperactive children treated with stimulants: is cognitive training a useful adjunct? *Archives of General Psychiatry* 42:953–961.

Achenbach, T. M. 1966. The classification of children's psychiatric symptoms: a factor-analytic study. *Psychological Monographs* 80(7, whole no. 615).

Braswell, L., and Kendall, P. C. 1987. Treating impulsive children via cognitive-behavioral therapy. In N. Jacobson, ed. *Psychotherapists in Clinical Practice: Cognitive and Behavioral Perspectives.* New York: Guilford.

Braswell, L.; Kendall, P. C.; Braith, J.; Carey, M.; and Vye, C. 1985. "Involvement" in cognitive-behavior therapy with children: process and its relation to outcome. *Cognitive Therapy and Research* 9:611–630.

Brown, A. L.; Bransford, J. D.; Ferrara, R. A.; and Campione, J. C. 1983. Learning, remembering, and understanding. In J. Flavell and E. Markman, eds. *Carmichael's Manual of Child Psychology,* vol. 1. New York: Wiley.

Dewey, J. 1938. *Experience and Education.* New York: Collier.

D'Zurilla, T. J. 1986. *Problem-solving Therapy: A Social Competence Approach to Clinical Intervention.* New York: Springer.

Elkind, D. 1967. Egocentrism in adolescence. In R. E. Muuss, ed. *Adolescent Behavior and Society: A Book of Readings.* New York: Random House, 1980.

Elkind, D. 1978. Understanding the young adolescent. *Adolescence* 13:127–134.

Flavell, J. H. 1977. *Cognitive Development.* Englewood Cliffs, NJ: Prentice-Hall.

Hinshaw, S. P.; Henker, B.; and Whalen, C. D. 1984. Self-control in hyperactive boys in anger inducing situations: effects of cognitive-behavior training and methylphenidate. *Journal of Consulting and Clinical Psychology* 52:739–749.

Hobbs, S. A.; Moguin, L. W.; Tyroler, M.; and Lahey, B. B. 1980. Cognitive-behavior therapy with children: has clinical utility been demonstrated. *Psychological Bulletin* 87:147–165.

Howard, B. L., and Kendall, P. C. 1988. Child intervention: having no peers? Philadelphia: Temple University. Typescript.

Hughes, J. 1988. *Cognitive-Behavioral Therapy with Children in Schools.* Oxford: Pergamon.

Ingram, R., and Kendall, P. C. 1986. Cognitive clinical psychology: implications of information processing perspectives. In R. Ingram, ed. *Information Processing Approaches to Clinical Psychology.* New York: Academic.

Kazdin, A. E.; Esveldt-Dawson, K.; French, N. H.; and Unis, A. S. 1987. Problem-solving skills training and relationship therapy in the treatment of antisocial child behavior. *Journal of Consulting and Clinical Psychology* 55:76–85.

Kendall, P. C. 1985. Toward a cognitive-behavioral model of child psychopathology and a critique of related interventions. *Journal of Abnormal Child Psychology* 13:357–371.

Kendall, P. C. 1989. *Stop and Think Workbook.* Available from the author, 238 Meeting House Lane, Merion Station, PA 19066.

Kendall, P. C., and Braswell, L. 1982. Cognitive-behavioral assessment: models, measures, and madness. In J. N. Butcher and C. D. Spielberger, eds. *Advances in Personality Assessment,* vol. 1. Hillsdale, N.J.: Erlbaum.

Kendall, P. C., and Braswell, L. 1985. *Cognitive-Behavioral Therapy for Impulsive Children.* New York: Guilford.

Kendall, P. C., and Finch, A. J., Jr. 1976. A cognitive-behavioral treatment for impulse control: a case study. *Journal of Consulting and Clinical Psychology* 44:852–857.

Kendall, P. C., and Finch, A. J. 1978. A cognitive-behavioral treatment for impulsivity: a group comparison study. *Journal of Consulting and Clinical Psychology* 46:110–118.

Kendall, P. C.; Howard, B. L.; and Epps, J. 1988. The anxious child: cognitive-behavioral treatment strategies. *Behavior Modification* 12:281–310.

Kendall, P. C., and Ingram, R. E. 1987. Future directions in the cognitive-behavioral assessment of anxiety: let's get specific. In L. Michelson and M. Ascher, eds. *Cognitive-Behavioral Assessment and Treatment of Anxiety Disorders*. New York: Guilford.

Kendall, P. C.; Kane, M.; Howard; and Siqueland, L. 1989. Cognitive-behavioral therapy for anxious children: treatment manual. Available from the author, 238 Meeting House Lane, Merion Station, PA 19066.

Kendall, P. C.; Padawer, W.; Zupan, B.; and Braswell, L. 1985. Developing self-control in children: the manual. In P. C. Kendall and L. Braswell, eds. *Cognitive-behavioral Therapy for Impulsive Children*. New York: Plenum.

Kendall, P. C., and Reber, M. 1987. Reply to Abikoff and Gittleman's evaluation of cognitive training with medicated hyperactive children. *Archives of General Psychiatry* 8:77–79.

Kendall, P. C.; Reber, M.; McCleer, S.; Epps, J.; and Ronan, K. R. in press. Cognitive-behavioral treatment of conduct disordered children. Cognitivek Therapy and Research.

Kendall, P. C., and Ronan, K. R. 1990. Assessment of children's anxieties, fears, and phobias: cognitive-behavioral models and methods. In C. R. Reynolds and R. W. Kamphaus, eds. *Handbook of Psychological and Educational Assessment of Children*. New York: Guilford.

Kendall, P. C.; Ronan, K. R.; and Epps, J. In press. Aggression in children and adolescents: cognitive-behavioral treatment perspectives. In D. Posler and K. Rubin, eds. *Development and Treatment of Childhood Aggression*. Hillsdale, N.J.: Erlbaum.

Kendall, P. C., and Siqueland, L. 1989. Child and adolescent therapy. In A. Nezv and C. Nezv, eds. *Clinical Decision Making in Behavior Therapy: A Problem-solving Perspective*. Champaign, Ill.: Research Press.

Kendall, P. C.; Stark, K.; and Adam, T. in press. Cognitive distortion versus cognitive deficits in childhood depression. Journal of Abnormal Child Psychology.

Kendall, P. C., and Wilcox, L. E. 1980. Cognitive-behavioral treatment for impulsivity: concrete versus conceptual training in non-self-controlled problem children. *Journal of Consulting and Clinical Psychology* 48:80–91.

Kendall, P. C., and Williams, C. L. 1986. Therapy with adolescents: treating the "marginal man." *Behavior Therapy* 17:522–537.

Kendall, P. C., and Zupan, B. A. 1981. Individual versus group application of cognitive-behavioral strategies for developing self-control in children. *Behavior Therapy* 12:344–359.

Marzillier, J. S. 1980. Cognitive therapy and behavioral practice. *Behavior Research and Therapy* 18:249–258.

Masten, A. S. 1979. Family therapy as a treatment for children: a critical review of outcome research. *Family Process* 18:323–335.

Meichenbaum, D. H., and Turk, D. C. 1988. *Facilitating Treatment Compliance: A Practitioner's Guidebook.* New York: Plenum.

Meyers, A. W., and Craighead, W. E. 1984. *Cognitive Behavior Therapy with Children.* New York: Plenum.

Overton, W. F. 1972. Piaget's theory of intellectual development and progressive education. In J. R. Squire, ed. *A New Look at Progressive Education.* Washington, D.C.: Association for Supervision and Curriculum Development.

Pelham, W. E., and Murphy, H. A. 1986. Attention deficit and conduct disorders. In M. Hersen, ed. *Pharmacological and Behavioral Treatment: An Integrated Approach.* New York: Wiley.

Piaget, J. 1954. *The Construction of Reality in the Child.* New York: Basic.

Schleser, R.; Cohen, R.; Meyers, A.; and Rodick, J. D. 1984. The effects of cognitive level and training procedures on the generalization of self-instructions. *Cognitive Therapy and Research* 8:187–200.

Spivack, G.; Platt, J.; and Shure, M. 1976. *The Problem-solving Approach to Adjustment.* San Francisco: Jossey-Bass.

Sprinthall, N. A., and Collins, W. A. 1984. *Adolescent Psychology: A Developmental View.* Reading, Mass.: Addison Wesley.

Steinberg, L., and Silverberg, S. B. 1986. The vicissitudes of autonomy in early adolescence. *Child Development* 57:841–852.

Tramontana, M. G. 1980. Critical review of research on psychotherapy outcome with adolescents: 1967–1977. *Psychological Bulletin* 88:429–450.

Turk, D. C., and Speers, M. A. 1983. Cognitive schemata and cognitive-behavioral interventions: going beyond the information given. In P. C. Kendall, ed. *Advances in Cognitive-Behavioral Research and Therapy*, vol. 2. New York: Academic.

Urbain, E. S., and Kendall, P. C. 1980. Review of social cognitive-problem solving interventions with children. *Psychological Bulletin* 88:109–143.

THE AUTHORS

JUDITH ABRAMOWITZ is Clinical Social Worker, Adolescent and Child Division, Chestnut Lodge Hospital, Rockville, Maryland.

E. JAMES ANTHONY is Clinical Professor of Psychiatry and Human Behavior, George Washington University School of Medicine; Director, Adolescent and Child Psychotherapy, Chestnut Lodge Hospital, Rockville, Maryland; and Training and Supervising Analyst, Washington Psychoanalytic Institute, Washington, D.C.

LINDA BETH BERMAN is Research and Editorial Assistant, Chestnut Lodge Research Institute, Rockville, Maryland.

SANDRA MCCRAE BOOTS is Clinical Assistant Professor of Psychiatry, Georgetown University School of Medicine; and Faculty Member, Washington School of Psychiatry, Child and Adolescent Psychotherapy Program, Washington, D.C.

ANDREW M. BOXER is Associate Director, Center for the Study of Adolescence, Michael Reese Hospital and the University of Chicago; and Faculty Member, Teacher Education Program, Institute for Psychoanalysis, Chicago, Illinois.

SUSAN JANE BRADLEY is Associate Professor, University of Toronto; Psychiatrist, the Hospital for Sick Children; and Consultant Psychiatrist, Clarke Institute of Psychiatry, Toronto, Canada.

DEXTER M. BULLARD, JR. is Medical Director, Chestnut Lodge Hospital, Rockville, Maryland.

DOUGLAS A. CHAVIS is Clinical Assistant Professor of Child Psychiatry, Georgetown University School of Medicine, Washington, D.C.

WAYNE FENTON is Staff Psychiatrist, Chestnut Lodge Hospital, Rockville, Maryland.

DENISE FORT is Faculty Member, Washington School of Psychiatry; and Staff Psychologist, Chestnut Lodge Hospital, Rockville, Maryland.

RICHARD C. FRITSCH is Clinical Assistant Professor of Psychology, Department of Psychology, George Washington University, Washington, D.C.; Research Coordinator, Adolescent and Child Division, Chestnut Lodge Research Institute; and Staff Psychologist, Chestnut Lodge Hospital, Rockville, Maryland.

CAROL S. FULLERTON is Research Assistant Professor, Department of Psychiatry, Uniformed Services, University of the Health Sciences, Bethesda, Maryland.

RICHARD A. GARDNER is Clinical Professor of Child Psychiatry, Columbia University College of Physicians and Surgeons, New York.

LAURA GOLD is a Postdoctoral Fellow in Psychiatry, University of Michigan, Ann Arbor.

HARVEY GOLOMBEK is Associate Professor, Department of Psychiatry, University of Toronto; and Coordinator of Psychotherapy Training, The Wellesley Hospital, Toronto, Canada.

DAVID GOODMAN, now in private practice, was Clinical Social Worker, Adolescent and Child Division, Chestnut Lodge Hospital, Rockville, Maryland.

WELLS GOODRICH is Clinical Professor of Psychiatry, Georgetown University School of Medicine; Director of Adolescent and Child Research, Chestnut Lodge Hospital; and Director, Intermediate Treatment Unit, Adolescent and Child Division, Chestnut Lodge Hospital, Rockville, Maryland.

SHEILA HAFTER GRAY is Clinical Professor of Psychiatry, University of Maryland School of Medicine, Baltimore; and Teaching Analyst, Washington Psychoanalytic Institute, Washington, D.C.

ROBERT W. HOLSTROM is Associate Professor, Department of Psychology, George Washington University, Washington, D.C.

WILLIAM HOPPE is Teacher and Group Psychotherapist, Chestnut Lodge School, Chestnut Lodge Hospital, Rockville, Maryland.

PHILIP KATZ is Professor, Department of Psychiatry, University of Manitoba; and President, American Society for Adolescent Psychiatry (1989–1990).

ALFRED KELLAM is Staff Psychologist, Outer River Drive Hospital, Lincoln Park, Michigan.

PHILIP C. KENDALL is Professor and Head, Division of Clinical Psychology, Temple University, Philadelphia, Pennsylvania.

ROBERT KING is Assistant Professor in Child Psychiatry, Yale Child Study Center, Yale University School of Medicine, New Haven, Connecticut.

MARSHALL KORENBLUM is Assistant Professor, Department of Psychiatry, University of Toronto; and Head, Adolescent Clinical Investigation Unit, C. M. Hincks Treatment Centre, Toronto, Canada.

NAOMI LOHR is Professor and Associate Chair, Department of Clinical Psychology; and Associate Director, Personality Disorders Program, University of Michigan, Ann Arbor.

DEMOSTHENES A. LORANDOS is Clinical Psychologist and Research Director, Michigan Psychological Services, Saginaw, Michigan.

SUSAN LOUGHMAN, now in private practice, was Clinical Social Worker, Adolescent and Child Division, Chestnut Lodge Hospital, Rockville, Maryland.

PAMELA LUDOLPH is Lecturer in Psychology and Supervising Psychologist, University Center for the Child and the Family, University of Michigan, Ann Arbor.

RICHARD C. MAROHN is Professor of Clinical Psychiatry, Northwestern University School of Medicine; and Faculty, Chicago Institute for Psychoanalysis, Chicago, Illinois.

PETER MARTON is Assistant Professor, Department of Psychiatry, University of Toronto; and Coordinator of Psychiatric Research, Department of Psychology, Sunnybrook Medical Centre, Toronto, Canada.

LAURICE MCAFEE is Staff Psychiatrist, Chestnut Lodge Hospital, Rockville, Maryland.

DEREK MILLER is Professor of Psychiatry; Director, Adolescent Psychiatry, Northwestern University School of Medicine, Chicago, Illinois; and President-Elect, International Society for Adolescent Psychiatry (1988–1992).

JOSEPH PALOMBO is Dean, Chicago Institute for Clinical Social Work; and Faculty Member, Child and Adolescent Psychotherapy Program, Chicago Institute for Psychoanalysis.

NICHOLAS PUTNAM is Associate Clinical Professor of Psychiatry, University of California at San Diego School of Medicine.

FRANK T. RAFFERTY is Clinical Professor of Psychiatry, Texas A. M. School of Medicine; and Vice President for Medical Affairs, Healthcare International, Austin, Texas.

REBECCA E. RIEGER is Clinical Professor of Psychiatry and Pediatrics, George Washington University School of Medicine; Senior Psychologist, Chestnut Lodge Hospital, Rockville, Maryland; and Faculty Member, Washington School of Psychiatry, Washington, D.C.

LILLIAN H. ROBINSON is Professor of Psychiatry and Pediatrics; and Training and Supervisory Analyst, Analytic Medicine Program, Tulane University School of Medicine, New Orleans, Louisiana.

KEVIN R. RONAN is a Doctoral Candidate, Division of Clinical Psychology, Temple University, Philadelphia, Pennsylvania.

KENNETH SILK is Clinical Associate Professor of Psychiatry, Department of Psychiatry, University of Michigan, Ann Arbor.

BERNARD A. STEIN is Associate Professor, Department of Psychiatry, University of Toronto; and Director of Psychotherapy, Division of Adolescent Psychiatry, Sunnybrook Medical Centre, Toronto, Canada.

MAX SUGAR is Clinical Professor of Psychiatry, Louisiana State University School of Medicine; Director, Children's Unit, Coliseum Medical Center, New Orleans; and a Senior Editor of this volume.

NANCY H. WEIL is Assistant Clinical Professor, Department of Psychiatry, University of Chicago; Attending Psychologist, Michael Reese Hospital and Medical Center; and Faculty Member, Teacher Education Program, Chicago Institute for Psychoanalysis.

DREW WESTEN is Adjunct Assistant Professor of Psychology, University of Michigan, Ann Arbor.

CAMILLE WOODBURY is Staff Psychiatrist, Chestnut Lodge Hospital, Rockville, Maryland.

BRIAN T. YATES is Associate Professor of Psychology; and Associate Dean for Graduate Affairs, College of Arts and Sciences, The American University, Washington, D.C.

CONTENTS OF VOLUMES 1–16

525

538

NAME INDEX

SUBJECT INDEX

Abuse, and violence, 421
Administrators, at Chestnut Lodge, 95,
   310, 315
Adoption
   frequency of, in hospitalized adoles-
      cents, 227, 239
   and patient subgroups, 213, 222
   running away and adoptive status, 293–
      94, 295, 296–97, 300
Affect, and personality functioning, 408,
   409–11
Affective disorders, and panic disorders,
   444–45
Affective education, in cognitive-
   behavioral therapy, 490
Alf, 63
American educational system. *See* Educational system
American Icarus syndrome, 335
The Analysis of the Self (Kohut), 338, 339
Anxiety, avoidant disorders and, 62
Asperger's syndrome, 53
Assessment
   of patients at Chestnut Lodge, 202–
      204, 204–207, 253
   see also Diagnosis
Attachment, as treatment process, 246–61
   borderline patients and, 259, 264–65
   brain-damaged patients and, 264–71
   case examples, impaired patients, 266–
      70
   containment and, 260
   diagnosis and, 253
   families of impaired children and, 265
   importance of, 257–59
   methods in study of, 250–53
   phases of treatment and, 247
   psychotic patients and, 259–60, 264–65
   results of study on, 253–57
   Scale of Symbiotic Relatedness, 251–
      53
   schizotypal patients and, 259

types of alliances, 249–50, 265
Attachment issues
   Chestnut Lodge treatment and, 96, 97,
      161–62, 232, 241, 317–18
   impaired patients and, 261–71
   outcome and, 246–61
   runaways and, 300
Avoidant disorders, anxiety and, 62

Back to the Future, 64–66
Behavioral therapy. *See* Cognitive-
   behavioral therapy
Biological factors, and violence, 422
Borderline adolescents vs. adults, 326,
   360–81
   affect tone of relationship paradigms in,
      364, 369, 370–71, 374, 375, 376,
      377, 378
   capacity for emotional investment in,
      364, 369, 370–71, 372, 374, 375,
      376, 377, 378
   complexity of representations of people
      in, 364, 368, 370–71, 374, 375,
      376, 377, 378
   developmental differences in, 377–80
   DIB in study of, 366
   families of patients, 364
   fixed period of development for disor-
      der, 362–63, 377–39
   gender ratio in study subjects, 373–74
   Kernberg on, 360, 361, 362
   Masterson on, 360–61, 362
   measures in study of, 367–73
   methods in study of, 365–73
   procedures in study of, 366–67, 373
   results in study of, 373–377
   roots of disorder, 360
   subjects in study of, 365–66
   TAT in study of, 364, 366–67, 369,
      372, 373, 374, 375, 377
   timing of effects of pathogenic influ-
      ences in, 363–64